Neurology Oral Boards Review

Neurology Oral Boards Review

A Concise and Systematic Approach to Clinical Practice

Eroboghene E. Ubogu, MD

*Louis Stokes Cleveland Veterans Affairs Medical Center
and Case Western Reserve University School of Medicine
Cleveland, Ohio*

Foreword by
Henry J. Kaminski, MD

*Louis Stokes Cleveland Veterans Affairs Medical Center
and Case Western Reserve University School of Medicine
Cleveland, Ohio*

HUMANA PRESS ✳ TOTOWA, NEW JERSEY

© 2005 Humana Press Inc.
999 Riverview Drive, Suite 208
Totowa, New Jersey 07512

humanapress.com

Due diligence has been taken by the publishers, editors, and authors of this book to assure the accuracy of the information published and to describe generally accepted practices. The contributors herein have carefully checked to ensure that the drug selections and dosages set forth in this text are accurate and in accord with the standards accepted at the time of publication. Notwithstanding, as new research, changes in government regulations, and knowledge from clinical experience relating to drug therapy and drug reactions constantly occurs, the reader is advised to check the product information provided by the manufacturer of each drug for any change in dosages or for additional warnings and contraindications. This is of utmost importance when the recommended drug herein is a new or infrequently used drug. It is the responsibility of the treating physician to determine dosages and treatment strategies for individual patients. Further it is the responsibility of the health care provider to ascertain the Food and Drug Administration status of each drug or device used in their clinical practice. The publisher, editors, and authors are not responsible for errors or omissions or for any consequences from the application of the information presented in this book and make no warranty, express or implied, with respect to the contents in this publication.

This publication is printed on acid-free paper. ∞
ANSI Z39.48-1984 (American Standards Institute) Permanence of Paper for Printed Library Materials.

Production Editor: Robin B. Weisberg

Cover design by Patricia F. Cleary

For additional copies, pricing for bulk purchases, and/or information about other Humana titles, contact Humana at the above address or at any of the following numbers: Tel.: 973-256-1699; Fax: 973-256-8341; E-mail: orders@humanapr.com; or visit our Website: www.humanapress.com.

Printed in the United States of America. 10 9 8 7 6 5 4 3 2 1

eISBN 978-1-59259-984-4

Library of Congress Cataloging-in-Publication Data

Ubogu, Eroboghene E.
  Neurology oral boards review : a concise and systematic approach to
clinical practice / Eroboghene E. Ubogu ; foreword by Henry J. Kaminski.
      p. cm.
  Includes bibliographical references and index.
  ISBN 978-1-58829-654-2 (alk. paper)
  1. Neurology--Case studies. 2. Neurologists--Licenses--United
States--Examinations--Study guides. I. Title.
  RC359.U26 2005
  616.8'0076--dc22
                                                              2005012358

Dedication

To my beloved wife, Anisa, our son, Oghenekome and all our family members whose encouragement, inspiration, love, patience, and support have made this book possible.

—E.E.U.

Foreword

It was 6 AM and the New Orleans Hilton lobby was dotted with young neurologists in suits wandering aimlessly, many mumbling to themselves, all with the eyes of a rough night on call. This was the morning of my Oral Board examination. Despite three years as a neurology resident, additional time as a fellow, and the experience of having performed probably more than 1000 neurological examinations by this time, I was deathly afraid of what this day would bring. The exam organizers had met with us the day before and given the overwhelming message to "RELAX." Certainly, this is sound advice prior to any examination, but the requisite for passing is knowing the material. This requires preparation, as well as practice.

An excellent first step is to use Eroboghene Ubogu's *Neurology Oral Boards Review* in the months before you begin studying for the Boards in earnest. A quick read will provide an internal assessment of your strengths and weaknesses, which should guide the study plan. The major neurology textbooks, which anyone sitting for the Boards should already have in their possession, should be studied. Finding a senior faculty member to quiz you is very helpful. There is no substitute for finding one of your former residency supervisors or a senior colleague in your group practice to perform a simulated Oral Board session. There is no substitute for feeling the sweat and sickness in your stomach during such a session, but it is far better to embarrass yourself in front of this sympathetic supporter then to receive a letter of failure from the Board. In the final weeks and days before THE DAY, use this *Neurology Oral Boards Review* again to solidify recollection of the stepwise approach to case-vignette discussion and to remind you of differential diagnoses, by using the text's excellent summaries. Such review will boost your confidence and make it easier for you to calm down, and stay calm, during the actual exam.

Henry J. Kaminski, MD
Professor and Vice Chair of Neurology
Case Western Reserve University School of Medicine
Chief, Neurology Service
Louis Stokes Cleveland Veterans Affairs Medical Center
Cleveland, Ohio

Preface

Neurology Oral Boards Review: A Concise and Systematic Approach to Clinical Practice is written specifically to assist neurologists preparing for the American Board of Psychiatry and Neurology (ABPN) Part II (Oral) Examination. This examination is clinically based, so a concise review of relevant topics and examination strategies to maximize one's chances of passing the examination is relevant. Most neurologists taking the Oral Boards are either in fellowship programs or in active clinical practice, so time constraints are usually a factor while attempting to prepare for the examination. This book will also be beneficial to the practicing general neurologist, neurology resident, or medical student looking for a concise and structured approach to clinical problem solving in neurology.

Neurology Oral Boards Review: A Concise and Systematic Approach to Clinical Practice is written in three parts: Part I provides a detailed description of the examination and advice on how to successfully approach it. This is important in an oral examination, as one's knowledge has to "shine through" the anxieties of the occasion. Having a systematic but thorough approach facilitates factual recall and allows the candidate to adequately cover the necessary points needed to pass this examination. There is also a recommended study approach that takes in mind the difficulties of dedicating a time block to prepare for the Oral Boards while in post-residency training or practice. This method provides a time frame for study review that would hopefully reduce the likelihood of incomplete preparation, resulting in loss of self-confidence.

Parts II and III provide clinical case vignettes similar to what the candidate is expected to deal with on the Oral Boards. The candidate is not always expected to obtain the diagnosis to the vignettecase since most are somewhat open-ended and subject to several differential diagnoses/therapeutic approaches. ABPN expects examinees to localize the plausible disease processes, provide reasonable differential diagnoses, indicate which investigations may help in establishing a diagnosis, deduce management/treatment plans, and provide information on prognosis, including patient/family counseling. These are fundamental aspects in the training and practice of neurologists that all candidates should be familiar with. Unlike in "real life," where the physician may have days, weeks, or months to consider several plausible explanations for a clinical presentation, the candidate has to quickly exhibit a broad knowledge of neurological practice. In fact, a large proportion of the vignettes have acute presentations and are potentially treatable, emphasizing the importance of early diagnosis. A synopsis is provided at the end of each case to highlight important points.

Parts II and III are divided into Emergencies and General Neurology, with each section divided based on topics. Having a separate section for emergencies was done in order to prepare the candidate to think critically when faced with a neurological emergency, putting resuscitation, patient safety, and rapid high-yield investigations at the top of the list, as expected by the examiners. Showing inadequate knowledge/approach in a neurological emergency may compromise a candidate's chances of passing the Oral Boards. The General Neurology section contains a broad range of topics that are likely to be tested on the Oral Boards. This section does not provide for all diagnoses in neurology, but covers a breadth as experienced in hospital and outpatient clinical settings.

The candidate can use this book as a concise review or self-assessment tool. The former approach would be useful for the busy neurologist with insufficient time to review reference texts who may be looking for "high-yield" information, whereas the latter approach may favor the candidate seeking a "last-minute" test prior to the examination. I suggest reading *Neurology Oral Boards Review: A Concise and Systematic Approach to Clinical Practice* initially as a study guide, as this may identify areas of relative weakness that would require more extensive study. The book can be subsequently used as an assessment tool in a format similar to the actual examination in the weeks prior to the test. A reference/bibliography list appears at the beginning of the book. This list is not exhaustive, but provides respected sources of information in neurology. These books can be used for more detailed information on the topics addressed in this book.

The ABPN Part II (Oral) Boards may sound daunting, but about 75 to 80% of candidates pass every year. The examiners are not trying to fail candidates and understand that the anxieties involved may affect true performance. All candidates, by virtue of completing residency training in neurology, are capable of passing the examination and have the knowledge to do so. The most important factor is being organized, systematic, and thorough. Remember, breadth of information and competence are being assessed. It is my sincere hope that candidates are able to reach their goals and pass the Oral Boards with the aid of this book.

Eroboghene E. Ubogu, MD

Acknowledgments

Special thanks to the faculty and residents, past and present, of the Department of Neurology, Case Western Reserve University School of Medicine and the Louis Stokes Cleveland Veterans Affairs Medical Center, who have taught and challenged me and supported my career in neurology. Thanks to the Division of Neuromuscular Disorders, Department of Neurology, Emory University School of Medicine for my subspecialist training and career development. Special gratitude and thanks goes to Dr. Henry Kaminski, my mentor and friend who has guided every step of my development as a neurologist and Dr. David Preston for their helpful criticisms and review of this book. Last, but surely not the least, I would like to give special thanks to the editors and publishing staff at Humana Press, especially Richard Lansing, for their enthusiasm, belief, and support for this project.

—*E.E.U.*

Contents

Abbreviations

ABG:	Arterial blood gas
ACA:	Anterior cerebral artery
ACE:	Angiotensin converting enzyme
ACh:	Acetylcholine
AChE:	Acetylcholinesterase
AChR:	Acetylcholine receptor
ACommA:	Anterior communicating artery
ACTH:	Adrenocorticotrophic hormone
AD:	Alzheimer's disease
AD:	Autosomal dominant
ADEM:	Acute disseminated encephalomyelitis
ADR:	Adverse drug reaction
ADLs:	Activities of daily living
AED:	Antiepileptic drug
AFB:	Acid-fast bacilli
AHC:	Anterior horn cells
AHI:	Apnea-hypopnea index
AI:	Arousal index
AICA:	Anterior inferior cerebellar artery
AIDP:	Acute inflammatory demyelinating polyradiculoneuropathy
AIDS:	Acquired immunodeficiency syndrome
ALD:	Adrenoleukodystrophy
ALS:	Amyotrophic lateral sclerosis
AMAN:	Acute motor axonal neuropathy
AMSAN:	Acute motor and sensory axonal neuropathy
ANA:	Anti-nuclear antibody
ANCA:	Anti-neutrophil cytoplasmic antibody
anti-ds-DNA:	Anti-double stranded DNA
AP:	Anterior-posterior
APC:	Activated protein C
aPL:	Anti-phospholipid antibodies
AR:	Autosomal recessive
ASA:	Aspirin
ASCS:	Anterior spinal cord syndrome
ASO:	Anti-streptolysin O
ATM:	Acute transverse myelitis
AVM:	Arteriovenous malformation
AZT:	Azidothymidine (zidovudine)

BA:	Basilar artery
BESAS:	Benign enlargement of the subarachnoid space
BFM:	Benign familial megalencephaly
BiPAP:	Bivalve positive airway pressure
BP:	Blood pressure
BPPV:	Benign paroxysmal positional vertigo
BUN:	Blood urea nitrogen
Ca^{2+}:	Calcium
CAD:	Coronary artery disease
C&S:	Culture and sensitivity
CBC:	Complete blood count
CBGD:	Cortical-basal ganglionic degeneration
CHF:	Congestive heart failure
CIDP:	Chronic inflammatory demyelinating polyradiculoneuropathy
CJD:	Creutzfeldt-Jakob disease
CK:	Creatine kinase
CMAP:	Compound motor action potential
CMV:	Cytomegalovirus
CN:	Cranial nerve
CNS:	Central nervous system
CO:	Carbon monoxide
CO_2:	Carbon dioxide
COMT:	Catechol-*O*-methyl transferase
COPD:	Chronic obstructive pulmonary disease
CPA:	Cerebellopontine angle
CPAP:	Continuous positive airway pressure
CPEO:	Chronic progressive external ophthalmoplegia
CPM:	Central pontine myelinolysis
CPT:	Carnitine palmitoyltransferase
Cr:	Creatinine
CRP:	C-reactive protein
CRPS:	Complex regional pain syndrome
CSF:	Cerebrospinal fluid
CT:	Computed tomography
CTA:	Computed tomography angiography
CTD:	Connective tissue disease
CTS:	Carpal tunnel syndrome
Cu^{2+}:	Copper
CVST:	Cortical venous sinus thrombosis
3,4-DAP:	3,4-diamino-pyridine
DBP:	Diastolic blood pressure
DBS:	Deep brain stimulation
DHE:	Dihydroergotamine
DLBD:	Diffuse Lewy body disease
DM:	Diabetes mellitus
DRPLA:	Dentatorubral pallidoluysian atrophy
DVT:	Deep venous thrombosis

DWI:	Diffusion-weighted imaging
EA:	Episodic ataxia
EBV:	Epstein-Barr virus
ECT:	Electroconvulsive therapy
EDH:	Epidural hematoma
EDS:	Excessive daytime somnolence
EEG:	Electroencephalogram
EKG:	Electrocardiogram
EMG:	Electromyography
ER:	Emergency room
ESR:	Erythrocyte sedimentation rate
FDA:	Food and Drug Administration
FISP:	Fast-in-flow steady state precession
FS:	Febrile seizure
FTA-ABS:	Fluorescent treponemal antibody-absorption test
FVC:	Forced vital capacity
GABA:	γ-aminobutyric acid
GBM:	Glioblastoma multiforme
GBS:	Guillain-Barré syndrome
GCA:	Giant-cell arteritis
GCS:	Glasgow Coma Scale
GI:	Gastrointestinal
GSD:	Gerstmann-Straussler disease
GTC:	Generalized tonic-clonic
GU:	Genitourinary
GVHD:	Graft-vs-host disease
HAART:	Highly active anti-retroviral therapy
Hb:	Hemoglobin
hCG:	Human chorionic gonadotrophin
HD:	Huntington's disease
HHV-6:	Human herpesvirus-6
HIE:	Hypoxic-ischemic encephalopathy
HIV:	Human immunodeficiency virus
HLA:	Human leukocyte antigen
HMSN:	Hereditary motor and sensory neuropathy
HNPP:	Hereditary neuropathy with liability to pressure palsies
HR:	Heart rate
HSAN:	Hereditary sensory and autonomic neuropathy
HSCT:	Hematopoietic stem cell transplantation
HSE:	Herpes simplex encephalitis
HSP:	Hereditary spastic paraparesis
HSV:	Herpes simplex virus
5-HT:	5-Hydroxytryptamine
HTLV:	Human T-cell lymphotropic virus
IAC:	Internal auditory canal
ICA:	Internal carotid artery
ICH:	Intracranial hemorrhage

ICU:	Intensive care unit
ICP:	Intracranial pressure
Ig:	Immunoglobulin
IgA:	Immunoglobulin A
IgG:	Immunoglobulin G
IgM:	Immunoglobulin M
IIH:	Idiopathic intracranial hypertension
INR:	International normalized ratio
i.m.:	Intramuscular
i.t.:	Intrathecal
i.v.:	Intravenous
IVIg:	Intravenous immunoglobulins
JME:	Juvenile myoclonic epilepsy
K^+:	Potassium
KP:	Korsakoff's psychosis
KSS:	Kearns–Sayre syndrome
LD:	Leukodystrophy
LEMS:	Lambert–Eaton Myasthenic syndrome
LFT:	Liver function test
LLN:	Lower limit of normal
LM:	Leptomeningeal metastases
LMN:	Lower motor neuron
LP:	Lumbar puncture
LSD:	Lysergic acid diethylamide
LV:	Left ventricle
MAG:	Myelin-associated glycoprotein
MAOI:	Monoamine oxidase inhibitor
MAP:	Mean arterial pressure
MCA:	Middle cerebral artery
MCTD:	Mixed connective tissue disease
MD:	Muscular dystrophy
MELAS:	Mitochondrial encephalopathy, lactic acidosis and stroke-like episodes
MERRF:	Myoclonic epilepsy with ragged red fibers
MFS:	Miller–Fisher syndrome
MG:	Myasthenia gravis
Mg^{2+}:	Magnesium
MI:	Myocardial infarction
MLF:	Medial longitudinal fasciculus
MMA:	Methylmalonic acid
MMSE:	Mini-mental status examination
MPS:	Mucopolysaccharidosis
MPTP:	1-Methyl-4-phenyl-1,2,3,6-tetrahydropyridine
MR:	Mental retardation
MRA:	Magnetic resonance angiography
MRC:	Medical Research Council
MRSA:	Methicillin-resistant *Staphylococcus aureus*
MRV:	Magnetic resonance venography

MRI:	Magnetic resonance imaging
MS:	Multiple sclerosis
MSA:	Multiple systems atrophy
MSUD:	Maple syrup urine disease
Na^+:	Sodium
NARP:	Neuropathy, ataxia, and retinitis pigmentosa
NASCET:	North American Symptomatic Carotid Endarterectomy Trial
NC:	Neurocutaneous
NCL:	Neuronal ceroid lipofuscinosis
NCS:	Nerve conduction studies
NF:	Neurofibromatosis
NHL:	Non-Hodgkin's lymphoma
NIF:	Negative inspiratory force
NIHSS:	National Institutes of Health Stroke Scale
NMDA:	N-Methyl-D-aspartate
NMJ:	Neuromuscular junction
NMS:	Neuroleptic malignant syndrome
NPH:	Normal pressure hydrocephalus
NSAID:	Nonsteroidal anti-inflammatory drug
OPCA:	Olivo-pontine cerebellar atrophy
OSA:	Obstructive sleep apnea
OSAHS:	Obstructive sleep apnea-hypopnea syndrome
PACNS:	Primary angiitis of the central nervous system
$PaCO_2$:	Arterial pressure for carbon dioxide
PAN:	Polyarteritis nodosa
PANDAS:	Pediatric autoimmune neuropsychiatric disorders associated with streptococcus
PCA:	Posterior cerebral artery
PCR:	Polymerase chain reaction
PCS:	Postconcussion syndrome
PCommA:	Posterior communicating artery
PCOS:	Polycystic ovarian syndrome
PD:	Parkinson's disease
PE:	Pulmonary embolism
PEF:	Positive expiratory force
PEG:	Percutaneous endoscopic gastrostomy
PET:	Positron emission tomography
PICA:	Posterior inferior cerebellar artery
PLEDs:	Periodic lateralizing epileptiform discharges
PLMS:	Periodic leg movements of sleep
PML:	Progressive multifocal leukoencephalopathy
PMJ:	Pontomedullary junction
PMP-22:	Peripheral myelin protein-22
PNS:	Peripheral nervous system
p.o.:	Orally
PaO_2:	Arterial pressure for oxygen
PO_4^{3-}:	Phosphorus (phosphate)

POTS:	Postural orthostatic tachycardia syndrome
PPD:	Purified protein derivative
PSA:	Prostate-specific antigen
PSP:	Progressive supranuclear palsy
PT:	Prothrombin time
PTH:	Parathyroid hormone
PTS:	Posttraumatic seizures
PTT:	Partial thromboplastin time
PVS:	Persistent vegetative state
QSART:	Quantitative sudomotor axon reflex test
RBC:	Red blood cells
RBD:	Rapid eye movement sleep behavior disorder
REM:	Rapid eye movement
RhA:	Rheumatic arthritis
RhC:	Rheumatic chorea
RhF:	Rheumatoid factor
RLS:	Restless legs syndrome
RNA:	Ribonucleic acid
RNS:	Repetitive nerve stimulation
RPR:	Rapid plasma reagin
RR:	Respiratory rate
r-tPA:	Recombinant tissue plasminogen activator
SAH:	Subarachnoid hemorrhage
SCA:	Spinocerebellar ataxia
SCA:	Superior cerebellar artery
SCLC:	Small-cell lung cancer
s.d.:	Standard deviation
SDH:	Subdural hematoma
SE:	Status epilepticus
SFEMG:	Single-fiber electromyography
SGPG:	Sulfonated glucuronyl paragloboside
SIADH:	Syndrome of inappropriate antidiuretic hormone secretion
SLE:	Systemic lupus erythematosus
SMA:	Spinal muscular atrophy
SMN:	Survival motor neuron
SNAP:	Sensory nerve action potential
SPECT:	Single-photon emission computed tomography
SSA:	Sjögren's syndrome A antibody
SSB:	Sjögren's syndrome B antibody
SSPE:	Subacute sclerosing panencephalitis
SSRI:	Selective serotonin reuptake inhibitor
SUNCT:	Short-lasting, unilateral, neuralgiform headache attacks with conjunctival injection and tearing
TB:	Tuberculosis
TCA:	Tricyclic antidepressant
TCD:	Transcranial doppler
TEE:	Transesophageal echocardiography
TENS:	Transcutaneous electrical nerve stimulator

TFT:	Thyroid function test
TGA:	Transient global amnesia
TIA:	Transient ischemic attack
TPE:	Therapeutic plasmapheresis
TSC:	Tuberous sclerosis
TST:	Thermoregulatory sweat test
TTE:	Transthoracic echocardiography
UMN:	Upper motor neuron
UPPP:	Uvulopalatopharyngoplasty
URI:	Upper respiratory tract infection
USS:	Ultrasound scan
VA:	Vertebral artery
VBD:	Vertebrobasilar dolichoectasia
VC:	Vital capacity
VDRL:	Venereal disease reference laboratory
VGCC:	Voltage-gated calcium channel
VLCFA:	Very-long chain fatty acids
VPA:	Valproic acid
VPL:	Ventral posterior lateral
VPM:	Ventral posterior medial
VZV:	Varicella zoster virus
WBC:	White blood cells
WG:	Wegener's granulomatosis

References/Bibliography

Most standard texts of neurology provide ample information in clinical practice to facilitate preparation for the Oral Boards. In addition, review articles in peer-reviewed journals or journal supplements provide recent summaries or practice guidelines to keep the practicing neurologist or neurologist-in-training updated. Sources utilized for this text include the following:

1. PubMed®: http://www.ncbi.nlm.nih.gov/entrez/query.fcgi
2. Clinical Pediatric Neurology. A signs and systems approach by G.M. Fenichel (4th ed.) published by W.B. Saunders Company.
3. Neurology for the Boards by J.D. Geyer, J.M. Keating and D.C. Potts (2nd ed.) published by Lippincott-Raven.
4. Neurology in Clinical Practice. The Neurological Disorders edited by W.G. Bradley, R.B. Daroff, G.M. Fenichel and J. Jankovic (4th ed. with updates on www.nicp.com) published by Butterworth-Heinemann.

PART I

INTRODUCTION

Test Description

The American Board of Psychiatry and Neurology (ABPN) Part II (Oral) Boards is a clinically based examination that consists of 3 hours of assessment divided into three 1-hour sections. Candidates would be scheduled to take the different sections of the examination in any order, and there is no advantage in having one section before the other, as each section is independent of the others.

There is a 1-hour "live patient" section in which the candidate is expected to take a complete history and perform a comprehensive neurological examination in the presence of two examiners. A senior examiner may come into the examining room for a short period of time to observe the examination. Thirty minutes are allocated for the history and physical examination and 15 minutes for case presentation and discussion of differential diagnoses, relevant investigations, management modalities, therapeutic measures, and prognosis. The ability to deduce a plausible differential diagnosis for the patient may best differentiate between passing and failing candidates. Adult neurology candidates are expected to evaluate an adult patient, whereas candidates for certification in child neurology would evaluate a pediatric patient. Fifteen minutes at the end are allocated for three clinical vignettes, each lasting 5 minutes on topics that are not related to the "live patient." These vignettes are similar to those assessed in the clinical vignette section of the examination, and may include a neurological emergency case. Candidates are allowed to take notes during the examination, but must submit all materials to the examiners before leaving the room.

One-hour clinical vignette sections are dedicated to cases in adult and pediatric neurology, respectively. These consist of six vignettes each, for which the candidate is allocated 10 minutes to read or have read, the clinical vignette and then provide information on localization, differential diagnoses, investigations, management/treatment, prognosis, and counseling. The vignettes cover a broad range of topics in adult and pediatric neurology. The Clinical Vignette section may include one or two neurological emergencies with four to five general neurology cases for assessment. Two adult or pediatric neurologists examine each section, with a senior examiner spending some limited time observing the examination. Examinees may also take notes on separate sheets of paper. These have to be submitted to the examiners on completion of the examination.

From: *Neurology Oral Boards Review:*
A Concise and Systematic Approach to Clinical Practice
By: E. E. Ubogu © Humana Press Inc., Totowa, NJ

For each section of the examination, the candidate is graded as pass or fail. To pass the Oral Boards, the candidate must receive a passing grade in all three sections. The "Live Patient" section (including the additional vignettes) provides 18 subsection grades (9 from each examiner; 6 for the patient evaluation and 3 for the vignettes), whereas the Clinical Vignette sections provide 12 subsection grades each (6 per examiner). Based on a recent report from ABPN,[1] 84% of adult neurology candidates passed the "Live Patient" section (88% for pediatric neurologists), 87% passed the adult Clinical Vignette section (92% for pediatric neurologists), and 79% passed the pediatric Clinical Vignette section (73% for pediatric neurologists). The average passing candidate demonstrated passing grades in 80–85% of subsections, with the average failing candidate receiving passing scores in 25–35% of subsections. This emphasizes that a broad knowledge base differentiates between passing and failing candidates on the Oral Boards.[1]

---

[1]Jones HR, Pascuzzi RM, Jull D, Scheiber SC. Performance on the ABPN Part II examination in neurology and child neurology. Neurology 2004; 62 (Suppl 5):A79–A80.

Study Approach and Testing-Taking Strategies

Congratulations on successfully completing Part I, the written part of American Board of Psychiatry and Neurology (ABPN) Board examinations. You can now focus on the art and science of clinical neurology as you prepare for the Oral Boards. As most neurologists have limited time to prepare for the Oral Boards, different approaches, such as Board Review Courses, group-study programs, and dedicated self-study have been used with success. This study guide provides some guidelines that the candidate may find useful in organizing a structured program of study that might facilitate retention of material and enhance one's chances of success. This guide is based on personal experience, and not on any published guidelines.

STUDY GUIDE

Three Months Before the Examination

This is a good time to start reviewing material for the Oral Boards. Depending on how much time the candidate has and how quickly a candidate can study, this time frame could be modified. An approach would be to review this book to identify areas of relative strength and weaknesses. The candidate can then refer to standard neurological texts and reference sources to review the material in greater depth. Focusing on more common neurological problems; generating tables, charts, or graphs that may enhance retention and recall; and speaking to recently successful candidates should be considered at this time.

The examination is designed for the general neurologist, so dedicating too much time to detailed subspecialist concepts is low yield. Remember, breadth not depth is required! Dedicating 2 hours every evening for study may be all that is needed at this point. It is important to pace one's self based on the study target goals in order to confidently cover the vast material in neurology. For the adult neurologist, this is a good time for an in-depth review of pediatric neurology and vice versa.

Two Months Before the Examination

You should receive your examination admission notice at least 6 to 8 weeks before the examination. Plan for your trip, including accommodations, transportation, and taking time off from work! One can save money by staying at a hotel a short walking distance from the examination hotel headquarters. Avoid

From: *Neurology Oral Boards Review:*
A Concise and Systematic Approach to Clinical Practice
By: E. E. Ubogu © Humana Press Inc., Totowa, NJ

planning to stay too far, as the last thing you want to worry about is transportation difficulties to the hotel headquarters or examination centers.

Focus on a general review of neurology by reading the clinically relevant sections of neurology review books, including what you studied for Part I. Updating on current management/therapeutic principles could be considered at this time. Consider reviewing a clinical textbook on disease localization or anatomy.

Practicing a comprehensive, but quick neurological examination would be useful in order to build up confidence that it can be systematically done in 5 to 10 minutes. Reviewing sections on clinical examination in standard neurological texts would be useful. Do not get engrossed in how to elucidate subtle signs, but focus on a comprehensive, general examination. Spend more time practicing aspects of the neurological examination that you do not usually perform in your everyday practice. For example, neurologists in fellowship training may neglect aspects of the general examination. Neurologists in clinical practice may have a skewed patient population and may have lost skills in portions of the examination. Generating or purchasing memory aids (e.g., cards) that contain the complete neurological examination should be considered.

One Month Before the Examination

This would be a good time to review again a concise review text for the Oral Boards for factual recall and as a self-assessment tool. Topics of relative weakness should be emphasized after a general review. Previously generated memory aids (e.g., differential diagnostic lists or tables) should be utilized to facilitate rapid recall. Avoid reading standard texts at this time as one may get distracted by less common diseases. This would be a great time to start memorizing drugs and dosing regimens required for neurological emergencies (adult and pediatric), as examiners would expect this. Writing these in an easily retrievable source for rapid review may aid the process. Knowledge of pharmacological and nonpharmacological therapeutic regimens is required for the general neurology vignettes, but precise dosing is not absolutely required.

Try to formulate an approach or technique for attempting to answer the Clinical Vignettes that allow categorization of disease entities into easily recalled headings. This would result in a structured and organized approach to answering the vignettes and allow you exhibit a broad knowledge of clinical neurology.

Spend time trying to outline the clinical history taking process for the "Live Patient" section to ensure that all aspects are covered. It is easy to forget the family, social history, or review of systems in a pressurized situation. These may be relevant to the case. By now you should know what style suits you best: writing notes while taking the history or afterward to only include the pertinent aspects. Practice whatever style that you are most comfortable with and aim to improve your speed so that a complete history is obtainable in 15 minutes. Also, practice a concise but comprehensive clinical examination when seeing patients. Having senior colleagues, faculty members, or attendings (who may examine or have examined on the Oral Boards) observe you in the outpatient clinic or hospital wards and provide feedback may be useful at this point.

One Week Before the Examination

Confirm that you have all the materials you need for the examination. Candidates are expected to bring their own instruments (tuning fork, pins, gloves, etc.) for the examination. Make sure that your ophthalmoscope is working and ensure that you are comfortable with its use! Recalling the Mini-Mental Status Examination (MMSE), Medical Research Council Motor Grading scale for example, would be useful.

Review your study materials, aids, and notes to enhance recollection. Selectively reviewing a concise text on the Oral Boards may help in focusing the thought process toward the examination format and candidate expectations. Repetitive review of neurological emergencies would be useful; in order to remain "on the ball," especially if you have not dealt with such problems in a while.

Ensure that you give yourself enough time to travel to the testing city and settle in. Some candidates arrive a week before and take Board-review courses, others arrive the morning of orientation/registration! It is advisable to arrive at least the evening before orientation/registration. You receive your official name badge and the examination and bus schedules after confirming your identification. You will receive a formal talk from the Board about the nature of the examination during orientation/registration. Make sure you can get to the examination hotel headquarters and know your bus schedule (provided by the Board, but you can make alternative arrangements) to the testing centers. It is imperative to arrive at the testing centers (usually a teaching hospital outpatient clinic center) on time.

The Night Before the Examination

Realize that you cannot know everything in neurology (nobody does and the examiners do not expect this!). Try to relax, have a decent meal, and good night's sleep. The knowledge you will exhibit the following day is an accumulation from medical school, through residency and fellowship or clinical practice. You have a better chance of performing better in a well-nourished and rested state. Review your history-taking and clinical examination techniques and ensure that all your instruments are in fine working condition. Also, focus on the general approaches to clinical problem solving in neurology, rather than on last-minute knowledge acquisition. Review emergency drugs and dosing regimens and your systematic approach to the Clinical Vignette sections, calling to mind the expected structural framework set out by ABPN.

The Morning of the Examination

Try to relax and think positively. Remember that you are equipped with the knowledge to pass the Oral Boards and be encouraged that the examiners are not trying to fail deserving candidates. Dress professionally (as you would do when attending an interview). You may wear a white coat but it is not mandatory. Ensure that you have all the equipment you need for the clinical examination and having a watch is useful to keep you on time. Do not forget to bring your ABPN-issued name badge, examination, and bus schedules. I do not believe that last-minute revision is particularly useful for the Oral Boards, as one is being tested on clinical knowledge and practice. A structured review of clinical neurology started early would be better than a last-minute rote-learning approach.

TEST-TAKING STRATEGIES

"Live Patient" Section

Perform the clinical history and physical examination concisely and thoroughly. Omission of formal evaluation of aspects of the neurological examination could result in failure. Ignore that two or three examiners are watching you and making notes. Imagine that you are in your practice/clinic seeing a friendly patient who has all the information you need to adequately diagnose and treat him or her. Maintain the usually expected professional and social etiquette. Use open-ended questions at the start of the interview.

Directed questioning (with "yes" or "no" answers) may be required if the patient loses focus or you are running short on time. This could be useful when trying to formulate a plausible diagnosis based on the presenting complaint or during the review of systems. Pertinent information in the history of presenting illness (HPI) is essential, but ensure that you cover past medical/past surgical/family/social/medication history (including allergies) as these may provide further insight to the disease. A broad review of systems may also uncover relevant detail you may have forgotten in the HPI. Aim to complete the history in 15 minutes.

Vital sign evaluations are not required during the physical examination. Cover mental status (including MMSE), higher cortical function, cranial nerve (II to XII), motor, sensory, reflex, coordination, and gait examinations. The examination should be complete, with more focus on the affected part of the nervous system as deduced from the clinical history if time permits. Ensure patient comfort during the examination by being gentle and exposing only relevant parts of the body. Perform the examination systematically in a well-rehearsed order. The average examinee has examined hundreds of neurological patients in training/practice; so do not panic if something unexpected occurs, such as observing ophthalmoparesis in a patient who did not inform you of diplopia. Focus on completing the examination and organizing the findings to support your differentials deduced from the history. Aim to complete the physical examination in 10 minutes.

Have 5 minutes to put your thoughts together and outline your presentation, case summary, and generate differential diagnoses for the patient. You may use this period to fill out any gaps or raise questions that you may have forgotten to ask. Having a watch helps keep you on time, however, you can ask for a warning 5 minutes before you are expected to complete your clinical evaluation. On completion of your evaluation, thank the patient. The patient will be escorted out of the room prior to your case presentation.

Present the case concisely, summarizing the information collected to support your hypothesis without leaving out important details. Aim to present the case in 5 to 10 minutes, depending on its complexity. Offer a differential diagnosis list, stating how parts of the history/examination support or refute those suggestions. An extensive "laundry list" may expose the candidate to being sidetracked by the examiner. Produce a reasonable differential of about five likely conditions that you feel comfortable discussing.

The remaining 5 to 10 minutes will be used by the examinees to discuss investigations, management options, and prognosis of this case and similarly related diagnoses. The examiners are not allowed to give feedback during the examination, and would attempt to assess the breadth not depth of your knowledge in particular topics. Do not be distracted by the examiner writing during the examination, especially after you may have provided a response to a question! Focus on commonly accepted practices and admit lack of knowledge on a certain topic after providing some insight to the examiner on how you would approach the problem and acquire information in clinical practice.

Clinical Vignette Sections

This discussion also includes the three 5-minute clinical vignettes at the end of the "Live Patient" section. The better approach is to read the vignette aloud, as reading and hearing may better facilitate recall than hearing the vignette alone. The candidate also has an opportunity to analyze symptom-complexes visually, as making visual associations while reading occurs during study. Expect at least one neurological emergency. Remember the principles of resuscitation (A-B-C), patient safety and rapid investigation during or after stabilization. The examiners are expecting an approach to the vignettes based on six principles: disease localization, plausible differential diagnosis, reasonable investigation, management modalities (including pharmacological and nonpharmacological methods), prognosis, and patient counseling. Some of these categories may have more relevance than others based on the vignette.

The vignettes are usually composed of about two to three sentences and usually allow a broad-thinking approach. Localize the site of pathology based on the symptoms and signs presented, mentioning the most likely localization (right/left cerebral hemisphere, cerebellum, brainstem, spinal cord, peripheral nerve, muscle). A single localization may not be possible, so provide reasons why you suggest your statements. A more precise localization may be required for certain disorders (e.g., right parietal stroke, temporal lobe seizures, frontotemporal dementia, progressive proximal myopathy, cervical myelopathy at or above C5-6 level). The more precise the information provided by vignette is, the more precise the localization should be.

Generate a list of five or six differential diagnoses based on the information provided. Mention your most likely diagnosis first, proving evidence from the vignette on why you believe this to be the case. Emergencies and potentially treatable conditions should be readily identified. Support your list of differential diagnosis based on the information provided in the vignette. The differentials may consist of neurological diseases or classes of disease, based on the nature of the vignette. If classes of disease are used, mention one or two disorders in each class. For example, a vignette of an akinetic-rigid syndrome results in a disease-based differential for parkinsonism (e.g., progressive supranuclear palsy, multiple systems atrophy, cortico-basal ganglionic degeneration), whereas a vignette of infantile hypotonia may result in a disease-class differential (e.g., anterior horn cell disease, polyneuropathy, congenital myopathy). Avoid mentioning diseases that you are not familiar with, as you may risk additional questions from the examiners.

Organized categorization of symptom-complex etiology would be a useful way of approaching a clinically vague vignette. For example, a differential list for progressive ataxia in a child could be divided into acquired and genetic causes. Acquired causes could be organized to include infectious/postinfectious, neoplastic, toxic-metabolic, drug ingestion, autoimmune/demyelinating, whereas genetic causes could be organized into degenerative and metabolic disorders.

In vignettes that clearly suggest a single diagnosis, mention your most likely diagnosis, supporting how you arrived at your inference. Provide a plausible list of differential diagnoses based on some of the symptoms and signs presented, but argue why the data does not support those diagnoses. Avoid stating that there are no other considerations, as such a statement may not support the open-mindedness required to be a thorough neurologist. This may also expose the candidate to a modified clinical scenario developed by the examiner in order to assess breadth of knowledge. Candidates are given a chance to demonstrate their knowledge base, so you are better off talking about what you know, as you are more likely receive questions on the statements you make.

Avoid a "shot-gun" approach to investigation. Mention confirmatory tests and which tests may help in differentiating between your differential diagnoses. Start with the simplest evaluations (e.g., blood/serum tests) and work up to more complex or invasive tests. In emergency cases, initially mention investigations that are critical for the initial management of the patient. Diagnostic/confirmatory tests can be performed once the patient is stabilized. Be prepared to discuss the utility/importance of the tests you mention in evaluating the case, and how the results would assist in diagnosis. Specialist referral outside neurology may be mentioned as part of the investigation, but the candidate should state why this is needed, and how such a referral may assist in diagnosis or management.

Patient management and therapeutics should remind you of your admitting orders for critically ill or hospitalized patients or care plan for outpatients. Organize your management strategy into acute and chronic, pharmacological and nonpharmacological, conservative and surgical/invasive, and so on, depending on the clinical vignette. Being organized demonstrates to the examiner that you have a thoughtful and thorough approach to patient care. Pharmacological care requires some knowledge of drugs administered, including their mechanism/duration of action, common side-effect profile, and contraindications. Drug-dosing regimens are required for the emergency neurology vignettes. Mention drugs or drug classes with which you are familiar or have experience. Stick to well-established or approved drugs/regimens and avoid controversy. Admit lack of precise knowledge and inform the examiners on how you would obtain the information in clinical practice.

Be aware of established criteria for surgical/invasive management. Have some knowledge of the procedures performed and potential short- and long-term complications. Do not spend too much time trying to learn these, but you should possess enough information to allow outpatient follow-up and patient counseling. Examples include vagal nerve stimulation for refractory epilepsy, deep brain stimulation for Parkinson's disease and endarterectomy for high-grade symptomatic carotid stenosis.

Prognosis should include established estimates for disease morbidity and mortality, including risks for disease progression and predictive factors for clinical improvement or deterioration. Having some knowledge on outcome data shows the examiner that you are knowledgeable enough to accurately counsel patients and their families. This is particularly important in pediatric neurology, as parents often want to know if there are any long-term sequelae associated with a particular disease. All candidates have been involved in prognostication and counseling of patients and family members during their residency or in practice, so are very capable of doing so on the Oral Boards. Being aware of numerical prognostic data estimates for common neurological problems, including emergencies, would be useful to pass the Boards and in clinical practice. Examples include the 1-year survival rates for glioblastoma multiforme, complete recovery rates from Guillain-Barre syndrome, risk of re-bleeding from aneurysmal subarachnoid hemorrhage, risk and timing of cerebral herniation post-stroke, and rate of disease progression in muscular dystrophies.

Counseling should be done in simple language, informing the examiners of what you would tell patients and their families. This may include issues such as diagnostic implications, medication compliance and side effects, alternative management options, genetic counseling, social concerns, and prognosis. Provide frank answers and admit lack of precise knowledge on certain unfamiliar issues. Mention how you may utilize patient information resources to enhance the counseling process.

PART II

CLINICAL VIGNETTES: EMERGENCIES

Cerebrovascular Disease

CASE 1

A 66-year-old right-handed man presented to the emergency room 2 hours after the onset of right-sided weakness and sensory loss, slurred speech, and visual disturbances. He had a known history of hypertension and diabetes mellitus (DM). Examination revealed a right hemiplegia and right hemisensory loss (mainly affecting the face and upper extremity), dysarthria, and a right visual field deficit.

Localization

Left cortical hemispheric dysfunction affecting the frontal and parietal lobes. Further clinical examination may decipher an inferior (parietal) or superior (temporal) quadrantanopsia. The clinical deficit most likely involves the left middle cerebral artery (MCA) vascular territory.

Differential Diagnoses

The differential diagnosis for a sudden onset of left cortical hemispheric dysfunction includes an *acute ischemic stroke, acute intracranial hemorrhage* (ICH; subarachnoid aneurysmal and nonaneurysmal/traumatic, intraparenchymal [e.g., secondary to hypertension or amyloid angiopathy], subdural or epidural), *post-ictal state following a seizure* (Todd's paralysis), *hemiplegic migraine, secondary to toxic-metabolic derangement associated with a remote infarct* (diagnoses of exclusion in the acute phase) or *hemorrhage into a brain tumor.* The clinical presentation most likely represents an acute vascular event that can be classified as a *brain attack* owing to its short duration at presentation (<3 hours). This is a neurological emergency as clinical outcomes depend on rapid evaluation and treatment. The history does not discriminate between ischemic and hemorrhagic strokes.

The history should be expanded to confirm the onset of neurological deficit, and assess for contraindications for thrombolysis (recent ICH, myocardial infarction [MI] or major surgery, seizure at stroke onset, gastrointestinal [GI] or genitourinary [GU] bleed within 3 weeks, stroke, or serious head injury within

From: *Neurology Oral Boards Review:*
A Concise and Systematic Approach to Clinical Practice
By: E. E. Ubogu © Humana Press Inc., Totowa, NJ

3 months). The clinical examination should be extended to deduce the patient's vital signs (especially blood pressure [BP] and heart rate [HR]/rhythm), as well as a formal evaluation of the National Institutes of Health Stroke Scale [NIHSS], Glasgow Coma Scale [GCS], and other aspects of the general examination.

Investigations

Investigations should include complete blood count (CBC) with differential, prothrombin time (PT)/partial thromboplastin time (PTT)/international normalized ratio (INR) and comprehensive metabolic panel. In patients younger than 45 years, "stroke in the young" work-up (Protein C, Protein S, antithrombin III, activated protein C [APC] resistance, factor V Leiden, rapid plasma regain [RPR]/fluorescent treponemal antibody-absorption test [FTA-ABS], antinuclear antibody [ANA] panel, antiphospholipid [aPL] and anticardiolipin antibodies, plasminogen, fibrinogen and homocysteine levels, hemoglobin [Hb] electrophoresis) should be considered. Toxicology screens should be considered with a suggestive history of substance abuse.

Noncontrasted computed tomography (CT) scan of the head should be emergently performed to exclude an ICH. The absence of an intracranial bleed and contraindications to thrombolysis in a patient with an NIHSS greater than 4 suggest that the patient is a candidate for recombinant tissue plasminogen activator (r-tPA) therapy. An intracranial bleed is an absolute contraindication, and surgical decompression may be required.

In cases of ischemic stroke, a magnetic resonance imaging (MRI) of the brain without gadolinium (including diffusion-weighted images [DWI]) and magnetic resonance angiography (MRA) of the intracranial and extracranial vessels should be performed once the patient is stable. This should confirm the extent of anatomical involvement and assist in deducing the probable etiology for the stroke (large-vessel occlusive, large-vessel thromboembolic, or small-vessel disease). If a high-grade stenosis of the carotid arteries is suggested on MRA, cerebral angiography is warranted (gold-standard). Carotid ultrasound scan (USS) and transcranial dopplers (TCDs) may be useful where magnetic resonance scans are not readily available.

Further investigations include electrocardiogram (EKG), cardiac holter monitor, or telemetry for atrial fibrillation, transesophageal echocardiography (TEE)/transthoracic echocardiography (TTE) to assess left ventricle (LV) function (<35% associated with stroke) and cardiac sources of emboli, such as mural thrombus, atrial septal defects with patent foramen ovale, valvular vegetations, or aortic arch atheroma.

Management

The initial management may involve BP control if BP is greater than 220/130 mmHg. Intravenous (i.v.) labetalol in escalating double doses, from 10 to 150 mg (maximum total dose 300 mg) can be administered every 10 to 20 minutes to keep BP below185/110 mmHg, especially prior to thrombolysis. Other options include i.v. nicardipine (5–15 mg per hour), captopril (0.625–1.25 mg every 6 hours), or nitroprusside (0.5–10 μg/kg per minute). Electrolyte abnormalities must be corrected.

Thrombolysis with r-tPA is administered at 0.9 mg/kg (maximum 90 mg) with 10% given as an i.v. bolus with the remaining 90% administered via i.v. infusion over 1 hour. This is the only Food and Drug Administration (FDA)-approved use for r-tPA in acute stroke. Other thrombolytics, such as streptokinase and glycoprotein IIb/IIIa antagonists, have not been approved.

The patient should be admitted to an intensive care or acute stroke unit for further management. Vital signs and neurological assessments should be taken every 4 hours. Bed rest for 24 hours, strict fluid balance with maintenance fluids (i.v. normal saline at 1–2 cc/kg per hour) and deep vein thrombosis (DVT) prophylaxis are necessary. Anti-pyretic treatment with acetaminophen should be used if body temperature is more than 37.5°C. Repeat head CT post-thrombolysis (within 24 hours) to exclude hemorrhage. Antiplatelet and anticoagulation therapy can be instituted more than 24 hours post-thrombolysis to prevent further stroke. Choice of drug depends on presumed etiology and may be contraindicated in large volume infarcts.

The use of i.v. unfractionated heparin (15–18 U/kg per hour, keeping PTT between 1.5 and 2.5 × baseline) and oral warfarin (to keep INR at 2–3) may be warranted in strokes associated with atrial fibrillation, arterial dissection, and cardiac sources of embolism. The utility of anticoagulant agents for other stroke etiologies is controversial but widely practiced in the United States and Canada despite lack of supporting data. Antiplatelet agents include aspirin (ASA) 81–325 mg per day, clopidogrel 75 mg per day, dipyridamole/ASA 100/25 mg twice a day or ticlopidine 250 mg twice a day. Common side effects (e.g., headache with dipyramidole/ASA, neutropenia with ticlopidine) should be noted.

Prognosis

Prognosis depends on the size and severity of stroke on presentation (NIHSS >15), age, co-morbidities, early administration, and response to thrombolysis and complications of the stroke and its treatments. A hyperdense MCA sign may confer a mortality rate of 80% in untreated cases. Greater than 50% MCA distribution ischemia within 5 hours of presentation or more than 66% involvement within 24 hours may confer a mortality owing to cerebral herniation (highest risk: 48–96 hours post-stroke) of about 80% despite treatment.

The administration of r-tPA reduces the odds of death and dependency at 3-month follow-up by 44%, but confers a three to four times increased risk of symptomatic and fatal brain hemorrhage within 7–10 days post-thrombolysis (overall risk of 6.4% vs 0.6% risk without r-tPA). In general, 15–20% of acute stroke patients die within the first month post-stroke (causes include heart attacks and dysrhythmias, pneumonia, DVT/pulmonary embolism [PE]), with 50% of survivors exhibiting some degree of disability. Severe disability at 1 month, despite acute rehabilitation, may predict long-term disability.

Counseling

Counseling should be tailored toward risk-factor modification, including smoking cessation, control of BP and diabetes, medication compliance, the use of stroke prophylaxis and early recognition of symptoms. If a high-grade (>70%) symptomatic carotid stenosis is present, discussion on carotid endarterectomy should be considered.

Based on the North American Symptomatic Carotid Endarterectomy Trial [NASCET] trial, surgery may confer a 70% relative risk reduction in ipsilateral stroke with an absolute risk reduction of 9% per year. However, a 1–5% risk of morbidity or mortality is associated with the procedure, and this should be emphasized to the patient. Timing of surgery after stroke is not well established. Two to six weeks may be necessary depending on stroke size and perceived risks of reperfusion injury. For patients younger than 45 years, identifying and managing potentially treatable/modifiable etiologies for stroke and genetic counseling would be necessary.

SUMMARY

- **Brain attack** is a neurological emergency as outcomes are dependent on resuscitation, especially BP management, excluding ICH and administering **r-tPA within 3 hours** if clinically indicated (**NIHSS >4** and no contraindications).
- **Differential diagnoses** for ischemic stroke include **ICH, post-ictal state** (Todd's paralysis), **hemorrhage into a tumor, hemiplegic migraine**, and **toxic-metabolic derangement**.
- For BP over 220/130 mmHg, give **labetalol** 10 mg i.v. over 1 to 2 minutes with escalating double doses (maximum 300 mg). Other options include **nicardipine, captopril**, or **nitroprusside**. Aim for stable BP **of less than 185/110 mmHg** before thrombolysis.
- Approved r-tPA dose is **0.9 mg/kg** (maximum 90 mg) i.v. with **10%** as bolus and remaining **90%** infused over 1 hour.
- Antiplatelet or anticoagulant medications can be administered when **more than 24 hours** following thrombolysis have elapsed.
- Prognostic information important for adequate counseling includes the risks and benefits of **r-tPA** or **carotid endarterectomy**.

CASE 2

A 33-year-old healthy woman who was 4 weeks postpartum suddenly developed generalized headache, vomiting, and mild bilateral lower extremity weakness 1 day ago. She had felt extremity tired over the past 48 hours, with poor fluid intake. The headache was refractory to over-the-counter (OTC) medications. Clinical examination revealed bilateral papilledema, mild paraparesis (Medical Research Council [MRC] 4/5), and hyperreflexia without sensory deficits.

Localization

A generalized headache with vomiting is nonlocalizing. Coupled with papilledema, these may indicate raised intracranial pressure (ICP). Signs of raised ICP are more likely to occur from ventricular outflow obstruction or reduced venous drainage, than excessive cerebrospinal fluid (CSF) production. Hyperreflexia suggests an upper motor neuron (UMN) cause for her weakness. Paraparesis localizes to the superior parasagittal frontal lobes, bilateral ventral brainstem from the midbrain rostrally, or bilateral central spinal cord lesions involving the corticospinal tracts bilaterally. The absence of sensory findings makes the first two options more likely. If further clinical evaluation excludes other signs and symptoms, bilateral parasagittal frontal lesions are more likely.

Differential Diagnosis

Cortical venous sinus thrombosis (CVST) is the most likely diagnosis, based on the acute clinical presentation and presence of risk factors for sino-occlusive disease (puerperium and dehydration). Other considerations include *tumor (meningioma) with hemorrhagic expansion, subdural hemorrhage involving the frontal convexity* (more common in older patients), *subarachnoid hemorrhage* (SAH) owing to rupture of an anterior communicating artery (ACommA) aneurysm with secondary meningeal irritation, *bilateral anterior cerebral artery (ACA) infarcts* (would not expect signs and symptoms of raised ICP) and *idiopathic intracranial hypertension* (IIH; especially if patient is obese with visual loss, but presentation is too acute and focal signs are unexpected).

Investigation

Investigation should include CBC with differential, PT/PTT/INR, and basic metabolic panel (sodium [Na^+], blood urea nitrogen [BUN]/creatinine [Cr] ratio may help with assessing dehydration). Emergent CT scan of the head without contrast should be performed to exclude ICH, space-occupying lesions, and hydrocephalus. Consider lumbar puncture (LP) if concerned about SAH or IIH. Opening pressure, CSF xanthochromia, CSF red blood cell (RBC)/white blood cell (WBC)/Protein with or without Gram stain are essential. If CVST is suggested (small ventricles, low-density infarcts, superficial petechial hemorrhages, cord/empty-δ signs on CT), a "thrombophilia" work-up can be ordered prior to initiating anticoagulation: antithrombin III, protein C, protein S, APC resistance, factor V Leiden, plasminogen, fibrinogen, aPL antibodies, ANA panel, cryoglobulins, homocysteine, or Hb electrophoresis.

Once stable, MRI of the brain without gadolinium with MRA and magnetic resonance venography (MRV) sequences or cerebral angiography should be performed to confirm the clinical suspicion and exclude aneurysms and arterial malformations.

Management

Rapid institution of i.v. fluids and heparin are warranted to prevent neurological deficit progression and worsening of ICP caused by venous outflow obstruction. Intravenous normal saline bolus of 1000 cc, followed by 2 to 3 cc/kg per hour should be given. Heparin i.v. infusion at 15–18 U/kg per hour without bolus should be started, keeping PTT 1.5–2.5 × above baseline. Hemorrhagic venous infarction or petechial hemorrhages are not an absolute contraindication, but caution is required. The efficacy of heparin has not been confirmed by randomized controlled trials. Bed rest and strict fluid balance (to ensure correction of water deficit appropriately) are necessary in the first 24–48 hours of admission. If a septic illness precedes neurological deficits, then broad-spectrum i.v. antibiotics should be administered. Oral anticoagulation with warfarin to keep INR 2–3 should be administered once the patient can tolerate oral intake. Symptomatic therapy of headache using analgesics (acetaminophen or mild opioids) and anti-emetics for nausea should be considered. Avoid non-steroidal anti-inflammatory drugs (NSAIDs).

The patient can be managed on a regular nursing floor with close neurological monitoring every 6 hours. Clinical deterioration requires intensive care. Progression in venous ischemia despite adequate anticoagulation may require local thrombolysis, although there are no controlled trials to demonstrate efficacy. Worsening in cognitive status would require repeat CT scanning (to exclude hemorrhage) and intubation for ventilatory support/airway protection. Severely elevated ICP may require ventriculostomy or hyperosmolar therapy if secondary to rare cerebral edema. The development of seizures would require appropriate aggressive therapy (*see* later sections on status epilepticus [SE]).

Prognosis

Survival and clinical recovery occurs in 80 to 90% of patients with CVST. Mortality and poor outcomes are associated with coma and ICP on presentation.

Relapses may occur in less than 10% of surviving patients and usually occur within the first 12 months. Prognosis is also dependent on underlying predisposing medical conditions (e.g., carcinoma, sepsis, congestive heart failure [CHF], polycythemia vera, etc.).

Counseling

The patient should be counseled on medication compliance, including the need for frequent INR checks. Dietary modifications (including alcohol intake) and medications that can modify INR should be discussed.

The suggested duration of oral anticoagulation therapy is 3–6 months in idiopathic cases and 6–12 months for acquired or inherited etiologies, to facilitate recanalization. These durations are empirical guidelines. Repeat MRI/MRV may guide the physician on when to cease therapy. The patient should be aware of the low risk of recurrence. For patients with seizures, antiepileptic drugs (AEDs) such as phenytoin are needed in the short-term (<1 year) and should be individually tailored. AED prophylaxis is not required in patients who do not initially present with seizures.

SUMMARY

- **CVST** is a neurological emergency, as outcomes depend on institution of **i.v. anticoagulation** and **fluids** before deterioration.
- Differential diagnoses for CVST include **tumor with hemorrhagic expansion, subdural/subarachnoid hemorrhages, arterial infarction, and IIH**.
- Etiologies include **idiopathic, primary inherited**, and **secondary acquired** causes.
- Treatment includes **heparin i.v. infusion at 15–18 U/kg per hour**, keeping PTT **1.5–2.5** × above baseline, and aggressive rehydration with **i.v. normal saline, 1000 cc bolus** with infusion at **2–3 cc/kg per hour**. Oral warfarin should be started to keep INR **2–3**.
- Complications, such as **seizures** and **raised ICP**, should be aggressively managed to prevent poor outcomes.
- Prognosis is generally **favorable (80–90%** survival and recovery).

CASE 3

A 53-year-old man with no known medical problems complained of a throbbing headache for more than 2 days. A few hours prior to presentation, he complained of severe vertigo, nausea with vomiting, imbalance, and inability to grasp objects with his right arm. Clinical examination showed a BP of 244/138 mmHg with poor responses to external stimuli, slurred speech, gaze-evoked nystagmus, and right-sided appendicular ataxia with intention tremor.

Localization

Right-sided appendicular ataxia with intention tremor, dysarthria, gaze-evoked nystagmus, vertigo, and imbalance (implying either gait or truncal ataxia) suggests dysfunction of the right cerebellar hemisphere with involvement of the midline cerebellum. These symptoms and signs may also localize to the right dorsolateral rostral medulla. If further history and examination do not reveal any sensory disturbances (ipsilateral facial sensory loss with contralateral loss of hemibody sensation), the right cerebellar hemisphere with midline involvement is the more likely localization.

Differential Diagnosis

Severe hypertension coupled with poor responses to external stimuli is worrisome for *hypertensive bleed with cerebellar expansion or herniation causing brainstem compression*. This is a neurological and neurosurgical emergency that requires prompt treatment.

Other differential diagnoses for acute right cerebellar dysfunction include *ischemic stroke* secondary to atherothrombotic or embolic disease affecting the posterior inferior cerebellar artery (PICA), anterior inferior cerebellar artery (AICA), or superior cerebellar artery (SCA) distributions (supplied by vertebral and basilar arteries), or dissection affecting the vertebral artery, *ICH* (secondary to hypertension, trauma, sympathomimetic drug use, bleeding disorders, anticoagulants, vascular malformation, aneurysm, or vasculitis), and *hemorrhage into a primary cerebellar tumor* (astrocytoma, medulloblastoma) or *metastatic disease* (lung, breast, metastatic melanoma, renal cell carcinoma, choriocarcinoma).

Acute cerebellar tonsillar herniation associated with an Arnold-Chiari malformation and *hypertensive encephalopathy* may cause poor levels of responsiveness and some nonlocalizing/midline cerebellar signs without hemiataxia and intention tremor. *A right dorsolateral medullary ischemic stroke* is still a diagnostic consideration.

Investigations

Immediate noncontrasted CT imaging of the head to evaluate for a cerebellar ICH is necessary. CBC, PTT/PT/INR, basic metabolic profile, urine/serum toxicology can be ordered *en route*. If the CT scan does not reveal a hemorrhage, MRI brain without gadolinium, with MRA of the intra- and extracranial vessels (including diffusion and dissection protocols, respectively) could be ordered for ischemic stroke evaluation once the patient is stable. MRI of the brain with and without gadolinium would be important for tumor evaluation. Cerebral angiography may be required to assess for vascular malformations.

Management

As a consequence of the reduction in responsiveness (document GCS) and the concern for brainstem compression, emergency intubation for airway support and mechanical ventilation should be performed. Keep head of bed at 30°, hyperventilate to keep arterial pressure for carbon dioxide ($PaCO_2$) at 25–30 mmHg and infuse mannitol 20% 1g/kg i.v. bolus over 30 minutes, then 0.25–0.5 g/kg every 4–6 hours to keep serum osmolarity between 300 and 320 mOsm/L (to reduce ICP). BP management should be initiated: labetalol i.v. in escalating double doses, from 10 to 150 mg (maximum total dose 300 mg) can be administered every 10–20 minutes to keep BP below 185/110 mmHg (or mean arterial pressure [MAP] <130). Other options include i.v. nicardipine (5–15 mg per hour), nitroprusside (0.5–10 µg/kg per minute), and captopril (0.625–1.25 mg every 6 hours). Precipitous reduction in BP should be avoided. Keep MAP at 70–120 mmHg.

On detecting a cerebellar ICH on CT, neurosurgery should be consulted for an emergency posterior fossa craniotomy for hemorrhage evacuation and brainstem decompression if hematoma diameter is greater than 3 cm, brainstem compression, hydrocephalus, or obliteration of the fourth ventricle or quadrigeminal cisterns is present. Clinical signs and symptoms of brainstem compression or coma require surgical referral independent of CT findings, even with ischemic cerebellar infarcts. The patient should be admitted to an intensive care unit (ICU) for pre- and postoperative care (regular neurological observations every 4 hours, ventricular drainage (shunt) and ICP monitoring, ventilatory support, DVT prophylaxis, wound healing). Long-term BP control should be initiated prior to discharge to an acute rehabilitation facility. Optimal medical and surgical treatment for ICH is not based on randomized control trials, but published guidelines.

Prognosis

Hypertension-induced ICH most likely occurs in the putamen (~35%), cerebrum (~25%), thalamus (~10–15%), cerebellum (~5–10%), caudate and pons (~5% each). Data for ICH associated with hypertension in general suggest a 1-month mortality of 30–50%, with death in the first 24–96 hours accounting for most cases. However, mortality increases with advancing age, degree of hypertension, low GCS on admission (<8), hematoma size, and intraventricular extension. Six-month death and severe disability rates could be as high as 75% in surgically treated and 90% in medically treated patients with ICH.

In cerebellar ICH that meet surgical criteria, failure to decompress the posterior fossa results in uniformly fatality. Recurrence rates for ICH are about 10% per patient-year if diastolic blood pressure (DBP) is more than 90 mmHg and less than 1.5% if DBP is less than 90 mmHg, emphasizing the need for adequate BP control. Prognosis also depends on intraoperative and postoperative surgical complications, as well as any pre-existing medical problems.

Counseling

Most surviving patients with ICH have some degree of disability and subsequent mortality rates are high. BP control is essential to preventing ICH recurrence. Anti-hypertensive drugs have been shown to reduce the risk of both ischemic and hemorrhagic stroke in large population trials. If medication noncompliance or illicit drug use are implicated, further counseling and detoxification should be considered. For cases associated with vascular malformations, surgical excision (if feasible without adverse sequelae) should be considered, weighing the risk–benefit ratio.

SUMMARY

- **Cerebellar ICH** is a neurological/neurosurgical emergency because survival is dependent on **rapid resuscitation, optimal medical management**, and **surgical decompression with hematoma evacuation.**
- If associated with hypertension, reduce BP to less than **185/100 or MAP to less than 130 mmHg**. Labetalol, nitroprusside, nicardipine, or enalapril can be used.
- The most emergent investigation is **head CT**. Surgical indicators include **hematoma diameter greater than 3 cm, hydrocephalus,** and **obliteration of quadrigeminal cisterns**. Signs of **brainstem compression** indicate surgery. **Mortality is approximately 100%** if not performed emergently.
- **Six-month mortality** and **severe disability** are as high as **75%** in ICH.
- **DBP greater than 90 mmHg** confers a hypertensive ICH recurrence of **10% per patient-year**. Long-term BP treatment is **essential**.

CASE 4

A 15-year-old girl with a 2-week history of intermittent fever, frontal headaches, and a purulent nasal discharge complained of double vision for 18 hours. Clinical examination revealed a lethargic girl with a temperature of 102°F, orbital congestion, proptosis, and near-complete ophthalmoplegia with a poorly reactive, dilated pupil on the left.

Localization

Orbital congestion and proptosis suggest left orbital involvement. Near-complete ophthalmoplegia with pupillary dilation suggest dysfunction of the muscles innervated by the left cranial nerve (CN) III (including the parasympathetic pupillary constrictors), IV, and VI. These findings suggest a process involving the cavernous sinus, superior orbital fissure, orbit, or a combination of these.

A patchy process involving the left midbrain and pons is unlikely if further clinical examination does not reveal any additional signs.

Differential Diagnosis

Cavernous sinus thrombosis is the most likely diagnosis given the history of preceding purulent sinus infection. Other considerations include *orbital inflammatory disease* (e.g., cellulitis, myositis), *orbital tumor* (e.g., optic glioma, dermoid cyst, hemangioma), and *orbital hemorrhage secondary to trauma.* Pain is likely with primary orbital disease. Thyroid ophthalmopathy (would not expect febrile illness and pupillary abnormalities), *cavernous sinus fistula* (would expect orbital bruit), *Tolosa-Hunt syndrome* (idiopathic granuloma of superior orbital fissure or cavernous sinus; usually more slowly progressive and associated with pain without proptosis, small pupils and marked CN V involvement), *Gradinego syndrome* (apical petrositis with unilateral CN VI and VII nerve palsies; degree of orbital disease and absence of facial droop make this unlikely) and *ophthalmoplegic migraine* (degree of orbital disease and absence of ipsilateral migraine-type headache associated with ocular signs reduces likelihood) are other possible, but rarer differentials.

Investigation

Investigations should include CBC with differential, PT/PTT/INR (to obtain baseline before LP, if needed to assess for meningitis; positive in 20%), basic metabolic profile, erythrocyte sedimentation rate (ESR)/C-reactive protein (CRP; does not discriminate between inflammatory conditions), thyroid function tests, blood (positive in 70%) and nasal cultures (causative organisms include *Staphylococcus aureus*, *Streptococcus pneumoniae*, Gram-negative bacilli, anaerobes, and fungi).

Head CT scan with thin cuts through the sinuses may identify source of infection and exclude hemorrhage. Coronal CT of the neck may identify cavernous sinus thrombosis. Consider MRI of the brain and orbits with and without gadolinium to exclude tumor, inflammatory disease, granuloma, and hemorrhage. Coronal MRI of the neck may be diagnostic if CT is equivocal. MRA may show reduced flow in cavernous portion of internal carotid artery (ICA). Cerebral angiography is rarely needed in equivocal cases, especially if carotid-cavernous fistula is suspected.

Management

This is a neurological emergency because early administration of broad-spectrum i.v. antibiotics and anticoagulation improve outcomes and may prevent irreversible neurological sequelae. Contralateral spread may occur 24–48 hours after ipsilateral orbital congestion if untreated. Broad-spectrum penicillins (or vancomycin if methicillin-resistant *S. aureus* [MRSA] suspected), third-generation cephalosporins and metronidazole i.v. can be used prior to blood culture and sensitivity results. Heparin i.v. (15–18 U/kg per hour without bolus, keep PTT 1.5–2.5 × baseline) should be started within 7 days of presentation, with conversion to oral warfarin (to keep INR 2–3). Treatment durations are empirical: 3–4 weeks for antibiotics and 4–6 weeks for anticoagulation. Aggressive i.v. hydration with normal saline to cover for insensible losses secondary to fever, antipyretics, and supportive care (e.g., regular nursing checks, adequate nutrition) are also necessary.

In refractory cases, surgical drainage of the cavernous sinus may be performed. Drainage of the precipitating infection (sinus, dental, orbital) is more commonly performed to facilitate recovery.

Prognosis

Mortality is as high as 80–100% with morbidity of 50–75% in survivors if untreated with antibiotics. Morbidity includes residual ocular motor deficits, blindness (retinal artery/vein occlusion, toxic optic neuropathy), seizures (cerebral abscess or meningoencephalitis), hemiparesis (ICA occlusion, CVST, cerebral abscess), and hypopituitarism (infarction or infection). With aggressive antibiotic therapy, mortality is about 20–30% with morbidity of about 20–25%. Anticoagulation may reduce morbidity (especially ocular motor sequelae) and mortality based on case series, but is untested by clinical trials.

Counseling

Patients should be aware of prognostic data, particularly the mortality rates despite adequate, aggressive treatment. The development of complications requires long-term supportive care and treatment (e.g., AEDs for seizures, hormonal replacement for hypopituitarism with implications for sexual maturation in prepubertal children, eye patches for ophthalmoparesis, physical/occupational therapy for hemiparesis). Early treatment of sinus or dental infections (and dental hygiene) should be emphasized.

SUMMARY

- **Cavernous sinus thrombosis** is a neurological emergency because outcomes depend on early institution of i.v. antibiotics and anticoagulation.
- **Ophthalmoparesis, proptosis,** and **orbital congestion** associated with **febrile illness** make diagnosis likely.
- **CT or MRI scans of the head and neck** are useful confirmatory tests that may exclude other potential differentials.
- Treatment involves **broad-spectrum i.v. antibiotics** to cover for *S. aureus, S. pneumoniae,* Gram-negative bacilli, and anaerobes.

- Anticoagulation should be given **within 7 days** of symptom onset.
- Duration of therapy: **3–4 weeks** for antibiotics and **4–6 weeks** for anti-coagulation.
- Mortality is **80–100%** without treatment, **20–30%** with treatment. Morbidity is **50–75%** without treatment, **20–25%** with treatment.

CASE 5

A 58-year-old woman had complained of a severe, nontraumatic, explosive headache 2 days ago. She subsequently developed persistent horizontal diplopia with right lateral gaze. About 6 hours ago, she experienced another headache associated with neck stiffness and severe nausea. In the emergency room (ER), her vital signs were normal. She was drowsy but able to appropriately answer simple questions and follow commands. Neurological examination revealed a fixed and dilated left pupil, moderate left ptosis, and adduction paresis without any further deficits. Brudzinski sign was present with neck flexion.

Localization

A left-sided temporal headache is nonlocalizing, but the subsequent development of meningismus (neck stiffness with positive Brudzinski sign) implies meningeal irritation. Horizontal diplopia on right lateral gaze associated with left ptosis, left adduction paresis, and pupillary dilation (reduced parasympathetic function) localizes to dysfunction of the left CN III. A left CN III palsy may be the result of nuclear lesion in the left midbrain or nerve lesion anywhere along its intracranial course (runs between SCA and posterior cerebral artery (PCA), then close to the medial temporal lobes to the cavernous sinus, to the superior orbital fissure into the orbit).

Reduced level of consciousness implies bilateral cerebral, diencephalic, or brainstem dysfunction. Isolated nausea could be indicative of raised ICP. In summary, the underlying process most likely diffusely affects the bilateral cerebral cortex with meningeal irritation and is associated with a left CN III palsy.

Differential Diagnosis

A severe explosive headache followed by meningismus and reduced level of consciousness is concerning for a subarachnoid hemorrhage (SAH). Early pupillary involvement with a CN III lesion is supportive of extrinsic compression. The most likely diagnosis in this case is an *aneurysmal SAH secondary to rupture of a distal left ICA or posterior communicating artery (PcommA) aneurysm with compression of the left CN III.* Other etiologies for SAH include arterial (carotid) dissection, cerebral or cervical arteriovenous malformations

(AVMs), dural arteriovenous fistulas, septic (mycotic) aneurysms, pituitary apoplexy, anticoagulant use, and cryptogenic (in about 15–20%).

Other differentials include *left midbrain ICH* (meningismus unlikely and other signs of midbrain dysfunction such as vertical gaze palsy, paralysis of accommodation, or contralateral hemiparesis would be expected), *acute left temporal subdural hematoma* (SDH; with transtentorial herniation and midbrain compression: would expect contralateral hemiparesis or hemisensory loss before ipsilateral CN III palsy), *left temporal cerebral abscess with intraventricular rupture* (headache would be more insidious and associated with focal deficits; e.g., receptive aphasia, inferior quadrantanopsia) or *hemorrhage into a primary or metastatic tumor* (with secondary cerebral herniation).

Investigations

A noncontrasted head CT scan should be performed immediately after the patient is stabilized. The sensitivity of CT for acute SAH is approximately 90–95% if performed within 24 hours and 75–80% if performed at 72 hours. LP should be performed if CT scan is negative. Opening pressure (determines ICP), CSF cell count (RBC >100,000/mm^3 with no reduction between tubes 1 and 4), protein and centrifugation (for xanthochromia: indicative of blood in CSF for >6–12 hours and supports diagnosis of SAH) should be performed. PT/PTT/INR should be checked before LP. Other initial laboratory tests include CBC with differentials, comprehensive metabolic panel, arterial blood gas (ABG), and type and screen. TCDs should be used to monitor for cerebral vasospasm (mean MCA velocity >120 cm per second indicates mild vasospasm, >200 cm per second indicates severe vasospasm).

Angiography should be performed to localize the ruptured aneurysm and establish its relationship to other vessels, size of its neck and to screen for other aneurysms. The gold standard is four-vessel digital subtraction contrast angiography (sensitivity of 85–98%), although MRA (sensitivity of ~85% if diameter >3 mm) or CT angiography (CTA) with three-dimensional (3-D) reconstruction (sensitivity 95%, specificity 85% if diameter >2.2 mm) can be performed initially, as these are less invasive with reduced associated risks.

Management

Endotracheal intubation should be performed if the patient loses consciousness or is unable to protect her airway. The severity of SAH should be graded based on either the Hunt and Hess scale (based on clinical features) or the World Federation of Neurologic Surgeons scale (based primarily on GCS). The principles of management are directed toward the most dreaded complications of SAH: rebleeding and cerebral ischemia secondary to vasospasm.

The patient should be admitted to an ICU with neurological checks every hour. Elevate the head of the bed to 30°. Low external stimulation, and reduced visitation, and noise levels should be observed. Analgesia should be provided for headache (acetaminophen–low-potency opioid combinations, steroids or opioids; avoid NSAIDs). BP should be kept between 120 and 160 mmHg systolic with i.v. normal saline at 1–2 cc/kg per hour (high BP increases risk for rebleeding, whereas low BP increases risk for cerebral vasospasm or cerebral salt-wasting).

Early surgical clipping or endovascular coiling appear to be the optimal methods of preventing rebleeding (performed within 72 hours), however, improved outcomes have not been conclusively demonstrated when compared to delayed surgery (10–12 days post-SAH). ε-Aminocaproic acid (Amicar®), an antifibrinolytic agent given as 10 g bolus with 2 g per hour i.v. infusion for 3–5 days, reduces the risk of rebleeding without improving short- or long-term outcomes in SAH (adverse drug reaction [ADRs]: hydrocephalus, vasospasm).

Following SAH, the risk of cerebral vasospasm is highest between days 4 and 14 post-bleed. Nimodipine, a calcium (Ca^{2+}) channel antagonist (60 mg po/ng every 4 hours for 21 days), has been shown to improve outcomes either via a neuroprotectant effect or mild reduction in cerebral vasospasm. The development of vasospasm requires hyperdynamic therapy ("triple H": hypervolemia, hypertension, and hemodilution) and vasodilatation via transluminal balloon angioplasty or intra-arterial papaverine (limited by its short-acting effect).

Additional supportive measures, for example, DVT/GI prophylaxis, stool softeners, strict fluid balance, mild sedation for anxiety, anti-emetics and seizure prophylaxis with phenytoin (controversial; given to reduce the potential risk of generalized tonic-clonic (GTC) seizure and its consequences with an unclipped aneurysm), are necessary. Raised ICP would require ventriculostomy, especially in more severely affected patients (to keep ICP 15–25 cm H_2O: associated with an increased risk of rebleeding).

Prognosis

The overall mortality from aneurysmal SAH is approximately 50%, with most deaths occurring within 30 days of presentation. About 10–15% of patients die before receiving medical attention. Of those reaching the hospital, approximately 8% die from progressive effects of initial bleed, whereas 7% die from the effects of cerebral vasospasm. Causes of morbidity and mortality include cerebral vasospasm with global ischemia (most significant cause in initial survivors), rebleeding with ICH (intraparenchymal in 20–40%, intraventricular in 15–30%, and SDH in 2–5%), acute hydrocephalus, myocardial infarction and cardiac dysrhythmias, SE (~3% of acute SAH patients develop seizures), and PE.

About 66% of survivors following successful aneurysmal clipping fail to return to their premorbid quality of life. Approximately 30–35% of survivors have moderate/severe disability, whereas about 20% have mild or minimal deficits at 4 months (improves to ~30% at 18 months). The risk of rebleeding is 4% on day 1, 1.5% per day for days 2–14, 15–20% within 2 weeks, and 50% within 6 months post-SAH. After 1 year, the risk becomes 3% per year with an annual mortality rate of 2%. Predictors of poor outcome include severity of neurological condition on initial admission, age greater than 70 years and amount of SAH on the initial CT.

Counseling

Patients and their families should be aware of the prognostic data and the implications for functional or independent recovery. Risk factors for developing SAH include hypertension, use of oral contraceptives, cigarette smoking, cocaine use, pregnancy and parturition, advancing age, positive family history, and medical conditions that predispose to cerebral aneurysms such as autosomal dominant (AD) polycystic kidney disease, connective tissue diseases (CTDs), Marfan's syndrome, atherosclerosis, and bacterial endocarditis.

The potential benefits of early surgical clipping need to be weighed against the risk of intraoperative aneurysmal rupture (~20%; associated with mortality/morbidity of ~30–35%). Without intraoperative rupture, the surgical risk of mortality is approximately 5% and morbidity approximately 12% following surgical clipping. Candidates for early surgical clipping include good premorbid medical condition, Hunt and Hess grade less than 3, large SAH, unstable BP or intractable seizures, signs of imminent or presence of early rebleeding, and a large ICH with mass effect associated with SAH.

In surgically unstable patients or individuals with failed clipping, endovascular coiling should be performed. More than 90% aneurysmal occlusion may occur in about 90% of patients with a 2% risk of aneurysmal perforation, 2–5% risk of procedure-related stroke, and approximately 1% peri-procedural mortality. This technique is particularly useful if there is a small aneurysmal neck or diameter less than 20 mm. There are no direct comparison controlled trials to ascertain whether surgical clipping or endovascular coiling is the better interventional procedure for ruptured aneurysmal SAH.

SUMMARY

- **Aneurysmal SAH** is a neurological emergency because of its **high early mortality rate** and outcomes are potentially modifiable by early medical and surgical intervention.
- Other etiologies for SAH include **arterial (carotid) dissection, cerebral** or **cervical AVMs, dural arteriovenous fistulas, septic aneurysms, pituitary apoplexy, anticoagulant use,** and **cryptogenic.**

- Differentials include **brainstem ICH, acute SDH with brainstem compression, cerebral abscess with intraventricular rupture**, and **hemorrhage into neoplasm**.
- Essential investigations include **CT head with or without LP** and **angiography (MRA, CTA, or digital subtraction contrast angiography)**. **TCD** is useful to monitor for cerebral vasospasm.
- Management is directed toward **prevention of rebleeding** (early surgical clipping or endovascular coiling, BP control, and ε-aminocaproic acid) and **cerebral vasospasm** (nimodipine). **Supportive care** and treating complications of SAH is essential.
- Overall mortality is approximately **50%**, with most deaths occuring within **30** days post-SAH. About **10–15%** die before receiving medical attention. The main causes of death and morbidity are related to **cerebral vasospasm** and **rebleeding**.
- **Severity on presentation, age older than 70** and **size of SAH** predict outcomes.
- Approximately **30%** of survivors are independent **18** months post-SAH.
- Comparative efficacy of surgical clipping vs endovascular coiling in ruptured aneurysmal SAH is **unknown**.

2

Epilepsy

CASE 1

A 32-year-old man was observed to suddenly become unresponsive followed by four episodes of generalized tonic-clonic convulsions of the upper and lower extremities while at work. Each episode lasted about 5–10 minutes and he failed to regain awareness after each episode. He was brought to the ER about 30 minutes after his first convulsion. Clinical examination revealed unresponsiveness to external stimuli, deep sighing breaths with respiratory rate of 24 per minute, BP of 155/100 mmHg, and HR of 118 per minute. Left lateral tonic head deviation and flexor contraction of the left upper extremity were observed before another episode of generalized convulsions in the ER.

Localization

Generalized convulsions suggest a global increase in cerebral activity, however, forced tonic head deviation to the left and flexor contraction of the left upper extremity prior to convulsions suggest a right frontal focus of cortical irritability.

Differential Diagnosis

Generalized convulsive SE is most likely. This is defined as a single generalized seizure lasting 5 minutes or more in adults, 10 minutes or more in children, or two or more seizures without fully regaining consciousness in between episodes. Etiologies include *abrupt AED withdrawal/noncompliance, alcohol withdrawal, metabolic derangement* (low/high Na^+, glucose, low Ca^{2+}, low magnesium [Mg^{2+}], uremia), *trauma, hypoxia, infection* (cerebral abscess, encephalitis), *neoplasms, vascular malformations, congenital malformations, genetic diseases* (children), *drug intoxication,* or *idiopathic.* Other diagnostic considerations include *anoxic encephalopathy with post-anoxic myoclonus, Wernicke's encephalopathy, malingering,* and *pseudoseizures.* However, the clinical presentation makes these differentials highly unlikely.

From: *Neurology Oral Boards Review:*
A Concise and Systematic Approach to Clinical Practice
By: E. E. Ubogu © Humana Press Inc., Totowa, NJ

Investigations

Investigations should include capillary (finger stick) glucose, CBC with differential, comprehensive metabolic profile, PT/PTT/INR (prior to LP if needed for septic work-up), thyroid function test (TFT), Mg^{2+}, phosphate ($PO_4{}^{3-}$), serum/urine toxicology, AED levels, and ABG (to assess for respiratory alkalotic compensation for metabolic acidosis). Lactate and prolactin levels may help differentiate SE from pseudoseizures. If convulsions are prolonged, creatine kinase (CK) is useful for assessing rhabdomyolysis. EKG (arrhythmias can occur during prolonged seizure or with treatment) should be performed.

Electroencephalogram (EEG) may also localize seizure focus post- or inter-ictally; continuous EEG monitoring may be necessary if the patient does not regain consciousness despite treatment (to evaluate for nonconvulsive SE) or to monitor comatose patient for electrographic seizure control. CT scan of the head without contrast should be performed when stable to exclude ICH. MRI of the brain with and without gadolinium (seizure protocol: thin cuts through temporal lobes) should be performed for a structural etiology.

Management

Generalized convulsive SE is a neurological emergency. The airways should be secured and adequate oxygenation provided. Intubation and mechanical ventilation in poorly responsive/comatose patients or if significant respiratory depression occurs is required. Adequate hydration with i.v. normal saline is necessary. Electrolyte abnormalities should be corrected. Give thiamine and glucose i.v. (can omit glucose if capillary or serum level is normal) in comatose patients of undetermined etiology.

Pharmacological treatment is as follows:

Lorazepam 0.05–0.20 mg/kg at 1–2 mg i.v. every 2 minutes (maximum about 8 mg in adults and 4 mg in children) or **diazepam** i.v. 0.15–0.25 mg/kg (adults) or 0.1–1.0 mg/kg (children) at maximum rate of 5 mg per minute. Maximum dose is 10 mg in adults and children.

Rectal diazepam 0.5 mg/kg (maximum dose 20 mg) can be given to children. There is a risk of SE recurrence approximately 30 minutes after administration, despite early onset of action with diazepam.

Phenytoin 20 mg/kg at 50 mg per minute (adults) or 1 mg/kg per minute (children) or **fosphenytoin** 20 mg/kg phenytoin equivalents at 150 mg per minute (adults) or 3 mg/kg per minute (children) should be given, even with SE cessation with lorazepam. Can give additional **phenytoin** 5–10 mg/kg at the same infusion rates for refractory cases (defined clinically as failure to respond to first and second-line agents), up to a total of 30 mg/kg. **Phenobarbital** (especially in children)

20 mg/kg at 50–100 mg per minute or **valproate** i.v. (in adults) 20–25 mg/kg over 60 minutes loading dose, then start at 10–15 mg/kg per day every 6 hours in divided doses can be used in addition to phenytoin in refractory cases.

If SE remains refractory, pharmacological coma with electrographic seizure cessation or "burst suppression" should be induced with anesthetics: **propofol** 1–2 mg/kg i.v. loading dose, then 2–10 mg/kg per hour, **midazolam** 0.2 mg/kg slow bolus, then 1–10 µg/kg per minute or **pentobarbital** (more commonly used in children) 5–15 mg/kg i.v. bolus over 1 hour, then 0.5–3.0 mg/kg per hour. Vasopressors may be required to maintain BP and cerebral perfusion while on these drugs. Maintenance doses of AEDs (e.g., phenytoin 3–5 mg/kg per day i.v. divided every 8 hours) should be instituted on cessation of SE. Check levels and titrate AED dose accordingly.

Hypotension, cardiac arrhythmias (particularly with phenytoin, less so with fosphenytoin), and respiratory depression (particularly with benzodiazepines and barbiturates) are common side effects of drug therapy in SE. There is an increased risk of infections with propofol (owing to its lipophilic nature). An "infusion syndrome" (rhabdomyolysis, severe metabolic acidosis, and cardiovascular collapse) rarely occurs in children treated with propofol, so it is contraindicated in this age group. Central nervous system (CNS) depression or paradoxical agitation is common in children treated with barbiturates. Midazolam undergoes tachyphylaxis after 24–48 hours, resulting in progressively increased doses for seizure control.

Prognosis

Prognosis after generalized convulsive SE depends on age of patient, duration (>30 minutes), and cause for SE. Mortality rates vary from 3 to 35% (average 25%), with children having lower mortality rates than adults. Morbidity is more difficult to estimate because of a lack of studies with neuropsychological evaluation. In SE, subtle-to-adverse effects on intellectual development in children and memory/cognitive deficits in adults may occur. Drugs used in treating SE may have toxic side effects that may influence morbidity.

Counseling

Patients should be counseled about AED compliance, alcohol and drug avoidance, and about the cognitive consequences of this disorder. Seizure triggers such as sleep deprivation or stress should be avoided. Long-term AEDs are not needed for SE secondary to metabolic etiologies. Structural and idiopathic etiologies require long-term management, with eventual AED cessation more likely in idiopathic cases. Having a medical alert bracelet should be suggested.

SUMMARY

- **Generalized convulsive SE** is a neurological emergency because outcomes are dependent on duration of seizures; with irreversible sequelae and death more likely for seizures **lasting more than 30 minutes**.
- **Cardiopulmonary support** may be required during treatment.
- Drug treatment may include the following:
    - First line: **lorazepam** 0.05–0.20 mg/kg at 1–2 mg i.v. every 2 minutes (preferred) or **diazepam** 0.15–0.25 mg/kg (adults) or 0.1–1.0 mg/kg (children) at a maximum rate of 5 mg per minute.
    - Second line: **Phenytoin** 20 mg/kg at 50 mg per minute (adults) or 1 mg/kg per minute (children) or **fosphenytoin** 20 mg/kg phenytoin equivalents at 150 mg per minute (adults) or 3 mg/kg per minute (children).
    - Third line: **Phenobarbital** (children/adults) 20 mg/kg at 50–100 mg per minute or **Valproate** i.v.(in adults) 20–25 mg/kg over 60 minutes.
    - Anesthetics: **propofol** 1–2 mg/kg i.v bolus, then 2–10 mg/kg per hour; **midazolam** 0.2 mg/kg bolus, then 1–10 µg/kg per minute or **pentobarbital** 5–15 mg/kg i.v. bolus over 1 hour, then 0.5–3.0 mg/kg per hour.
- Mortality is **3–35%**: depends on **age, cause,** and **duration** of SE.

3

Neuromuscular Disorders

CASE 1

A 42-year-old woman had complained of intermittent double vision, difficulty chewing, and easy fatigability in her arms for a month. She was brought to the ER complaining of severe dyspnea, which she thought was related to a recent respiratory tract infection. On examination, she had a respiratory rate (RR) of 28 per minute and she was unable to complete a short sentence in one breath. There was bilateral fatigable ptosis, bilateral abduction paresis, nasal speech, facial diplegia, and proximal weakness (MRC 4/5) that worsened with exercise (MRC 2/5).

Localization

Ptosis, diplopia with bilateral abduction paresis, difficulty chewing, dysarthria, and facial diplegia suggest a disorder involving the CN III, V, VI, VII, or the muscles innervated by these nerves. Proximal weakness can be caused by disorders affecting anterior horn cells (AHC), nerve roots (C5–C8 and L2–S2), upper brachial/lumbar plexi, peripheral nerves, neuromuscular junction, or muscle. Exercise-induced fatigability, as well as the constellation of manifestations, suggests the neuromuscular junction is the most likely site of localization.

Differential Diagnosis

The most likely diagnosis is *respiratory failure secondary to myasthenia gravis* (MG; i.e., *myasthenic crisis*). Other diagnostic considerations include *cholinergic crisis* owing to overdosage with cholinesterase inhibitors (rare; history should indicate if patient was receiving these agents for MG, signs of cholinergic excess; e.g., miosis, sialorrhea, diarrhea, fasciculations, or muscle cramps may occur), *organophosphate poisoning* (would expect signs of cholinergic excess), *botulism* (would expect pupillary abnormalities in 50% and signs of autonomic dysfunction, such as dry mouth or constipation), *diphtheria* (toxin can cause an acute to subacute demyelinating polyneuritis of cranial and peripheral nerves; sensory findings, dysautonomia and pseudomembranous

From: *Neurology Oral Boards Review:*
A Concise and Systematic Approach to Clinical Practice
By: E. E. Ubogu © Humana Press Inc., Totowa, NJ

pharyngitis occur), *Lambert-Eaton Myasthenic Syndrome* (LEMS; rarely causes respiratory weakness, ocular signs usually mild, autonomic features present and strength may improve initially after exercise), *tick paralysis* and *snake envenomization* (cobra venom, krait venom [α-bungarotoxin, β-bungarotoxin]; would expect exposure and multiorgan involvement).

Investigations

Investigations should include CBC with differential, comprehensive metabolic panel, Mg^{2+}, PO_4^{3-}, PT/PTT/INR (prior to placement of wide-bore canula for plasma exchange), TFT, acetylcholine receptor (AChR) antibodies (positive in 80–90% with generalized MG and 50% with pure ocular MG), ESR/CRP, autoimmune screen (ANA panel, rheumatoid factor [RhF], anti-double stranded [anti-ds] DNA, etc.), serum immunoglobulin A (IgA) (prior to intravenous immunoglobulin [IVIg]), purified protein derivative (PPD) prior to steroids. Septic screen (chest X-ray, urinalysis with or without blood cultures) required if infection suspected.

Chest CT scan for thymoma evaluation should be performed once stable. Tensilon test may be considered in patients with suspected MG crisis. Electromyography (EMG) with repetitive nerve stimulation (RNS) distinguishes between pre- and post-synaptic neuromuscular junction (NMJ) disorders (MG shows decrement at 2–5 Hz, no increment at 30–50 Hz) and single-fiber electromyography (SFEMG; increased jitter, sensitive but not specific for MG) adds diagnostic yield if AChR antibodies are negative.

Management

Myasthenic crises is a neurological emergency because respiratory failure can ensue secondary to respiratory muscle fatigue. Oxygenate via high-flow nasal canula or mask and breathing bag if dyspnea is more severe. Close respiratory monitoring in an ICU every 2–4 hours is needed. Intubate if forced vital capacity (FVC) is less than 12–15 mL/kg or less than 1 L, negative inspiratory force (NIF) is more than –20 cm H_2O, positive expiratory force (PEF) is less than 40 cm H_2O, tidal volume is less than 5 mL/kg, and maximal breathing capacity is three times tidal volume or for airway protection from aspiration. Oxygen desaturations and blood gas changes occur late. Guidelines are not absolute and the overall clinical picture needs to be considered. Stop all cholinesterase inhibitors and offending drugs (e.g., aminoglycosides). Treat underlying infections (avoid antibiotics that affect NMJ) and correct electrolyte abnormalities, especially low potassium (K^+) and PO_4^{3-}. Avoid incentive spirometry (causes respiratory muscle fatigue).

Therapeutic plasmapheresis (TPE) should be initiated at 40–50 mL of plasma/kg every other day for five to six exchanges (total of 200–250 mL/kg).

IVIg at 0.4 g/kg infused daily for 5 days (total 2g/kg) is an alternative to TPE. High-dose corticosteroids (e.g., prednisone 1–1.5 mg/kg per day) may be started once the patient responds to immunomodulating therapy, but this agent at high doses may exacerbate weakness. Supportive care (e.g., pulmonary toilet, DVT prophylaxis, prevention of decubitus ulcers, nutritional support) is also required.

Prognosis

Median duration of hospitalization is 30 days with 50% spent in the ICU. With treatment, 25% of patients are extubated by day 7, 50% by day 13, and 75% by day 31. Prolonged intubation is dependent on age over 50 years, preintubation serum bicarbonate of 30 mg/dL or more and peak vital capacity at more than 7 days post-intubation less than 25mL/kg. Patients intubated for more than 2 weeks have 75–80% functional dependence at discharge; if less than 2 weeks, functional dependence is 35–40%. Morbidity may be influenced by complications of prolonged hospitalization: atelectasis, *Clostridium difficile* colitis, anemia and CHF, or adverse reactions to therapy with TPE (cardiac arrhythmias, hypotension, catheter-related infection, bleeding caused by loss of clotting factors) or IVIg (flu-like illness, renal failure, hyperviscosity, headache).

Mortality is about 3–5%. Surviving patients make significant recovery. About 70% of patients are normal or have mild deficits at 3–5 years after immunosuppressant and surgical therapy.

Counseling

Rapid clinical improvement occurs in 75–100% and 50–100% of patients treated with TPE and IVIg respectively. Prognostic data should be discussed with patients. Long-term therapy with corticosteroids with or without steroid-sparing immunosuppresants such as azathioprine, cyclosporine, or cellcept is required for remission.

Cholinesterase inhibitors should be used for symptomatic therapy. Avoidance of precipitating conditions (emotional stress, infection, surgery) and drugs should be discussed. Such drugs include β-blockers, aminoglycoside, and polymyxin antibiotics, anti-arrhythmics, and *d*-penicillamine. Patients should be aware of early signs of exacerbation. Thymectomy should be considered once stable, especially in patients with thymoma (mandatory), severe generalized MG without thymoma if younger than 60 or life expectancy is greater than 10 years.

SUMMARY

- **MG crisis** is defined as an **MG exacerbation with respiratory or bulbar compromise** requiring intubation.
- Indications for intubation include: **FVC less than 12–15 mL/kg or less than 1 L, NIF greater than –20 cm H$_2$O, PEF less than 40 cm H$_2$O,**

> tidal volume less than 5 mL/kg, and maximal breathing capacity three times the tidal volume or for airway protection from aspiration.
> - Diagnostic considerations include cholinergic crisis, organophosphate poisoning, botulism, diphtheria, severe LEMS, tick paralysis, and snake envenomization.
> - Treatment includes TPE 40–50 mL of plasma/kg every other day for five to six exchanges (total of 200–250 mL/kg) or IVIg at 0.4 g/kg infused daily for 5 days (total 2 g/kg). Prednisone 1–1.5 mg/kg per day can be administered when stable.
> - 75–100% of patients rapidly improve with TPE; 50–100% with IVIg.
> - Outcomes depend on duration of intubation, complications of prolonged hospitalization, adverse effects of therapy, and underlying disease. The mortality rate is 3–5%.
> - Long-term management requires immunosuppresants and cholinesterase inhibitors for symptomatic therapy.
> - Thymectomy should be considered in all patients with a thymoma, generalized MG younger than 60 or with more than 10 years life expectancy.
> - Approximately 70% of patients are highly functional at 3–5 years with immunosuppressant and surgical therapy.

CASE 2

Three days ago, a 15-year-old boy complained of progressive numbness and tingling in his feet that was restricted to his legs. He had noticed weakness in his lower extremities that initially affected his feet and progressed proximally over 24 hours. On examination, there was mild bilateral abduction paresis, facial diplegia, quadriparesis with MRC 4/5 in the upper extremities and 3/5 in the lower extremities, mild sensory loss to vibration, and pinprick in a stocking distribution and areflexia.

Localization

Bilateral abduction paresis and facial weakness suggest involvement of CN VI and VII at the level of the nuclei (pons), nerves directly or muscles innervated by these nerves. Quadriparesis with areflexia could localize to bilateral descending corticospinal tracts (early), AHC/nerve roots (cervical: C5–T1 and lumbosacral: L2–S2 roots), brachial and lumbosacral plexi, peripheral nerves, NMJ, or muscle. Distal sensory loss and parasthesias in the feet/legs localize to the lumbosacral nerve roots (L4–S1), plexus, or peripheral nerves. Based on the constellation of signs and symptoms, the most likely localization is a polyradiculoneuropathy affecting peripheral and cranial nerves.

Differential Diagnosis

The most likely diagnosis for a rapid progressing quadriparesis with mild sensory and cranial nerve involvement is *Guillain-Barré syndrome* (GBS). The most common variant in the Western hemisphere is acute inflammatory demyelinating polyradiculoneuropathy (AIDP), with acute motor and sensory axonal neuropathy (AMSAN) and acute motor axonal neuropathy (AMAN) being more common in China and Japan. Other possible differentials include *acute neuropathies* (critical illness neuropathy, porphyria, diphtheria, toxins such as arsenic, thallium, fish and shellfish poisoning, e.g., saxitoxin, vasculitis, infectious myeloradiculopathies, e.g., cytomegalovirus [CMV] and Lyme; and tick paralysis), *disorders of NMJ transmission* (MG, botulism), *fulminant myopathies* (polymyositis, dermatomyositis, critical care myopathy, low K^+/PO_4^{3-}), *AHC disease* (polio, West Nile virus), and *early CNS disorders* (basilar artery thrombosis, brainstem encephalitis, acute transverse myelitis [ATM]).

Further clinical history would help in differentiating these disorders.

Investigations

Investigations should include CBC with differential, comprehensive metabolic panel, PT/PTT/INR (prior to LP), Mg^{2+}, PO_4^{3-}, CK, human immunodeficiency virus (HIV) titer, and ESR. Check serum IgA level before IVIg. Based on history, the following may be considered: ANA, RhF, anti-ds DNA, Lyme titer, serum and urine porphyria screen, 24-hour urine for heavy metals. Check EKG. LP may be needed to evaluate for albuminocytologic dissociation (LP may be normal during first week and in approximately 10% of all patients; consider CT head to exclude mass lesion before LP. LP may show elevated cell count in HIV seroconversion).

In atypical cases, MRI of the brain and spinal cord may be necessary to exclude CNS disease. EMG/nerve conduction studies (NCS) may show diffuse primary demyelinating or axonal features; earliest finding is prolonged F- and H-wave responses. RNS can be performed to exclude NMJ disorder if clinically indicated. Muscle and nerve biopsy should be performed if vasculitis is highly suspected.

Management

GBS is a neurological emergency because progression to involve respiratory muscles may occur, causing respiratory failure. Early fatal cardiac arrhythmias and severe dysautonomia may also occur. Monitoring in an ICU or telemetry unit (for continuous cardiac monitoring and FVC/NIF evaluations every 4–6 hours) is needed. Intubation should be performed for clinical or objective evidence of worsening respiratory function or airway protection (similar for MG crises; *see* criteria on p. 38). Tracheostomy should be considered if patient is intubated for more than 7–10 days. Aggressive i.v. hydration is needed for dysautonomia. Supportive care (DVT prophylaxis, nutritional support, artificial tears, analgesia, e.g., neurontin, tricyclic antidepressants [TCAs], NSAIDs, opioids for back/radicular pain, and regular repositioning) is needed.

Pharmacological treatment consists of IVIg at 0.4 g/kg infused daily for 5 days (total 2 g/kg) or TPE 40–50 mL of plasma/kg every other day for five to six exchanges (total of 200–250 mL/kg). Both treatments are equally efficacious, and have been shown to reduce the duration of progression and time to recovery. These therapies may be alternatively used if the other is contraindicated in a particular patient (e.g., dysautonomia for TPE and CHF for IVIg). IVIg is preferred because of ease of administration and widespread availability. In-patient rehabilitation is needed on completion of acute medical management.

Prognosis

Children have a more favorable prognosis than adults. In general, 10–20% of patients develop respiratory failure requiring intubation. Of all patients, 65–75% fully recover (70% by 12 months, 85% by 2 years), approximately 20–30% have residual motor deficits, and death occurs in about 5%. Causes of death include cardiac arrest, PE, and infections. Poor outcomes are predicted by age over 60 years, ventilatory support, rapidly progressive course with maximum deficit within 7 days, low compound motor action potential (CMAP; <20% lower limit of normal [LLN]) on NCS. Outcomes may also be influenced by complications of therapy. Recurrence may occur in 3–5% of patients following initial recovery.

Counseling

Prognostic data should be discussed with the patient. The monophasic nature of GBS should be emphasized. Encouragement and supportive devices (e.g., orthoses) may reduce burden on patient and assist recovery.

SUMMARY

- **GBS** is a neurological emergency because of the potential for respiratory compromise and severe dysautonomia.
- Differential diagnoses include **acute neuropathics, NMJ transmission disorders, fulminant myopathies, AHC disease,** and **CNS disorders.**
- Intubation may be needed in **10–20%** of patients.
- Treatment consists of **IVIg at 0.4 g/kg daily** for 5 days **(total 2 g/kg)** or **TPE 40–50 mL of plasma/kg every other day** for five to six exchanges (total of **200–250 mL/kg**). IVIg is generally preferred.
- Outcomes depend on **age, rate of clinical progression,** and **low CMAPs (<20% LLN) on NCS.**
- Mortality is approximately **5%.** Complete recovery is seen in **65–75%** of cases, with residual motor deficits in **20–30%.** Recurrence occurs in **3–5%.**

CASE 3

A 4-month-old girl was brought to the ER because of generalized weakness and failure to thrive for 36 hours. Her mother said the baby was constipated a week ago and had a poor suck. Examination showed pupillary dilation with sluggish responses to light, ptosis, weak cry, dysphagia to liquids, and generalized hypotonia with hyporeflexic quadriparesis.

Localization

Pupillary dilation and sluggish light responses with ptosis suggest involvement of the autonomic and motor CN III fibers. Poor suck, weak cry, and dysphagia suggest CN VII, IX, X and XII involvement, or their nuclei (pons and medulla) or muscles innervated. Generalized hypotonia with hyporeflexic quadriparesis suggest a lower motor neuron disorder (AHC, nerve roots, plexus, peripheral nerve, NMJ, or muscle) affecting the cervical and lumbosacral myotomes. This disorder localizes to the peripheral nervous system (PNS) with involvement of muscle (craniobulbar, cervical, and lumbosacral) and autonomic end organs.

Differential Diagnosis

The most likely diagnosis is *infantile botulism,* which is usually secondary to ingestion of *Clostridium botulinum* spores and exotoxin. Wound botulism is more common in adults, who present with blurred vision, dysphagia/dysarthria, and generalized weakness. Other considerations include *diphtheria* (febrile illness, pseudomembranous pharyngitis, sensory involvement), GBS (rare in children younger than 12 months, pupillary involvement unlikely), *infantile spinal muscular atrophy* (SMA 1: Werdnig-Hoffman disease; would not expect early craniobulbar or autonomic features and course is more progressive) or *generalized MG* (autonomic features and hyporeflexia not expected). In adults, causes of rapidly progressive quadriparesis (*see* p. 41) should be considered, although further clinical history and examination may help in diagnostic differentiation.

Investigation

Stool sample for *C. botulinum* isolation and detection of botulinum toxin is required. Colonic irrigation with normal saline may be needed in constipated infants to obtain a sample. Wound cultures should be done in adults. Serum assay for botulinum toxin (children and adults should be considered). In equivocal cases, laboratory tests described in evaluating MG and GBS could be considered (*see* pp. 38 and 41). Survival motor neuron (SMN) gene analysis on chromosome 5 may be considered in atypical cases.

EMG with RNS should be performed to demonstrate a presynaptic disorder in NMJ transmission (reduced CMAPs, increment with 20–50 Hz, persistent post-tetanic facilitation without exhaustion; note that hypermagnesemia may show similar findings). EMG/NCS may help differentiate from GBS or diphtheria (sensory involvement). SFEMG shows increased jitter, but this is not specific for botulism and would be difficult to perform in a child or uncooperative adult.

Management

The mainstay of therapy is supportive. However, the potential for respiratory failure (sudden apnea) and fatal dysautonomia make botulism a neurological emergency and warrants ICU admission for respiratory (every 4 hours) and continuous cardiac monitoring. Intubation should be performed for evidence of respiratory compromise (*see* p. 38) or airway protection. In children, loss of protective airway reflexes (e.g., gag, cough) indicates intubation. Signs of respiratory distress (e.g., sighing, tachypnea, paradoxical breathing) may occur later. Nasogastric feeding, i.v. fluid support, DVT prophylaxis, and decubiti prevention should be performed. In-patient rehabilitation would be required on discharge to promote recovery.

Pharmacological treatment for adult botulism consists of divalent (A and B) or trivalent (A, B, and E) botulinum antitoxin. Antibiotics are not effective, but may be used to treat the underlying wound infection. Because of the self-limiting nature of infantile botulism, neither antitoxin nor antibiotics are indicated. There is a risk of anaphylaxis with antitoxin and risk of worsening NMJ transmission with antibiotics, owing to direct effects of lysis of bacteria causing more release of toxin in the gut. However, a recent study of treatment of infants with human-derived antitoxin (botulinum-immune globulin) showed reduced hospitalization, need for intubation, and nasogastric feedings, making this the option of choice in this age group.

Prognosis

The prognosis of botulism is excellent. Mortality rate is approximately 2%, secondary to respiratory or cardiac arrest. Infantile botulism is a self-limiting disease of about 2–6 weeks duration. Recovery is slow (over several months) but usually complete in adult and infantile forms. In infantile botulism, average duration of hospitalization is 44 days, with mean duration of intubation of 23 days. Return to oral intake takes an average of 51 days from admission. Morbidity may be influenced by complications such as infections or syndrome of inappropriate antidiuretic hormone secretion (SIADH). Relapse rate is about 5% and occurs within the first month after discharge.

Counseling

Honey, corn syrup, and home-canned foods should not be given to children younger than 12 months old. Eradication of dusty environment or removal of infants from construction or agricultural sites should be considered. Wounds should be treated early and aggressively in adults. If i.v. drug use is a concern, detoxification and cessation counseling are important. Parents should be aware of the prognostic data.

SUMMARY

- **Infantile botulism** is usually caused by **ingestion**, whereas **adult botulism** is usually secondary to **wound colonization**.
- Botulism is a neurological emergency because of the potential for **sudden respiratory or cardiac arrest**. ICU admission is required.
- Differential diagnoses include **diphtheria, GBS, MG, SMA** (infants), or causes of **rapidly progressive quadriparesis** (adults).
- Diagnose with **stool/wound cultures, serum for botulinum toxin**, and **RNS**.
- Treatment: **supportive** with **antitoxin (adults)** or **botulinum-immune globulin (infants)**. Antibiotics are non-efficacious.
- Mortality rate is approximately **2%**. Recovery takes many **months** and is **complete**.
- Preventative measures, especially in infants, are important.

Case 4

A 55-year-old man complained of a 3-week history of low back pain, associated with some low-grade fevers and generalized malaise. Over the last 6 hours, he developed urinary and fecal incontinence, progressive loss of sensation in his perineum and thighs, with some difficulty walking. Clinical examination revealed point tenderness at the T12–L1 spinal level, mild (MRC 4/5) weakness in ankle dorsiflexion and plantarflexion, symmetrical saddle anesthesia to pinprick, and absent ankle jerks bilaterally.

Localization

Weakness in ankle dorsiflexion (L4–L5), plantar flexion (L5–S1), and absent ankle jerks (S1) bilaterally suggest diffuse involvement of the AHC or nerve roots derived from these spinal levels. Urinary and fecal incontinence with saddle anesthesia suggest involvement of autonomic (Onuf's nucleus) and sensory nerves or nerve roots (S2–S4). However, early centrally located lesions of the CNS affecting the corticospinal tracts, descending autonomic tracts or ascending sensory tracts (anterior lateral/spinothalmic system) in the spinal cord may cause similar symptoms. Focal tenderness at the T12–L1 level may localize the process to the conus medullaris or cauda equina, with involvement of spinal levels L4–S4.

Differential Diagnosis

The differential diagnosis consists of *conus medullaris syndrome* and *cauda equina syndrome*. These are anatomical diagnoses and have several etiologies. The sudden presentation, early bladder/bowel involvement with symmetrical saddle anesthesia without radicular pain and mild bilateral lower extremity weakness makes conus medullaris syndrome the more likely diagnosis. Hyporeflexia can be seen in both conus medullaris (early) and cauda equina syndromes.

Cauda equina syndrome is associated with more radicular pain, late bladder/bowel involvement and is more gradual and asymmetrical in presentation. Dissociated sensory loss is more common with conus medullaris syndrome (impaired pain and temperature, light touch spared), whereas all modalities are affected with cauda equina syndrome. Spastic hyperreflexia may develop later on in the course of conus medullaris syndrome, whereas more widespread involvement of muscles innervated by L4–S2 nerve roots is expected with cauda equina syndrome (e.g., hip extension, knee flexion).

Causes of conus medullaris syndrome include *trauma* (direct injury or indirect from vertebral fractures, epidural hematoma, acute disc prolapse), *tumors* (epidural metastasis from lung, breast, prostate; intradural extramedullary lesions like meningioma; intradural intramedullary lesions like ependymoma [children], astrocytoma [adults] or metastases), *epidural abscess* (e.g., following osteomyelitis secondary to *S. aureus*, tuberculosis [TB]), *infarction* (vascular occlusion secondary to emboli, vasculitis, or spinal AVMs) and *inflammation* (secondary to multiple sclerosis [MS], collagen vascular diseases like systemic lupus erythematosus [SLE] or postinfectious following rubella, varicella).

The preceding history of low back pain with a febrile systemic illness makes *epidural abscess* or *metastases* the most likely etiology for the clinical presentation of conus medullaris syndrome.

Investigations

Emergent MRI of the thoracic and lumbar spine with and without gadolinium should be performed to evaluate for the etiology of the conus medullaris syndrome. Compression by epidural abscess, hematoma or metastases, extradural or intradural tumors, or herniated discs can be seen. MRI would also reveal intrinsic spinal cord tumors, evidence for inflammation, or infarction. AVMs may be difficult to detect without angiography.

If MRI is not readily available, CT myelography should be performed. If epidural metastases are suspected, MRI of the entire spine should be performed to exclude more widespread disease. Further investigation should be tailored toward potential etiologies: CBC with differential, ESR/CRP, blood cultures, prostate-specific antigen (PSA), CT chest, mammography, ANA panel, RhF, anti-ds DNA, LP for oligoclonal bands, for example.

Management

Conus medullaris syndrome secondary to compression is a neurological emergency because recovery and prevention of irreversible sequelae depend on rapid institution of therapy. High-dose corticosteroids; methylprednisolone 30 mg/kg i.v. bolus, then 5.4 mg/kg per hour for 24–48 hours followed by prednisone taper or dexamethasone 100 mg i.v. bolus, then 24 mg orally (p.o.)/i.v. every 6 hours for 48 hours followed by taper over 10–14 days, should be started within 8–12 hours of neurological deficit. Underlying etiology should be treated concurrently. Radiotherapy should be considered for metastatic disease. Emergent surgical decompression may be required for compressive lesions if the patient is medically stable with symptoms of less than 24-hour duration. Intravenous antibiotics would be required following decompression of epidural abscess. Spinal immobilization is necessary for trauma.

General supportive care (e.g., bowel and bladder hygiene with pharmacological and nonpharmacological measures, DVT prophylaxis, frequent repositioning, and active rehabilitation are essential. The patient should be managed in a spinal cord or acute neurological unit with expertise in caring for patients with acute and chronic spinal cord disease.

Prognosis

Outcomes depend on the underlying disease, time from neurological deficit to treatment and severity of neurological deficit at presentation. In traumatic spinal cord injury, outcomes (independent ambulation, neurological recovery) were improved if treated within 8 hours (<3 hours more favorable), whereas with spinal epidural metastases, treatment within 12 hours results in more favorable outcomes, including pain control. Of non-ambulatory patients, 50% walk with adequate treatment. Patients are less likely to completely recover if they present with paraplegia, severe bladder/bowel dysfunction, or saddle anesthesia. Mortality does not occur as a direct consequence of conus medullaris syndrome, but may be associated with its etiology and the complications of its neurological sequelae.

Counseling

Patients should be aware that residual neurological deficits are common despite adequate treatment, but chances of recovery are improved by early aggressive medical and surgical intervention, depending on the etiology. Inpatient rehabilitation may improve recovery. Patients should be taught self-catherization and bowel hygiene. Dependent patients may require walking aids or wheelchairs. Quality and length of life of patients with metastatic epidural metastases are dependent on early steroid and radiation therapy, so these therapies should be encouraged.

SUMMARY

- **Conus medullaris syndrome** is a neurological emergency as prevention of long-term sequelae is dependent on instituting therapy.
- Differential diagnosis includes **cauda equina syndrome**. Etiologies include **trauma, tumor, epidural abscess, infarction,** or **inflammation**. **MRI** is the diagnostic test of choice.
- Treatment includes high-dose steroids: **methylprednisolone 30 mg/kg i.v. bolus,** then **5.4 mg/kg per hour** for **24–48 hours** followed by prednisone taper or **dexamethasone 100 mg i.v. bolus,** then **24 mg p.o./i.v. every 6 hours** for **48 hours** followed by taper over 10–14 days.
- Treatment should be instituted **within 8–12 hours** of deficit.
- **Emergency surgery** should be considered for compressive etiologies, especially if **medically stable** with **deficits of less than 24 hour duration**.
- Underlying cause should be treated concurrently.
- Outcomes depend on **underlying disease, severity of deficit at presentation** and **timing of treatment**. Residual deficits are common.

4

Herniation Syndromes

CASE 1

A 16-year-old girl was hit by a pitch while playing softball. It was estimated that the ball traveled at about 60 miles an hour and hit the left side of her head. About 3 hours after the incident, she became somnolent. On arrival to the ER 15 minutes later, she was responding minimally to external stimuli. Clinical examination revealed a dilated left pupil with sluggish reaction to light and a Babinski sign on the right.

Localization

Reduced level of arousal is nonlocalizing, but suggests global cerebral dysfunction. A poorly reactive dilated left pupil suggests a left CN III lesion involving the Edinger-Westphal nucleus in the midbrain or parasympathetic fibers innervating the pupillary constrictors. Further clinical examination would address if there was ophthalmoparesis indicative of involvement of the oculomotor fibers of CN III.

A Babinski sign on the right suggests an upper motor neuron lesion on the left (motor cortex, subcortical white matter, internal capsule, cerebral peduncles, or pyramidal tracts). The most likely localization is the left midbrain with bilateral cerebral cortex involvement.

Differential Diagnosis

A posttraumatic left midbrain deficit with mental status changes is most likely the result of a *left-sided ICH with transtentorial herniation of the left temporal lobe against the midbrain.* ICH could be an epidural hemorrhage owing to a skull fracture, subdural hemorrhage, intraparenchymal hematoma, or traumatic SAH. The history is most supportive of an *epidural hemorrhage.*

Other diagnostic considerations include *ischemic stroke* (i.e., Weber syndrome secondary to PCA or penetrating vessel disease: uncommon in children and would not expect mental status changes so early in the course without more extensive neurological deficit or cytotoxic edema following large temporal lobe stroke;

From: *Neurology Oral Boards Review:*
A Concise and Systematic Approach to Clinical Practice
By: E. E. Ubogu © Humana Press Inc., Totowa, NJ

would expect this to occur 48–96 hours after initial stroke), *temporal lobe tumor* (e.g., cystic astrocytoma or brain metastasis: would expect a slower clinical progression, unless there is an acute hemorrhage into the tumor), *aneurysm* (e.g., PCommA, basilar tip, PCA: would not expect acute course unless aneurysmal rupture occurred) or *infection* (e.g., herpes simplex encephalitis [HSE] with secondary temporal lobe edema: clinical presentation is too acute and febrile illness with a behavioral prodrome is more likely). A *toxic-metabolic encephalopathy* would cause global cerebral deficit without lateralizing signs, but could be superimposed on an underlying focal pathogenic process.

Investigations

An emergent noncontrasted CT scan of the head should be performed to evaluate for an ICH, as well as skull fracture. Other space-occupying lesions, foreign bodies, and hydrocephalus can be diagnosed. If etiology is unclear and mass lesions have been excluded, LP (for CSF RBC/WBC/Protein/herpes simplex virus-polymerase chain reaction [HSV-PCR]/xanthochromia) should be considered. If an aneurysmal rupture is suspected, four-vessel cerebral angiography should be performed for potential diagnostic and therapeutic purposes (e.g., coiling).

MRI of the brain may be useful following nondiagnostic CT scans in detecting shearing injuries, nonhemorrhagic cerebral contusions, and posterior fossa pathology. Laboratory investigations (e.g., CBC, comprehensive metabolic profile, PT/PTT/INR, urine/blood toxicology, blood cultures) may be performed to exclude a superimposed toxic-metabolic encephalopathy, especially in patients with limited histories or to obtain baseline values.

Management

Intubation and mechanical ventilation should be instituted for airway protection and for hyperventilation to treat raised ICP. Hyperventilation should be performed to keep $PaCO_2$ 25–30 mmHg. Osmotic diuresis with mannitol 20% should be started: 1 g/kg i.v. bolus over 30 minutes, then 0.25–0.5 g/kg every 4–6 hours. Keep serum osmolarity below 300–320 mOsm/L. The head of the bed should be elevated to 30°. Electrolyte abnormalities should be corrected.

If an ICH causing more than a 5 mm midline shift is present or neurological deterioration is refractory to medical management, decompressive craniotomy and surgical hematoma evacuation should be performed emergently because outcomes depend on the prevention of irreversible brain damage. Temporal lobe or posterior fossa hematomas with any degree of midline shift may require early surgery because of high herniation risk. Craniectomy may be required to reduce medically refractory ICP (this is controversial).

Postoperative care should be performed in an ICU with ICP monitoring. General supportive measures such as frequent neurological checks (every 1–2 hours),

pressor and volume support, surgical wound care, DVT and stress ulcer prophylaxis, seizure prophylaxis (controversial; to prevent early seizures, i.e., <7
days), and decubitus ulcer prevention are necessary. In-patient rehabilitation
would be required to improve functional status on discharge.

Prognosis

The prognosis of posttraumatic transtentorial herniation is dependent on
age, level of consciousness, and residual upper brainstem function on admission. Children have a more favorable outcome. A mortality rate of 60%, with
good recovery in 9%, moderate disability in 9%, severe disability in 11%, and
persistent vegetative state (PVS) in 11% may occur irrespective of cause. The
prognosis of acute traumatic extradural hemorrhage is better than intracere-
bral hemorrhage and depends on its cause and severity, GCS less than 8 on
presentation, presence of multiple intracranial lesions, concurrent medical
factors, time to surgical decompression and postoperative care (including
management of ICP), and the development of complications during ICU stay.
The mortality of extradural hemorrhages ranges from 5 to 12%.

An outcome study on traumatic epidural hemorrhage at hospital discharge
(average 28 days) showed 46% with good recovery (defined as return to normal life with minor residual deficits), 31% moderately disabled, 10% severely
disabled, 4% in PVS, and 9% dead. With acute SDH, decompression accom-
plished within 4 hours may result in 30% mortality, whereas after 4 hours
results in 90% mortality rate. SDH with more than a 15 mm midline shift is
also highly associated with late deterioration and death.

Counseling

Patients should be aware of prognostic data. Aggressive management of
early posttraumatic transtentorial herniation improves chance of survival.
Posttraumatic seizures (PTS) occur more commonly in children than adults. In
general, 5% of patients with acute head injury develop early PTS, 30% of
which occur within the first hour of injury and may evolve into SE. Twenty
percent of patients with epidural hematomas develop late PTS (>7 days); about
50% of which occurs within the first year. Posttraumatic amnesia for more
than 24 hours, early PTS, focal brain injuries, and dural lacerations increase
the risk.

SUMMARY

- **Acute posttraumatic transtentorial herniation** is a neurological
  emergency as outcomes are dependent on clinical signs on presentation
  and early treatment of ICP.
- Most likely etiology is **ICH** (epidural, subdural, SAH, or parenchymal).

- Differential diagnoses include **ischemic stroke, temporal lobe tumor, aneurysmal compression,** or **infection (HSE).** A toxic-metabolic encephalopathy may be superimposed.
- **Emergent CT of the head** is required to evaluate for skull fracture and ICH.
- Management consists of hyperventilation to keep **PaCO$_2$ 25–30 mmHg,** osmotic diuresis with **mannitol 20% 1g/kg i.v. bolus,** then **0.25–0.50 g/kg every 4–6 hours.** Elevate head of bed to 30°.
- **Surgical evacuation** and **decompressive craniotomy** may be required for ICH if indicated.
- Mortality from posttraumatic transtentorial herniation is **60%.** Outcomes are dependent on **age, level of consciousness,** and **residual upper brain stem function** on admission.
- Mortality from acute epidural hemorrhage is **approximately 10%.** Good outcomes may occur in **46%** of patients on discharge from hospital.

CASE 2

A 63-year-old smoker was brought to the ER with abnormal breathing and poor responsiveness. His wife stated that he had progressive weakness in the left face and upper extremity with milder involvement of the lower extremity for about 3 weeks. He had denied any problems and was not aware of his weakness. On examination, the patient responded intermittently to external stimuli. He exhibited Cheyne-Stokes respiration, bilateral small and reactive pupils, absent reflexive vertical gaze, left spastic hemiplegia, generalized hyperreflexia, and bilateral Babinski signs.

Localization

Poor responsiveness is a nonlocalizing sign that suggests global cerebral dysfunction. Cheyne-Stokes respiration is also nonlocalizing, as it may be seen in bilateral hemispheric, diencephalic, or brainstem dysfunction. The clinical history of anosognosia, left-sided neglect with spastic hemiplegia on examination localizes the initial lesion to the right fronto-parietal lobes. Generalized hyperreflexia and bilateral Babinski signs suggest bilateral upper motor neuron dysfunction (cerebral cortex, subcortical white matter, internal capsule, cerebral peduncles, pyramidal tracts, or spinal cord).

Bilateral small, reactive pupils suggest dysfunction of the pupillodilator sympathetic fibers and absent reflexive vertical gaze suggests dysfunction of supranuclear gaze control in the midbrain. These findings suggest dysfunction of the bilateral diencephalon and midbrain, which could be secondary to the initial lesion.

Differential Diagnosis

The most likely explanation for a progressive, subacute right fronto-parietal lesion with central herniation is an *expanding brain tumor with surrounding edema*. This could be a *primary* (anaplastic astrocytoma, glioblastoma multiforme [GBM], primary CNS lymphoma, etc.) or *secondary* (e.g., lung, breast, liver, testicular metastases) intraparenchymal lesion. A *parasagittal meningioma* could cause a similar presentation, as symptoms may only occur at a large tumor size. Other differentials include *cerebral abscess* (e.g., toxoplasmosis, *S. pneumoniae*, mucormycosis), *subdural hematoma, tumor-like MS,* or a *toxic-metabolic encephalopathy* superimposed on a remote right MCA stroke.

Investigations

Emergent CT scan of the head should be performed to diagnose a mass lesion and to exclude an ICH. Once stable, an MRI of the brain with and without gadolinium should be performed to elucidate the nature and size of primary lesion, degree of cerebral edema, and extent of brainstem involvement. LP should not be performed if a mass lesion is suspected.

Laboratory investigations (such as CBC, comprehensive metabolic profile, PT/PTT/INR, urine/blood toxicology, blood cultures) may be performed to exclude a superimposed toxic-metabolic encephalopathy such as low Na^+ from SIADH or cerebral salt-wasting. A diagnostic brain biopsy may be considered once the patient is stable, as that may direct therapy for intraparenchymal neoplasms.

Management

An altered level of consciousness, respiratory distress, and early signs of central herniation warrant emergent intubation and mechanical ventilation. ICU admission is required. The head of the bed should be raised to 30°. Ventriculostomy should be considered as a therapeutic modality for raised ICP and for ICP monitoring. Tumor-induced vasogenic brain edema is treated with dexamethasone 10 mg i.v. stat, then 4 mg i.v. every 6 hours (can also be given every 12 hours to achieve a total of 16 mg per day) until clinical improvement occurs (usually more than 48 hours required). Slow taper over 7–10 days should be carried out using i.v./p.o. doses. Mannitol has no role in treating vasogenic edema, but may reduce ICP.

Depending on the accessibility of the primary lesion causing central herniation, a diagnostic and therapeutic craniotomy or stereotactic radiosurgery can be performed, especially for solitary lesions. Whole-brain radiation therapy, chemotherapy, or both should be considered as well, and may be the only option for multiple or nonaccessible neoplastic lesions. These modalities are useful depending on the type of brain tumor. Treat any electrolyte abnormalities.

General supportive care, such as frequent neurological checks (every 1–2 hours), ICP monitoring, pressor and volume support, surgical wound care, DVT and stress ulcer prophylaxis, and decubitus ulcer prevention is necessary. A neuro-oncology consultation for specific treatment protocols should be sought to maximize recovery. The development of seizures requires aggressive management with AEDs, avoiding phenytoin if cranial irradiation is planned or ongoing (can cause fatal Stevens-Johnson syndrome). Rehabilitation would be required to improve functional status.

Prognosis

The prognosis from nontraumatic cerebral herniation depends on its cause, degree of brainstem dysfunction, and level of consciousness on admission. Data specifically for tumor-induced herniation is sparse, however, there is 61% mortality in nontraumatic coma at 1 year, with good recovery (independent with or without mild disability) occurring in 16%, moderate to severe disability after regaining consciousness in 11%, and PVS in 12%. Prognosis would be modified by the degree of recovery of brainstem reflexes within 7 days and the natural history of the brain tumor.

An autopsy study of patients with supratentorial glioblastomas showed that cerebral herniation was directly associated with lack of *ante mortem* diagnosis, presence of multifocal tumors and brainstem invasion by tumor and indirectly associated with *ante mortem* cranial irradiation. Sudden death was most likely caused by acute cerebral herniation. The development of complications during ICU stay also influences outcomes. The use of dexamethasone for brain metastasis results in clinical resolution in 50%, mild improvement in 15% and lack of any appreciable benefit in 35%.

Counseling

Patients should be aware of prognostic data. Seizure prophylaxis is not warranted in patients with brain tumors. Treatment should be instituted on developing seizures. Survival data for the underlying brain tumor and treatment options should be discussed, as well as the complications of therapy (e.g., radiation necrosis, postoperative hemorrhage, or adverse effects of chemotherapy). Hospice care may be needed for patients with poorly prognostic tumors or significant brain damage from herniation. Information about support groups should be provided.

SUMMARY

- **Tumor-induced cerebral herniation** is a neurological emergency because survival and recovery depend on preventing irreversible brainstem dysfunction.
- Differential diagnosis for a subacute, progressive lesion causing central herniation includes **primary/secondary intraparenchymal brain**

tumor, meningioma, cerebral abscess, subdural hematoma, tumor-like MS, or **a toxic-metabolic encephalopathy** superimposed on a remote stroke.

- For glioblastoma, herniation is most likely to occur with **multifocal lesions, brainstem invasion,** and **undiagnosed cases**.
- **Emergent CT** is important to exclude ICH and show mass lesion. **MRI** better delineates pathology and extent of involvement.
- Treatment includes **ventriculostomy** and **dexamethasone 10 mg i.v. stat,** then **4 mg i.v. every 6 hours for more than 48 hours** until clinical improvement.
- Prognosis depends on **cause, degree of brainstem dysfunction,** and **level of consciousness** on admission.
- Mortality could be **greater than 60% at 1 year,** but dexamethasone use early can improve chances of recovery.

5

Infectious Diseases

CASE 1

A 21-year-old college student was found poorly responsive in her room. She had complained of a headache for about 4 days that was refractory to OTC NSAIDs. In the ER, temperature was 39.5°C, with BP 145/100 mmHg, HR of 112 per minute and RR of 18 per minute. She partly responded to verbal commands, localized symmetrically to noxious stimuli, and moaned incoherently. Neurological examination showed nuchal rigidity, and normal brainstem reflexes, with symmetric hyperreflexia and flexor plantar responses.

Localization

Altered level of consciousness with symmetrical hyperreflexia suggests global cerebral dysfunction with corticospinal tract involvement. Nuchal rigidity suggests diffuse meningeal irritation. Further history may be required to assess for any focal symptoms prior to unresponsiveness. Clinical examination for focal signs should be carried out in more depth as mental status improves.

Differential Diagnosis

The most likely diagnosis is *community-acquired meningitis*. This could be *bacterial* or *viral* in origin (fungal tends to be more chronic). In this age group, *Neisseria meningitides* and herpes simplex should be highly considered. Other considerations include *S. pneumoniae, H. influenzae, S. aureus,* mycoplasma, listeria for bacteria, whereas enteroviruses (coxsackie, echo), arborviruses, HIV, and other herpes viruses should be considered for viral etiologies. Brain abscess and subdural empyema would expectedly cause focal signs.

Other differentials include *SAH* (aneurysmal rupture or trauma can cause preceding headache and blood in CSF is a meningeal irritant), *carcinomatous meningitis* (unlikely in this age group), *drug intoxication, toxic-metabolic encephalopathy* (fever less likely, e.g., uremia, hepatic failure, low/high Na+ or glucose, thyrotoxicosis), *vasculitis* (primary angiitis or secondary to connective

From: *Neurology Oral Boards Review:*
A Concise and Systematic Approach to Clinical Practice
By: E. E. Ubogu © Humana Press Inc., Totowa, NJ

tissue disorders such as SLE, polyarteritis nodosa [PAN], Sjögrens syndrome), or *sarcoidosis*.

Investigations

Emergent noncontrasted CT scan of the head should be performed to exclude mass lesions that contraindicate LP. LP should be performed for CSF WBC (with differential), RBC, protein, glucose, Gram stain (positive in 50–60%), fluid clarity (turbulence, xanthochromia), culture and sensitivity (C&S; positive in 70–80%), bacterial latex agglutination, HSV-PCR, and cytology (if indicated). Opening pressure should be measured. Laboratory investigations including CBC with differential, comprehensive metabolic profile, PT/PTT/INR (before LP), blood cultures (plus sputum Gram stain, C&S, and chest X-ray if preceding respiratory illness), HIV titer (if appropriate), nasal discharge for glucose/chloride to exclude posttraumatic CSF leak, should be considered based on the clinical history. If LP is nondiagnostic, MRI of the brain with and without contrast with or without meningeal biopsy may be required, especially if primary angiitis of the CNS (PACNS) is suspected.

Management

Intravenous antibiotics should be started immediately (as soon as diagnosis is considered) as early treatment improves survival and reduces neurological sequelae. This can be started 24 hours before LP. Administration of dexamethasone (0.15 mg/kg i.v. every 6 hours for 4 days or 0.4 mg/kg every 12 hours for 2 days, with the first dose prior to antibiotic) should be considered in all children older than 6 months. In adults its role is debatable, but 0.15 mg/kg i.v. every 6 hours for 4 days (maximum 10 mg i.v. every 6 hours) can be administered, especially if patient is immunocompetent and there are signs of raised ICP. Its role in nosocomial meningitis (including Gram-negative bacteria, following neurosurgical procedures or trauma) is uncertain.

Initial empirical antibiotic regimen in the patient's age group should include ceftriaxone 2 g i.v. every 12 hours (or cefotaxime 2 g i.v. every 4 hours) and vancomycin 500 mg i.v. every 6 hours. In children (3 months to 18 years), doses are ceftriaxone 50–100 mg/kg i.v. every 12 hours and vancomycin 10 mg/kg i.v. every 6 hours. If patient is less than 3 months old, substitute ampicillin 50 mg/kg i.v. every 8 hours or add 2 g i.v. every 4 hours if patient is over 50 years of age. Consider herpes coverage with acyclovir 10 mg/kg i.v. every 8 hours. The patient should be managed in hospital, on a regular nursing floor. Antibiotic regimens should be modified based on CSF C&S. Rifampin prophylaxis (600 mg p.o. daily) should be provided for the patient's social contacts if meningococcus isolated.

Supportive care including frequent neurological checks (every 4 hours), i.v. hydration, nutritional support, DVT and stress ulcer prophylaxis (especially with high-dose steroids), and decubitus ulcer prevention is necessary. Infectious disease consultation should be considered for atypical or refractory cases. Neurological deterioration requires aggressive management and possible ICU transfer.

Prognosis

Mortality from bacterial meningitis varies from 10 to 30%, despite advances in antibiotics and critical care. Half of all deaths occur within the first week, with 66% within 2 weeks of admission. Coma, septic shock, and intractable seizures are the most common causes of immediate death. Age over 60 years, seizures within 24 hours of admission, and low level of consciousness on admission are possible risk factors.

The risk of death and neurological sequelae in acute community-acquired bacterial meningitis (*H. influenzae*, pneumococcus, and possibly meningococcus) is significantly reduced with dexamethasone in both children and adults, with minimal adverse effects. About 25–50% of survivors have permanent neurological sequelae attributable to stroke (secondary to thrombophlebitis), hydrocephalus, seizures, cranial nerve dysfunction, hearing loss, growth retardation, and arrest of mental development (children), cognitive/behavioral changes and chronic fatigue and insomnia (in epidemics).

Counseling

Patients should be aware of prognostic data, especially the likelihood of permanent neurological sequelae following survival. The potential behavioral and cognitive sequelae should be emphasized, especially in children. Treating infections early and aggressively (especially sites contiguous to the brain, e.g. inner ear, sinuses) and adequate prophylaxis for neurosurgical procedures should be advised. The use of *H. influenzae* b vaccine has reduced the incidence of meningitis attributable to this microbe, and should be encouraged in children. Administration of the meningococcal vaccination (subgroups A and C) when traveling to epidemic areas should be considered. Patients (and their families) should be encouraged to identify social contacts for rifampin prophylaxis following meningococcal meningitis.

SUMMARY

- **Acute bacterial meningitis** is a neurological emergency because survival and the prevention of neurological sequelae depend on instituting therapy **early**.
- Differentials include **viral meningitis, SAH, carcinomatous meningitis, drug intoxication, toxic-metabolic encephalopathy, vasculitis,** and **sarcoidosis.**

- Treatment includes empirical antibiotics: **ceftriaxone 2 g i.v. every 12 hours** (or **50–100 mg/kg i.v. every 12 hours** in children) and **vancomycin 500 mg i.v. every 6 hours** (or **10mg/kg i.v. every 6 hours** in children). **Acyclovir** coverage for herpes (**10 mg/kg i.v. every 8 hours**) may be required.
- **Dexamethasone 0.15 mg/kg i.v. every 6 hours** for 4 days or **0.4 mg/kg every 12 hours** for 2 days should be given to **children older than 6 months** and considered in **adults** (maximum dose: **10 mg i.v. every 6 hours**).
- Mortality varies from **10 to 30%**. **Fifty percent** occurs within the **first week,** and **66%** within **2 weeks**.
- Of survivors, **25–50%** have permanent neurological sequelae secondary to **stroke, seizures, cognitive–behavioral deficits, hearing loss, arrest of development** (children), and **chronic fatigue and insomnia** (in epidemics).

CASE 2

A 49-year-old man developed a headache associated with fever, personality changes with increased irritability, poor comprehension and memory of recent events over the last 5 days. He was brought to the ER after an episode of staring with facial grimacing and forced head deviation to the left lasting about 2 minutes. On examination, temperature was 38°C with normal BP/HR. Neurological examination revealed an alert man with a receptive aphasia, mild right hemiparesis (MRC 4/5) and right hemisensory deficit.

Localization

Personality changes with increased irritability and poor memory of recent events suggest bilateral fronto-temporal dysfunction. Poor comprehension could represent a receptive aphasia (left temporal lobe) or poor attention (bifrontal dysfunction). Forced head version to the left, coupled with an episode of facial grimacing and staring suggest a left temporal lobe focus, which is further supported by the receptive aphasia. Right hemiparesis and hemisensory deficit support dysfunction in the left frontal and parietal lobes, respectively. The initial process localizes to bilateral frontal and temporal lobes, whereas the seizure localizes to the left temporal lobe with post-ictal involvement of the left frontal and parietal lobes.

Differential Diagnosis

The most likely diagnosis of a febrile illness with bilateral fronto-temporal disease and temporal lobe seizures is *viral encephalitis*. The most likely etiology is *HSV 1*, which causes oral herpes and HSE; HSV 2 causes genital disease, congenitally acquired neonatal encephalitis and aseptic meningitis. Other etiological agents include enteroviruses, arborviruses, measles, mumps, CMV, varicela zoster virus (VZV) and human herpesvirus (HHV)-6.

Other differential diagnoses include *parainfectious/postinfectious encephalitis,* such as subacute sclerosing panencephalitis (SSPE), *brain abscess* (e.g., anaerobic or polymorphic bacteria following dental abscess; fungal: cryptococcus, aspergillosis, mucormycosis; parasitic: toxoplasmosis, cysticercosis, etc.), *subdural empyema, cranial epidural abscess, Reye's syndrome* (in children), *bacterial endocarditis, toxic-metabolic encephalopathy, drug intoxication* (cocaine, amphetamines), *septicemia, vasculitis* (primary angiitis or secondary to collagen vascular diseases), *cerebral venous sinus thrombosis,* and *mitochondrial encephalopathy* (e.g., MELAS).

Investigations

CBC with differential, comprehensive metabolic panel, PT/PTT/INR (before LP), septic screen (blood/urine cultures, chest X-ray), ESR/CRP, autoimmune panel (e.g., ANA titer, RhF, Sjögren's syndrome (SS)A/SSB antibodies depending on history) and serum/urine toxicology can be considered.

Noncontrasted CT of the head to exclude mass lesions should be performed prior to LP. LP should be sent for CSF WBC/RBC, protein, glucose, Gram stain, bacterial C&S, viral cultures and PCR (especially HSV-PCR: >95% sensitive and ~100% specific), India ink stain and cryptococcal antigen if cerebral abscess suspected. EEG may assist with seizure focus localization (post-ictal slowing), to exclude nonconvulsive SE following prolonged post-ictal state and may show characteristic patterns for HSE (periodic lateralizing epileptiform discharges [PLEDs]) or SSPE (periodic slow-wave complexes) or nonspecific encephalopathy (diffuse slowing).

MRI of the brain with and without contrast, with thin cuts through the temporal lobes, may show bilateral temporal and orbitofrontal signal changes with or without hemorrhages as seen in HSE (highly sensitive). MRI will also further assess for potential differential diagnoses. In atypical cases, MRV, cerebral angiography, and brain biopsy may be necessary.

Management

The mainstay of therapy is acyclovir 10 mg/kg i.v. every 8 hours for 14 days. Its major adverse effect is reversible renal insufficiency. Vidarabine 15 mg/kg slow i.v. infusion every 24 hours for 14 days can be used for acyclovir-allergic patients or resistant strains. Treatment should be instituted immediately as mortality rates are high in untreated cases. Therapy may be stopped if HSV-PCR is negative. The patient can be managed on a regular nursing floor.

Seizures can be treated with phenytoin 20 mg/kg i.v. loading dose at 50 mg per minute (or 1 mg/kg per minute in children), then 3–5 mg/kg per day in divided doses every 8 hours i.v. or extended-release capsules at bedtime. Other options include valproate 20–25 mg/kg loading, then 10–15 mg/kg per day in divided doses every 6 hours i.v. or twice daily divalproex sodium tablets. Titrate AED to seizure control without toxicity, so daily levels may be required at the onset. If the patient presents in generalized convulsive SE, management should be performed as described on pp. 34–35. Long-term seizure management would be needed.

General supportive care, including regular nursing observations (a sitter or restraints may be needed), nutritional and fluid support, antipyretics, DVT prophylaxis, speech and language therapy would be adjunctive. Relapses may infrequently occur, and require brain biopsy to confirm the diagnosis. Treatment includes acyclovir 15 mg/kg i.v. every 8 hours and vidarabine infusion for 21 days.

Prognosis

The mortality rate of HSE is 20–30% (70–90% without treatment). Common causes of death include SE and transtentorial herniation. Coma on presentation increases the likelihood of demise. Recovery usually takes several weeks. About 30–50% of patients fully recover with no or mild neurological sequelae, such as personality change. About 20–50% may have moderate to severe neurological deficits such as the Klüver-Bucy syndrome (hyperorality, hypersexuality, visual agnosia, and loss of fear with aggression), amnesia, apathy, depression, poor attention span, emotional lability, and hypermetamorphosis (continued over-attention to external stimuli). The neuropsychological complications of HSE can be very disabling.

Counseling

It is important to note that HSE is the most common cause, but accounts for only 10–20% of acute viral encephalitides. Adults usually acquire the disease by reactivation of latent virus (about 60–70% of cases), whereas 75–80% of children acquire the virus by primary contact (respiratory or saliva). Patients and their families should be aware of the survival data and neuropsychological sequelae for HSE. Relapses should be aggressively treated in hospital and causes of immunocompromisate sought after.

Loss of previous employment and functional status may occur in survivors. Long-term care with supervision may be required in severely affected survivors. The development of epilepsy would require chronic AED therapy. Cognitive and behavioral training can be considered to improve functional status in mild-to-moderately affected survivors.

SUMMARY

- **Herpes simplex encephalitis** is a neurological emergency because survival and outcomes depend on instituting therapy early.
- Differentials include other **viral encephalitides, postinfectious/parainfectious encephalitis, brain abscess** (bacterial, fungal or parasitic), **subdural empyema, cranial epidural abscess, Reye's syndrome** (in children), **bacterial endocarditis, toxic-metabolic encephalopathy, drug intoxication, septicemia, vasculitis, cerebral venous sinus thrombosis,** and **mitochondrial disease**.
- In adults, **60–70%** acquire the disease by latent virus reactivation; **70–80%** of children acquire the disease by primary contact.
- **MRI of the brain** and **HSV-PCR** provide highest diagnostic yield.
- Treatment includes **acyclovir 10 mg/kg i.v. every 8 hours** (preferred) or **vidarabine 15 mg/kg slow i.v. infusion every 24 hours** for **14 days**.
- Mortality is **20–30%** if treated. If untreated, mortality is **approximately 70–90%**.
- **Approximately 30–50%** of patients fully recover with no or mild neurological sequelae. About **20–50%** may have moderate to severe neurological deficits (neuropsychological) that are disabling.

6

Spinal Cord Disease

CASE 1

A 17-year-old boy fell from a horse while riding at about 40 miles an hour approximately 1–2 hours ago. He hit the ground head first with associated neck flexion. He complained of inability to move his arms or legs and some difficulty breathing. On examination, temperature was 37.2°C, BP 75/40 mmHg, HR was 48 per minute with RR at 30 per minute. Neurological examination showed intact mental status and cranial nerve function. Motor examination showed flaccid quadriplegia apart from MRC 1/5 strength in shoulder abduction and elbow flexion bilaterally. Sensory examination revealed a sensory level to pinprick at the level of the clavicles with normal light touch examination. There was generalized areflexia with extensor plantar responses.

Localization

The normal mental status and cranial nerve function reduces the likelihood that there is bilateral involvement of the cerebral cortex and brainstem. However, extensor plantar responses suggest that an upper motor neuron process is present. Bradycardia and hypotension are most likely the result of neurogenic shock secondary to disruption of the sympathetic innervation to the heart.

The sensory level to pinprick localizes to the C4 dermatome, which may represent spinal levels C2–C6. Respiratory difficulties are associated with C3–C5 dysfunction. Residual strength in the deltoid and biceps muscles suggests that the process localizes at the C5–C6 spinal level. Sparing of dorsal column function localizes the lesion to the anterolateral aspects of the spinal cord. Flaccid quadriparesis and generalized areflexia can occur secondary to spinal shock.

Differential Diagnosis

The most likely diagnosis is an *acute anterior spinal cord syndrome* (ASCS) at the C5 level. This is an anatomical diagnosis with several etiologies. The preceding history of trauma suggests that this is the most likely cause. *Trauma* can

From: *Neurology Oral Boards Review:*
A Concise and Systematic Approach to Clinical Practice
By: E. E. Ubogu © Humana Press Inc., Totowa, NJ

cause direct injury to the spinal cord (contusion, hemorrhage, transection: more commonly seen in children than adults) or indirect injury from vertebral fractures/dislocations, acute disc herniation, or epidural hematoma.

Other causes of ASCS include *nontraumatic arthropathies* (spondylosis, canal stenosis, ankylosing spondylitis, disc herniation: more common in adults), *tumors* (epidural metastasis from lung, breast, prostate; intradural extramedullary lesions like meningioma; intradural intramedullary lesions like ependymoma [children], astrocytoma [adults] or metastasis: would expect a preceding history of back pain), *epidural abscess* (e.g., following osteomyelitis secondary to *S. aureus*, TB), *infarction* (vascular occlusion secondary to emboli, vasculitis or spinal AVMs: less common in children), and *autoimmune/demyelination* (secondary to MS, collagen vascular diseases like SLE or postinfectious diseases following rubella, varicella).

Nutritional deficiencies or *toxins* (e.g., vitamin B_{12} or folate deficiency and nitric oxide inhalation) tend to cause subacute to chronic posterior column and corticospinal tract dysfunction. *Infections* (e.g., viral infections such as HIV, HTLV, VZV) can cause subacute to chronic disease, whereas Lyme disease causes an acute myeloradiculitis. The clinical presentation would be more progressive and may exhibit more systemic features.

Investigations

Investigations should include emergent plain radiographs of cervical spine (anterior-posterior [AP], lateral, and oblique) to exclude bony injury. If clinically indicated, thoracolumbar films may be needed to assess for noncontiguous injury. MRI of spinal cord (with particular attention to the cervical spine) with and without gadolinium should be performed emergently following immobilization to deduce the etiology for the ASCS. If MRI is not readily available, CT myelography may be performed. Any suggestion of head injury requires a noncontrasted CT scan of the head to exclude hemorrhage and bony trauma.

Further investigations should be tailored toward potential etiologies (especially in atypical cases) and complications. Chest X-ray, CBC with differential, ESR/CRP, blood cultures, PSA, CT chest, mammography, ANA panel, RhF, anti-ds DNA, vitamin B_{12} levels, RPR, HIV titer, human T-cell lymphotropic virus (HTLV) antibodies, LP for oligoclonal bands, immunoglobulin (Ig)G index, viral PCR, or Lyme IgM/IgG may be considered. Blood should be typed and screened for potential transfusion prior to or during surgery.

Management

Traumatic ASCS is a neurological emergency because the prevention of irreversible sequelae depends on rapid institution of therapy. Furthermore, respiratory and cardiovascular compromise require resuscitation.

Immobilization with a halo or tongs is required to prevent further cord injury. Intubation (with care) and mechanical ventilation should be performed if RR is more than 30 per minute, vital capacity (VC) less than 500 cc, PaO_2 less than 70 mmHg, $PaCO_2$ more than 45 mmHg, evidence of increased work of breathing, abnormal breathing patterns, or for airway protection from aspiration. Chest-tube insertion would be required for pneumothorax or hemothorax. Circulatory support should be performed using a central line with infusion of crystalloid or colloid to achieve normotension. Central venous pressure or pulmonary wedge pressure should be monitored. Vasopressors would be required if fluid resuscitation were insufficient. Intravenous atropine would be indicated for severe bradycardia. Acute spinal realignment should be attempted on confirming the cause of traumatic ASCS.

Methylprednisolone 30 mg/kg i.v. bolus, then 5.4 mg/kg per hour for 24–48 hours followed by prednisone taper over 10–14 days, should be started within 8 hours of spinal cord injury. Emergent surgical decompression or debridment should be considered in ASCS to release a vital cervical nerve root (e.g., C3–C5), for compound fracture or penetrating spinal cord injury, unreducible fracture dislocations causing spinal cord compression or incomplete lesions with progression in neurological deficit despite reduction or bony fragments/ soft-tissue elements within the spinal canal. Emergency surgery is contraindicated for complete spinal cord injury more than 24 hours duration, in a medically unstable patient and central cord syndrome without cord compression.

General supportive care (e.g., regular nursing checks every 1–2 hours, nasogastric tube for paralytic ileus and gastric dilatation, urinary catherization, temperature control, nutritional support, GI and DVT prophylaxis, frequent repositioning, analgesia, traction, and active rehabilitation) is essential. The patient should be transferred from ICU to a spinal cord unit with expertise in caring for such patients once stable.

Prognosis

Outcomes depend on the underlying disease, anatomical localization of spinal cord injury, severity of neurological deficit at presentation, time from spinal cord injury to treatment, and the presence of multiple trauma. In general, mortality from acute spinal cord injury could be as high as 50%, with 80% of deaths occurring before or on arrival to the hospital. For patients surviving to reach the hospital, mortality rates vary from 5 to 20%. Functional motor recovery occurs in 10–20% of ASCS, 50% of central cord syndrome, and approximately 90% of Brown-Séquard's syndrome (spinal cord hemitransection). Outcomes are better with incomplete spinal cord injuries than complete.

Treatment with high-dose methylprednisolone within 8 hours of presentation (<3 hours more favorable) is associated with better functional outcomes (independent ambulation, neurological recovery) at 6 weeks, 6 and 12 months after injury. Mortality is more common with high cervical lesions (owing to cardiorespiratory compromise) and the presence of multiple trauma (e.g., cerebral contusion, flail chest, appendicular bony fractures) with systemic hypotension and hypoxia.

Counseling

Patients should be aware that residual neurological deficits are common despite optimal treatment. Chances of recovery are improved by early aggressive medical intervention and spinal cord stabilization. Early surgical decompression (<72 hours) may improve outcomes, but this has not been confirmed by randomized controlled trials.

Active rehabilitation may improve recovery. Patients should be taught self-catheterization and bowel hygiene, and ambulatory patients may require walking aids. Nonambulatory patients would require wheelchairs. Chronic mechanical ventilation would be required for high cervical injuries and tracheostomy should be performed if intubated for more than 7 days. Highly dependent patients would require hospital beds to prevent decubiti and significant caregiver support for nutritional and hygiene needs.

SUMMARY

- **ASCS** is a neurological emergency because prevention of long-term sequelae is dependent on instituting therapy early.
- Etiologies include **trauma, nontraumatic arthropathies, tumor, epidural abscess, infarction, autoimmune** or **inflammation, nutritional deficiencies, toxins, and infection**.
- **Plain radiographs** and **MRI** are the diagnostic tests of choice.
- Acute **spinal stabilization** and **realignment** are necessary.
- Pharmacological treatment should be instituted **within 8 hours** of injury.
- Treatment consists of **methylprednisolone 30 mg/kg i.v. bolus**, then **5.4 mg/kg per hour** for **24–48 hours**, followed by prednisone taper over 10–14 days.
- **Emergency surgery** is contraindicated in **complete spinal cord injury more than 24 hours duration, medically unstable patients**, and **central cord syndrome without cord compression**.
- Mortality is approximately **50%** before or on arrival to the hospital in acute spinal cord injury. Death occurs in **5–20%** of initially surviving patients.
- Outcomes depend on **underlying etiology, anatomical localization of injury, severity of deficit at presentation, timing of treatment, and presence of multiple trauma**. Residual deficits are common in survivors.
- Functional motor recovery occurs in only **10–20%** of ASCS.

CASE 2

A 33-year-old man suddenly developed back pain with weakness in both legs about 12 hours ago. This had progressed to difficulty with micturition and defecation. There was no history of trauma. On examination, temperature was 38°C with normal mental status and cranial nerve examinations. Motor examination revealed normal strength in the upper extremities, with MRC 3–4/5 strength in the lower extremities. Sensory examination showed a sensory level to pinprick and light touch at the umbilicus. Hyperreflexia was present in the lower extremities with extensor plantar responses. Bladder catherization produced 350 cc of clear urine.

Localization

The normal mental status, cranial nerve, and upper extremity examinations suggest that the process localizes below the T1 spinal cord or nerve root level. Hyperreflexic weakness with extensor plantar responses implies an upper motor neuron lesion, suggesting that the process is in the thoracolumbar spinal cord. A sensory level at T10 suggests that the process could localize between spinal levels T8–T12. The fact that both light touch and pinprick are impaired suggests a diffuse process affecting the low thoracic spinal cord.

Differential Diagnosis

Acute diffuse spinal cord involvement with a low-grade fever makes *acute transverse myelitis* (ATM) the most likely diagnosis. The absence of trauma by history makes traumatic spinal cord injury very unlikely, however *nontraumatic arthropathy* is possible (e.g., spondylosis, canal stenosis, etc.: less likely in this age group). *Spinal cord infarction* (secondary to embolism, vasculitis, dissection, AVM, venous occlusion, hypotension, etc.: progression is usually >4 hours), *spinal cord tumor* (e.g., gliomas: expect slower, more chronic progression, but may acutely present), *epidural hematoma* (would expect some preceding trauma unless there is a history of inherited or acquired bleeding diathesis), and *epidural abscess* (would expect a more prolonged history of back pain secondary to osteomyelitis and point tenderness on examination; should be excluded in febrile individuals) are other diagnostic considerations.

Etiologies for ATM include *autoimmune/postinfections* such as MS (may present asymmetrically; check for prior CNS involvement), neuromyelitis optica (would expect signs of optic neuritis), or acute disseminated encephalomyelitis (ADEM; postviral: brain involvement commonly associated), *infectious*: viral (coxsackie, echovirus, HSV, Epstein-Barr virus [EBV], VZV, CMV), bacterial (mycoplasma, Coxiella, *M. tuberculosis*), spirochete (Lyme disease), *parainfectious/postimmunization* (e.g., mumps), *connective tissue disorders* (SLE, mixed connective tissue disease [MCTD], aPL syndrome, Sjögren's syndrome, Behçet's disease), *sarcoidosis, postradiation therapy, mitochondrial disorders* (Leigh's disease, also known as subacute necrotizing encephalomyelopathy: abnormal movements such as tremor, ataxia, chorea with respiratory dysfunction, external ophthalmoplegia, and paralysis of deglutition), and *idiopathic* (about 20–40% of all cases of ATM).

Investigations

MRI of the spinal cord with and without gadolinium is the diagnostic test of choice for ATM. MRI of the brain with and without contrast can be performed if there are signs of brain involvement clinically. MRI would exclude compressive lesions and may show hyperintense cord signals that enhance. If MRI is not available, CT myelography should be performed. LP should be performed to evaluate for MS (oligoclonal bands, IgG ratio and index), infectious (CSF WBC/RBC/Protein/glucose, CSF gram/acid-fast bacilli [AFB] stain, CSF viral and bacterial cultures, PCR for herpesviruses, Lyme IgM/IgG) and neoplastic causes (cytology).

Based on the history, further laboratory tests may be required such as CBC with differential, PT/PTT/INR (before LP and if bleeding diathesis suspected), ESR/CRP, ANA panel, anticardiolipin antibodies, aPL antibodies, anti-ds-DNA antibodies, SSA and SSB antibodies, complement and angiotensin-converting enzyme (ACE) levels. In atypical and refractory cases, a spinal cord biopsy may be rarely required, especially if a neoplastic lesion is highly considered. Angiography may be required for vascular causes, especially AVM.

Management

The acute management of ATM is directed toward reducing spinal cord inflammation and treating the underlying cause. High-dose corticosteroids are used acutely for spinal cord inflammation. Methylprednisolone 1 g i.v. every 24 hours (as a single slow infusion or divided every 6 hours) in adults or 580 mg/m^2 per day in children is commonly administered, followed by 1 mg/kg per day of prednisone for 2–3 days followed by titration over 10–14 days. Further immunosuppresants would be required for connective tissue disorders, antimicrobials for infectious causes, and immune modulators for autoimmune causes.

General supportive care (e.g., regular nursing checks every 4–6 hours, bladder/bowel hygiene with nonpharmacological and pharmacological methods, nutritional and fluid support, glucose checks while on steroids, GI and DVT prophylaxis, frequent repositioning, analgesia (avoid opioids: aggravate urinary retention and constipation), and active rehabilitation are essential. The patient should be managed in a spinal cord unit or general neurology floor with expertise in caring for patients with spinal cord disease.

Prognosis

Outcomes in ATM may depend on age (especially in children), severity of symptoms on presentation, rate of symptom progression, and the underlying cause. The role of high-dose steroids is debatable. This therapy has been shown to improve functional recovery in some series, but it has not been formally assessed in a randomized control trial. Full recovery occurs in 35–45% of patients, with mild deficits occurring in 30–35% and moderate/severe deficits in 20–35% of patients. Of patients with complete ATM, 7–10% develop MS, whereas 70–90% of patients with partial/incomplete ATM subsequently develop this disease.

Counseling

Patients should be aware of the prognostic data. As many as 20–40% of cases of ATM are idiopathic, so patients should not be surprised by a failure to ascertain a cause for ATM. Sphincter dysfunction is the most resistant to recovery, so long-term therapies for detrusor instability (bladder hyperactivity) may be needed, such as anticholinergics or intermittent catherization. Patients should be taught about bladder/bowel hygiene. Acute rehabilitation may aid in recovery, so this should be encouraged. Relapsing ATM more commonly occurs with autoimmune and connective tissue disorders, so a more thorough work-up may be required with a subsequent episode, aimed at finding a cause.

SUMMARY

- **ATM** is a neurological emergency because early diagnosis and intervention may prevent long-term sequelae.
- Differentials include **nontraumatic spinal cord injury, cord infarction, spinal cord tumor, epidural hematoma,** and **epidural abscess**.
- Etiologies include **autoimmune/postinfectious, infections, parainfectious/postimmunization, connective tissue disorders, sarcoidosis, postradiation therapy, mitochondrial disease,** and **idiopathic**.
- **MRI** of the **spinal cord** with or without gadolinium is the test of choice.
- Management consists of **methylprednisolone 1 g i.v. every 24 hours** (in adults) or **580 mg/m^2 per day** (children), followed by **1 mg/kg per day of prednisone** for 2–3 days, then titration over 10–14 days.
- Full recovery occurs in **35–45%**, mild deficits in **30–35%** and moderate/severe deficits in **20–35%**.
- Outcomes may depend on **age, severity at presentation, rate of disease progression,** and **underlying cause**.
- Of patients with complete ATM, **7–10%** develop MS, whereas **70–90%** of patients with partial/incomplete ATM develop this disease.

7

Movement Disorders

CASE 1

A 24-year-old man with schizophrenia was admitted with agitation and psychosis. He had received several doses of haloperidol for symptom control. Over the previous 36 hours since his last dose, he had become confused and rigid. Clinical examination revealed a temperature of 39.8°C, HR 114 per minute, BP 165/100 mmHg, and RR of 22 per minute with shallow breaths. Neurological examination showed fluctuating level of consciousness with normal brainstem reflexes, lead-pipe rigidity in all limbs, symmetrical facial grimacing to deep noxious stimuli, and generalized hyperreflexia.

Localization

Mental status changes with normal brainstem reflexes suggest bilateral cerebral cortical dysfunction. Hypertonia, lead-pipe rigidity, and hyperreflexia in all limbs further support an upper motor neuron dysfunction (cerebral cortex, basal ganglia, or spinal cord). Dysautonomia and hyperpyrexia could suggest dysfunction of the hypothalamus or its central projections. Based on the findings, bilateral cerebral cortex, basal ganglia, and hypothalamus are the most likely localizations. Concurrent spinal cord involvement is also possible.

Differential Diagnosis

The most likely diagnosis based on the history of fever, dysautonomia, lead-pipe rigidity, and mental status changes following haloperidol use is *neuroleptic malignant syndrome* (NMS). This is an idiosyncratic adverse reaction to dopamine antagonists or sudden withdrawal of dopaminergic agents.

Other differentials include *heat stroke* (can be induced by neuroleptics or antihistamines owing to anticholinergic effects: there is usually a history of higher than normal heat/humidity exposure with or without exercise; skin is dry), *malignant hyperthermia* (associated with inhalational anesthetics or succinylcholine: occurs rapidly after exposure), *central anticholinergic syndrome* (dry eyes, dry mouth, dilated pupils, urinary retention, and delirium), and

From: *Neurology Oral Boards Review:*
A Concise and Systematic Approach to Clinical Practice
By: E. E. Ubogu © Humana Press Inc., Totowa, NJ

serotonin syndrome (usually associated with selective serotonin reuptake inhibitors [SSRIs], especially with concurrent use of TCAs or monoamine oxidase inhibitors [MAOIs]: tremors and myoclonus more common, whereas fever, rigidity and rhabdomyolysis less common).

Further diagnostic considerations include *drug-induced states and overdose* (such as amphetamines, cocaine, phencyclidine, lysergic acid diethylamide [LSD]), *acute lethal catatonia* (usually have stereotypical choreiform movements, primitive hyperkinesias, torsion spasm before akinetic state), *thyrotoxicosis* (anxiety, insomnia, tremors; look for lid lag and infrequent blinking), *pheochromocytoma* (usually hypertension, diaphoresis, and palpitations, with muscle rigidity and fever less likely), *acute psychosis with agitation*, and *CNS or systemic infections,* including sepsis.

Investigations

Investigations should include CBC with differential, comprehensive metabolic panel, CK (elevated in ~70% of patients), serum/urine toxicology, urinalysis (for myoglobin) and ABGs. CT scan of the head should be performed if there are any focal signs and prior to LP. LP should be performed to exclude CNS infection. Check PT/PTT/INR before LP. In atypical cases, TFT and serum/urine catecholamine levels may be required to exclude an endocrinopathy; EEG may be required to exclude catatonia (normal background activity). Septic screen (chest X-ray, blood cultures, and urinalysis) may be required to exclude systemic infection.

Management

NMS is considered a neurological emergency because death may occur from cardiovascular instability or respiratory failure if not treated early. Intubation and mechanical ventilation should be instituted if there are signs of respiratory failure or for airway protection. Intravenous hydration with normal saline should be started to prevent renal failure from rhabdomyolysis, adequately hydrate the patient and facilitate cooling and treat dysautonomia. All neuroleptic agents should be discontinued.

Pharmacological therapy consists of bromocriptine 2.5–10 mg i.v. every 8 hours. Increase by 5 mg per day until clinical improvement is seen. Continue for at least 10 days after NMS control and then taper slowly. Bromocriptine can cause hypotension. Alternatives include dantrolene (drug of choice for malignant hyperthermia), start at 0.25 mg/kg i.v. every 6–12 hours, increasing to 3 mg/kg per day for 2–3 days. Oral dantrolene therapy (50–600 mg per day) may be continued for several days afterward. Watch for hepatic toxicity. Bromocriptine and dantrolene may be safely combined in severe cases. Amantadine 100–200 mg p.o. twice a day may also be effective. Diazepam 2–10 mg i.v. every 4–6 hours when necessary (maximum 60 mg) helps reduce muscle rigidity and control agitation if present.

Electroconvulsive therapy (ECT) with neuromuscular blockade can be used in pharmacologically refractory cases. ECT helps fever, diaphoresis, and reduced level of consciousness. Succinylcholine should not be used (can cause hyperkalemia and cardiac arrhythmias in patients with rhabdomyolysis or dysautonomia).

Supportive care (e.g., frequent nursing checks, decubitus prevention, DVT prophylaxis, active cooling with blankets and antipyretics, strict fluid balance, nutritional support, and rehabilitation) is necessary. Patients should be managed in an ICU if dysautonomia is present or respiratory support required. Otherwise, a regular nursing floor should be adequate. Hemodialysis may be required to treat acute renal failure.

Prognosis

Mortality rate is approximately 5–10% despite previous therapeutic measures. Serious sequelae may occur in a further 20%. Complete recovery occurs in more than 70% of patients. Mortality rates have declined from 15 to 25% 20 years ago because of earlier recognition and aggressive pharmacological and supportive care. Factors adversely affecting mortality are development of acute renal failure and core temperature higher than 40°C. Causes of death include cardiorespiratory arrest, hepatorenal failure, pneumonia, PE, and sepsis. Serious sequelae include seizures, extrapyramidal or cerebellar deficits, and chronic renal failure.

Counseling

Patients should be aware of prognostic data. Risk for developing NMS includes dehydration, agitation, prior NMS, high-dose, rapid increase or intramuscular administration of neuroleptics. Recurrence of NMS may occur with reintroduction of high-potency neuroleptics, but less commonly with atypical agents. For patients medically dependent on these agents, slow reintroduction may be necessary later than 2 weeks after treating NMS. Chronic renal failure from rhabdomyolysis would require appropriate therapy (referral to a nephrologist prudent for optimal management). Seizures would require long-term AEDs. Muscle relaxants may be required for long-term management of residual hypertonia.

SUMMARY

- **NMS** is a neurological emergency because outcomes are dependent on rapid institution of pharmacological and supportive therapy.
- Differentials include **heat stroke, malignant hyperthermia, central anticholinergic syndrome, serotonin syndrome, drug-induced states and overdose, acute lethal catatonia, thyrotoxicosis, pheochromocytoma, acute psychosis with agitation,** and **CNS/systemic infections.**

- Investigations are nonspecific, but **CK is elevated in approximately 70%**. Other potential causes of hyperthermia must be excluded.
- Pharmacological therapy: **Bromocriptine 2.5–10 mg i.v. every 8 hours**, increase by 5 mg per day until clinical improvement, then for more than 10 days and/or **dantrolene 0.25 mg/kg i.v. every 6–12 hours**, increasing to 3 mg/kg per day for 2–3 days, then oral therapy (50–600 mg per day).
- Respiratory and cardiovascular support may be required.
- Aggressive hydration is necessary to prevent acute renal failure
- Mortality is approximately **5–10%**. Severe sequelae in approximately **20%** with full recovery in more than **70%**. Development of **acute renal failure** and **core temperature over 40°C** increase risk for death.

CASE 2

An 85-year-old woman with diabetic neuropathy on nortryptiline became severely depressed following the death of her husband of 60 years. She was started on sertraline 50 mg p.o. daily about 6 hours ago. She was noticed to be confused and tremulous. On examination, temperature was 37.2°C, HR 108 per minute, BP 165/90 mmHg, and RR 14 per minute with mild diaphoresis. Neurological examination revealed fluctuating levels of consciousness with mydriasis, spontaneous, nonpurposeful muscle jerks, and symmetrical withdrawal to noxious stimuli in all limbs. Generalized hyperreflexia and intentional tremor with appendicular ataxia were also present on examination.

Localization

Mental status changes suggest bilateral cerebral cortical dysfunction. Mydriasis, tachycardia, and mild hypertension suggest sympathetic overstimulation or parasympathetic outflow dysfunction. Generalized hyperreflexia suggests upper motor neuron dysfunction, whereas myoclonus may be secondary to dysfunction in the brainstem or spinal cord. Intentional tremor and appendicular ataxia localize to the lateral cerebellar hemispheres (or central connections) bilaterally. Based on the clinical features, there is bilateral dysfunction in the cerebral and cerebellar hemispheres, possibly with brainstem and spinal cord disease.

Differential Diagnosis

The most likely diagnosis for the clinical presentation occurring after administration of an SSRI to a regimen with a TCA in an elderly woman is *serotonin syndrome*. This is a predictable adverse effect of serotonergic drug use owing to overstimulation of serotonin receptors in the brainstem and spinal cord associated with therapeutic or toxic doses of serotonergic drugs or reduced metabolism of these agents.

Differentials include *NMS* (slower onset; requires institution or dose increase of dopamine antagonists or withdrawal from dopamine agonists; muscle rigidity with rhabdomyolysis, hyperthermia, severe dysautonomia are more common in NMS), *delirium tremens* (should have a preceding history of alcohol use more than 48 hours prior, hallucinations common), *sympathomimetic/anticholinergic drug overdose, stiff-person syndrome* (mental status usually preserved), *heat stroke* (exertional or nonexertional), *acute lethal catatonia, malignant hyperthermia, drugs/toxins* (e.g., lithium, cocaine, strychnine), *metabolic encephalopathy* (e.g., anoxia, hepatic/renal failure) or *systemic* and *CNS infections.* (*see* pp. 73–74 for differentiating features.)

Investigations

Investigations are nonspecific and are performed to exclude other potential causes. CK is usually normal, unless there is severe muscle rigidity. Tests are similar to those performed in NMS (*see* p. 74). The clinical history is the most important diagnostic tool.

Management

Serotonin syndrome is considered a neurological emergency because death could ensue from cardiopulmonary arrest or acute renal failure; however, withdrawal of the offending drugs with supportive care may be all that is required in less severe cases. Intubation should be performed for airway protection in comatose patients. Cardiac arrhythmias and dysautonomia should be aggressively treated. Intravenous hydration should be started.

Pharmacological treatment consists of cyproheptadine (a nonspecific 5-hydroxytryptamine [5-HT] receptor antagonist) 4–8 mg p.o./n.g. stat, then 2–4 mg p.o./n.g. every 8 hours until clinical resolution (improvement usually occurs within 12–24 hours). This is based on case series and not on randomized controlled trials. Other options include β-blockers (that block 5-HT_1 and/or 5-HT_2 receptors, e.g., propranolol, pindolol), benzodiazepines (e.g., diazepam or lorazepam; probable inhibitors of serotonergic transmission, useful for myoclonus and muscle rigidity; avoid over-sedation), chlorpromazine 50–100mg intramuscularly (i.m.) (antagonism of dopamine, 5-HT_{1A} and $5HT_2$ receptors), and methysergide (nonselective 5-HT receptor antagonist). Rarely, dantrolene or bromocriptine or both have been used successfully for severe rigidity with hyperthermia (*see* section on NMS for doses). Supportive care is similar to that required for NMS (*see* p. 75).

Prognosis

Mortality from serotonin syndrome is 1–3%; main causes of death include cardiac and respiratory arrest and renal failure secondary to rhabdomyolysis. Less common complications include disseminated intravascular coagulation, leukopenia, thrombocytopenia, tonic-clonic seizures, and multiorgan failure.

These occur less commonly than in NMS. Withdrawal of the offending agent with or without pharmacotherapy usually results in clinical recovery in 60–70% within 24 hours. Approximately 40% of patients require ICU care, 25% of whom may undergo intubation. Full recovery is expected in more than 90% of cases, with mild sequelae (e.g., residual hypertonia, seizures) present in approximately 5%.

Counseling

Patients should be aware of the risk factors for developing serotonin syndrome: institution or increased dosage of serotonergic drug, singly or in combination with other serotonergic agents, especially in the elderly or individuals with predisposing factors for adverse effects including cardiac, pulmonary, or hepatic disease (may have endogenously reduced MAOI and cytochrome *P450* activity, with resultant reduction in metabolism).

Offending drugs include SSRIs, MAOIs, TCAs and tetracyclic antidepressants, dopamine serotonin receptor agonists, opioids, L-tryptophan, and amphetamine derivatives. The introduction of an SSRI should occur 2–4 weeks after discontinuing MAOIs. Serotonergic agents should be administered to the elderly in lower doses with gentler titration. Patients should be aware of prognostic data and overall good recovery.

SUMMARY

- **Serotonin syndrome** is an **iatrogenic** adverse effect of hyperserotoninemia, which may cause cardiorespiratory/renal failure.
- Diagnosis requires **cognitive–behavioral changes, dysautonomia**, and **neuromuscular hyperexcitability**.
- Differential diagnoses are **similar to those for NMS**.
- Treatment includes **removal of offending agents, supportive care**, and **cyproheptadine 4–8 mg stat**, then **2–4 mg every 8 hours** until resolution.
- Other options include β**-blockers, benzodiazepines, dantrolene/ bromocriptine, chlorpromazine**, and **methysergide**.
- Mortality is **1–3%**. Full recovery is expected in more than **90%** of patients; **60–70%** recover within **24 hours**. Mild sequelae are uncommon.

8

Toxic-Metabolic Disorders

CASE 1

A 48-year-old man was brought to the ER with a 1-week history of confusion with marked lethargy for 24 hours. He had a history of chronic alcohol use and poor nutrition. On examination, he was poorly responsive to external stimuli with intermittent eye opening to commands. Cranial nerve examination revealed sluggish pupillary light responses, vertical nystagmus on upgaze, and abduction paresis with horizontal end-gaze nystagmus on lateral gaze bilaterally. Further neurological examination revealed symmetrical localization to noxious stimuli in all limbs with severe truncal ataxia in a sitting position.

Localization

Mental status changes suggest bilateral dysfunction in the cerebral cortex or diencephalon (e.g., thalamus). Sluggish bilateral pupillary light responses (direct and consensual) suggest retinal or optic nerve disease or dysfunction of optic tracts in the posterior commissure or CN III nucleus in the midbrain or parasympathetic pupilloconstrictor fibers. Vertical nystagmus on upgaze suggests dysfunction in the supranuclear or vestibular modulation of CN III.

Abduction paresis is the result of CN VI dysfunction in the pons, whereas horizontal end-gaze nystagmus suggests dysfunction in the supranuclear or vestibular modulation of CN VI. Truncal ataxia suggest vestibular or midline cerebellar dysfunction. The clinical picture suggests involvement of the cerebral cortex and brainstem (possibly with midline cerebellum) bilaterally.

Differential Diagnosis

The most likely diagnosis for mental status changes, ophthalmoparesis, truncal ataxia, and nystagmus occurring acutely in a malnourished, chronic alcohol user is *Wernicke's encephalopathy*. This is caused by thiamine (vitamin B$_1$) deficiency. Although chronic alcoholism is the most likely etiology, nonalcoholic patients with poor nutritional state (inadequate intake, malabsorption, or increased metabolic requirement) are susceptible. Associated conditions include

From: *Neurology Oral Boards Review:*
A Concise and Systematic Approach to Clinical Practice
By: E. E. Ubogu © Humana Press Inc., Totowa, NJ

systemic malignancy, GI surgery, anorexia nervosa, acquired immunodeficiency syndrome (AIDS), hyperemesis gravidarum, and refeeding after prolonged fasting/starvation.

Other differentials include other *metabolic encephalopathies* (uremia, dialysis, hypo/hypernatremia, hypo/hyperglycemia, hypomagnesemia, etc: oculomotor paresis would be unusual except if associated with DM), *hypoxic-ischemic encephalopathy* (HIE; e.g., postcardiac arrest), *drug intoxication/withdrawal* (e.g., phenytoin, TCAs, benzodiazepines, anticholinergics), *brainstem encephalitis* (paraneoplastic or infectious, i.e., viral), brainstem stroke (e.g., basilar artery thrombosis: course more acute, with corticospinal tract findings), *systemic infections/sepsis, meningitis/encephalitis* (especially fungal: causes basal meningitis with CN signs; course more chronic. Carcinomatous meningitis may also affect cranial nerves), *CNS vasculitis* (primary/secondary: brainstem findings unexpected), *SAH, post-ictal state, hydrocephalus* (acutely presents with coma; normal pressure hydrocephalus [NPH] chronically causes dementia, gait ataxia, and urinary incontinence) and *central pontine myelinolysis* (CPM).

Investigations

Investigations are clinically tailored to exclude other diseases. Laboratory tests include CBC with differential, comprehensive metabolic panel, serum/urine toxicology, drug levels (if ingestion known), and septic screen (chest X-ray, blood, and urine cultures). Head CT scan should be performed for focal signs or history of preceding trauma. LP may be performed to exclude meningoencephalitis or SAH.

Brain MRI with and without gadolinium (with DWI) may show hyperintensity or enhancement in the thalami, mammillary bodies, periaqueductal gray matter, and adjacent to the third and fourth ventricles. MRI would also exclude brainstem disease and CNS vasculitis (if suspected, biopsy may be necessary). EEG may show focal slowing suggestive for a recent seizure focus. Serum thiamine levels and RBC transketolase may be reduced, with elevated serum pyruvate in thiamine deficient individuals with or without Wernicke's encephalopathy. Clinical history is the most important diagnostic tool in establishing the diagnosis.

Management

The mainstay of therapy is the parenteral administration of thiamine. The exact dose and duration of therapy has not been conclusively established. Thiamine 100 mg i.v./i.m. every 24 hours for 3–5 days (or until oral intake is possible), then 100 mg p.o. daily until clinical resolution and correction of the underlying etiology (if possible). Thiamine should be administered prior to i.v. glucose in patients with hypoglycemia or refeeding after prolonged fasting/starvation to prevent precipitating this syndrome. If there is evidence of respiratory compromise or need for airway protection, intubation and mechanical ventilation should be instituted. Circulatory support would be necessary for patients with dysautonomia (from dysfunction of hypothalamic/brainstem autonomic pathways).

Supportive care (e.g., frequent nursing checks, decubitus prevention, DVT prophylaxis, active warming with blankets for hypothermia, strict fluid balance, gradual nutritional support, and rehabilitation) is necessary. Benzodiazepines may be required to prevent delirium tremens. The patient should be managed in an ICU for dysautonomia/respiratory support; otherwise, a regular nursing floor should be adequate. Underlying causes and electrolyte abnormalities should be addressed.

Prognosis

Mortality is 10–20% despite thiamine treatment. Causes of death include bronchopneumonia, sepsis, and pancreatitis. Irreversible brain damage may contribute to mortality. Of the survivors, 15–20% recover fully and 80–85% develop Korsakoff's psychosis (KP). The majority of ocular signs resolve within an hour of treatment, with residual fine horizontal nystagmus persisting in approximately 60% of patients. Gait/truncal ataxia is relatively resistant to treatment, with more than 33% of patients with ambulatory problems months after illness.

Lethargy and confusion gradually improve over days to weeks, with residual amnesia (KP). Of the patients with KP, approximately 20% show complete recovery; approximately 25% significant recovery, approximately 30% only slight improvement and approximately 25% no improvement. Recovery may take from 2 months to 10 years. Twenty-five percent of patients with KP require long-term care.

Counseling

The classic symptoms of Wernicke's encephalopathy only occur in 10–20% of patients, so clinicians should have a low threshold to treat. Chronic alcoholism should be addressed through medical counseling and supportive groups (e.g., Alcoholics Anonymous). Malnutrition (and any predisposing conditions) should be treated. Chronic vitamin supplements may be needed. Patients and their families should be aware of the prognostic data and likely progression to KP. KP and Wernicke's encephalopathy should be considered part of a single disease spectrum.

SUMMARY

- **Wernicke's encephalopathy** occurs as a consequence of **vitamin B$_1$ (thiamine) deficiency** and is potentially reversible.
- Differentials include other **metabolic encephalopathies, HIE, drug intoxication/withdrawal, brainstem encephalitis/stroke, systemic/CNS infection, SAH, CNS vasculitis, post-ictal, hydrocephalus**, and **CPM**.

- Clinical history is vital. Note that only **10–20%** of patients present classically.
- Treatment consists of **thiamine 100 mg i.v./i.m daily** for 3–5 days, then **100 mg p.o. daily** until resolution. Alcohol cessation and improved nutrition should be emphasized. Associated causes should be concurrently treated.
- Mortality is **10–20%**. Of survivors, **approximately 15–20%** fully recover and **approximately 80–85%** develop KP.
- Of patients with KP, **approximately 20%** show complete recovery; **approximately 25%** show significant recovery, **approximately 30%** only slight improvement, and **approximately 25%** show no improvement. Recovery takes **2 months to 10 years**.

CASE 2

A 57-year-old woman was brought to the ER in a confused and agitated state. She had a history of chronic alcohol use and had been missing for about 72 hours. In the ER, she stated that "small pink animals" attacked her that morning. Restraints were needed to control her violent behavior. On examination, temperature was 38.5°C, HR 122 per minute, BP 170/95 mmHg, and RR 16 per minute. The patient was diaphoretic with a supple neck. Neurological examination showed waxing and waning levels of consciousness with intermittent agitation. There was generalized tremulousness without any focal signs on examination.

Localization

Delirium is nonlocalizing and suggests bilateral dysfunction of the cerebral cortex. Agitation could occur owng to bilateral limbic (mesial frontal or temporal) dysfunction. Generalized tremors may be seen with bilateral basal ganglionic (rest, i.e., parkinsonian), midbrain (postural, i.e., rubral), or cerebellar (intentional) disorders.

Visual hallucinations can be caused by dysfunction in the visual pathways from the retina to the occipital lobe. Well-formed hallucinations may occur with occipito-temporal lesions. Hyperpyrexia and signs of adrenergic excess could imply lesions in the hypothalamus or descending autonomic pathways. This process localizes diffusely to the cerebral and cerebellar cortices with possible hypothalamic involvement bilaterally.

Differential Diagnosis

The most likely diagnosis for the clinical presentation of agitated delirium with vivid visual hallucinations of small animals, hyperpyrexia, adrenergic excess, and tremulousness about 3 days after last presumed alcohol intake is *delirium tremens.* This is an alcohol withdrawal syndrome that could be fatal if untreated. A similar syndrome may occur with benzodiazepines/barbiturate withdrawal.

Other differentials include *metabolic encephalopathies* (hepatic, uremic, hypo/hyperglycemia, hypo/hypernatremia, hypo/hypercalcemia, hypo/hypermagnesemia), *endocrinopathies* (thyrotoxicosis, hypo/hypercortisolemia), *vitamin deficiencies* (thiamine, vitamin B_{12}, nicotinamide), *industrial toxins* (carbon monoxide [CO], carbon disulfide, organic solvents), *heavy metal intoxication* (mercury, lead, manganese), *drug intoxications* (opiates, phencyclidine, anticholinergics, sympathomimetics, anticonvulsants), *infections* (CNS and systemic), *epilepsy* (ictally, inter-ictally, or post-ictally), *infarction* (strokes, e.g., right MCA/left or bilateral PCA, hypotension, hypoxia, hypertensive encephalopathy, SAH, CNS vasculitis), *perioperative* (may be related to metabolic/electrolyte, hypoperfusion or drug effects), *neoplasia* (brain tumors, metastases, paraneoplastic limbic encephalitis), *psychiatric* (manic or psychotic disorders), and *sensory deprivation.*

Investigations

CBC with differential, comprehensive metabolic panel, TFT, PT/PTT/INR (prior to LP), Mg^{2+} levels, vitamin B_{12}/folate levels, ESR/CRP, serum/urine toxicology (serum alcohol levels may be normal), ABG, heavy metal screen, septic screen (chest X-ray, blood/urine cultures), and LP (to exclude CNS infection or inflammation) are recommended. Autoimmune screen (e.g., ANA panel, RhF) is necessary if vasculitis is suspected. CT head without contrast should be performed emergently to exclude ICH. EKG to exclude cardiac arrhythmia (may need longer term monitoring) and EEG to evaluate for possible subclinical seizures or recent seizure focus should be performed.

MRI of the brain with and without gadolinium (or with and without DWI, MRA, MRV) may be required in atypical cases, if a focal lesion is suspected or there is evidence of brainstem dysfunction clinically. The collaborative history is the most important factor in tailoring diagnostic tests, so it should be performed thoroughly.

Management

The mainstay of treatment involves the administration of benzodiazepines. These agents reduce the signs and symptoms of withdrawal. A fixed-dose regimen is required for delirium tremens. Lorazepam 2 mg i.v./i.m. every 6 hours for four doses, then 1 mg i.v./i.m. every 6 hours for eight doses should be administered. Titrate by 30–50% per day after 48 hours. Other options (at the same frequency) include: diazepam 10 mg then 5 mg i.v., oxazepam 30 mg, then 15 mg p.o. or chlordiazepoxide 50 mg, then 25 mg p.o. Excessive sedation may occur in the elderly and those with liver disease.

Adrenergic excess should be treated with β-blockers (e.g., atenolol 25–100 mg p.o. once daily to twice daily, titrated to HR) or clonidine (0.1–0.3 mg p.o. twice a day). Electrolyte abnormalities should be treated. Thiamine 100 mg i.v.

every day for 3 days should be administered to prevent Wernicke's encephalopathy, especially prior to glucose administration. Underlying medical conditions must be treated.

Patients should be managed on nursing floors with cardiac monitoring or ICU if there is evidence of cardiac arrhythmias. The room should be quiet and well lit. Restraints, which may make agitation worse, should b avoided but may be required for patient and staff protection and to facilitate medical care. Intravenous fluids and antipyretics should be administered. Folic acid 1 mg p.o. daily, daily multivitamins, and adequate nutrition should be provided. General supportive care, including regular nursing checks, DVT prophylaxis, decubitus prevention in sedated/intubated patients, and active cooling with blankets should be provided.

Prognosis

Mortality is 1–5% with treatment and approximately 20% without treatment. Complications of delirium tremens and potential causes of death include cardiac arrhythmias, sepsis, aspiration pneumonia, volume depletion, and electrolyte disturbances. Complete recovery is expected in surviving patients. This may take days to weeks. Risk factors for developing delirium tremens include chronic alcohol use, age over 30 years, low socioeconomic status, number of days since last drink (can occur up to 2 weeks after intake), concurrent acute medical illness, malnutrition or dehydration, and previous history of an alcohol withdrawal syndrome.

Counseling

Patients and their families should be aware of the risks of chronic alcohol use. Prognostic data should be discussed. Alcohol cessation programs and counseling should be offered on recovery. Malnutrition (and any predisposing conditions) should be treated. Chronic vitamin supplements may be needed, especially thiamine. Patients should be aware of the risks of delirium tremens recurrence with continued alcohol use.

SUMMARY

- **Delirium tremens** is a neurological emergency because outcomes depend on appropriate early treatment.
- Differentials include **benzodiazepine/barbiturate withdrawal, metabolic causes, endocrinopathies, vitamin deficiencies, industrial toxins, heavy metal intoxication, drug intoxication, infections, epilepsy, infarction, neoplasia, perioperative, psychiatric**, and **sensory deprivation**.
- **Collaborative history** most useful in establishing diagnosis. Other causes of agitated delirium should be excluded.

- Treatment includes **benzodiazepines: lorazepam 2 mg** i.v./i.m. **every 6 hours for four doses**, then **1 mg** i.v./i.m **every 6 hours for eight doses**, with taper by **30–50%** every day after 48 hours. Other options include **diazepam, oxazepam**, and **chlordiazepoxide**.
- Treat adrenergic excess with β-**blockers/clonidine**.
- Hydration, vitamin supplementation, antipyretics are needed.
- **Quiet, well-lit** environment helps reduce delirium.
- Mortality is **1–5%**. It is **approximately 20%** without treatment.
- Risks for delirium tremens depend on **age, demographics, duration from last drink, concurrent acute medical illness, malnutrition/dehydration**, and **previous history of an alcohol withdrawal syndrome**.
- **Complete recovery** is expected in survivors.

CASE 3

A 29-year-old man with chronic low back pain following a work-related injury was brought to the ER in an unresponsive state. Temperature of 35.6°C, HR 44 per minute, BP 80/35 mmHg, and RR of six to eight breaths per minute were obtained. There were no responses to external stimuli and no spontaneous verbal output. Neurological examination revealed bilateral pinpoint pupils with minimal responses to light. Motor examination revealed no spontaneous or reflexive movements with reduced tone and increased reflexes.

Localization

The patient is clinically in coma. Coma indicates bilateral cerebral dysfunction. Bilateral pinpoint or miotic pupils is indicative dysfunction of the descending sympathetic pathways from the hypothalamus to the spinal cord (at C8–T1) or at the level of the pupillodilator muscles in the eyes. Increased parasympathetic innervation to the pupilloconstrictor muscles can also cause these eye findings.

Bilateral thalamic lesions also cause pinpoint pupils. Further support for sympathetic tract dysfunction comes from the presence of hypothermia, hypotension, and bradycardia. However, lesions of medulla could cause circulatory failure, as well as respiratory suppression as seen in this case. In the absence of further findings on examination, this process diffusely localizes to the bilateral cerebral cortex and brainstem.

Differential Diagnosis

The most likely diagnosis for a comatose patient with pinpoint pupils, cardiorespiratory suppression, and a history of chronic back pain is *opioid overdose*. However, an assumption is made of access to narcotic analgesics. Further collaborative history is required.

Other differentials include any *metabolic encephalopathy* (e.g., hepatic, uremic, hypo/hyperglycemia (nonketotic), hypo/ hypernatremia, hypo/hypercalcemia, hypermagnesemia, Addisonian crisis), *HIE, carbon dioxide (CO_2) narcosis, cholinergic syndrome* (e.g., organophosphates, cholinesterase inhibitors: would expect muscarinic-nausea, vomiting, abdominal cramps, increased bronchial secretions and nicotinic-weakness, fasciculations, tachycardia, signs; severe toxicity presents similarly to opioid overdose), *bilateral pontine infarction* (e.g., hemorrhage or ischemia from basilar occlusion: would expect other signs such as gaze palsies, motor weakness, etc., and may be initially asymmetric), or *bilateral thalamic infarction* (bilateral; from hemorrhage or ischemia, i.e., top of the basilar syndrome or CVST; would expect other signs of thalamic dysfunction and usually presents asymmetrically). *Acute bilateral lateral medullary infarctions* can cause Horner's syndrome (ptosis, miosis, and anhydrosis), but coma would not be expected unless there was cardiorespiratory failure from bilateral midline involvement.

Investigations

Naloxone administration is diagnostic and therapeutic in opioid overdose. Emergent CT scan of the head should be performed to exclude an ICH, which may occur concurrently with opioid overdose, especially if the drug was illicitly combined with a sympathomimetic or there was head trauma. Capillary blood glucose should be checked to exclude hypo- or hyperglycemia. Serum/urine toxicology (positive for commonly used opioids 2–5 days after use) is required.

Laboratory investigations should be broad to evaluate for possible causes of coma, especially if there is no response to naloxone: CBC with differential, comprehensive metabolic panel, TFT, PT/PTT/INR (prior to LP), Mg^{2+} levels, ABG, septic screen (chest X-ray, ESR/CRP, blood/urine cultures: hypothermia may occur with sepsis), LP (to exclude CNS infection or inflammation). Autoimmune screen (ANA panel, RhF etc.) if vasculitis suspected. MRI of the brain (with DWI, MRA/MRV) may be required if infarction is suspected (clinical signs, asymmetrical onset, etc.) or to evaluate HIE.

Management

Respiratory failure in a comatose patient requires emergent intubation and mechanical ventilation. Circulatory failure requires insertion of a central line for i.v. fluids/pressor support. The patient requires ICU admission for treatment and close monitoring. The mainstay of therapy for opioid overdose is naloxone (an opiate antagonist) 2 mg i.v./i.m. every 2–3 minutes (total of 10–20 mg). This immediately reverses coma and respiratory depression (within 10 minutes); however, repeated bolus or infusion may be required due to its short half-life (1–4 hours) during the acute illness. Electrolyte abnormalities should be treated. Potential co-intoxicants should be searched for and reversed if possible. The patient can be transferred to the regular floor once stable.

Supportive care, including frequent nursing checks, decubitus prevention, DVT prophylaxis, active warming with blankets for hypothermia, strict fluid balance, gradual nutritional support, is required. Methadone or opium are used to treat naloxone-induced opioid withdrawal in chronic users (may be prevented by gradual titration in naloxone while treating respiratory depression).

Prognosis

Mortality from opioid overdose is approximately 1% if treated early and as high as 12% if unrecognized. Risk factors for death include male sex, single marital status, unemployed, chronic use/dependency, i.v. use, and concomitant use of CNS depressants (alcohol, benzodiazepines). Causes of death include cardiorespiratory failure, acute noncardiogenic pulmonary edema, cardiac arrhythmias, acute cardiomyopathy, pneumonia, acute renal failure secondary to rhabdomyolysis, hepatic failure, or seizures. Overdose accounts for approximately 50% of deaths in heroin abusers. About 3–7% of patients seen in the ER require hospitalization for further treatment or sequelae (excluding 24-hour observation after acute reversal), most of whom recover completely with minimal sequelae if they survive the initial overdose. Nonfatal overdose occurs in 20–35% of chronic heroin users within a given year; 70% during duration of use.

Counseling

Patients should undergo drug counseling and chronic detoxification. Opioid withdrawal is unpleasant, but not life-threatening in itself. Methadone 20 mg p.o. once or twice a day (with clonidine to suppress autonomic features), with gradual titration by 10–20% every 1–2 days over several weeks, would be useful for dependent patients. Because chronic polysubstance abuse is common in patients who abuse opioids (as high as 60–70% use other drugs, including alcohol), the following issues should be addressed: detoxification, medical counseling, health maintenance, and thiamine supplementation. Suicidal ideation or intention if present, should be addressed urgently.

Patients (and families or close associates) should be aware of signs of overdose in order to alert medical services. Routine administration of naloxone in comatose patients by trained ambulance services may prevent prehospital mortality with minor adverse effects. The underlying disorder requiring chronic opioid use should be addressed and adequately treated.

SUMMARY

- **Opioid overdose** is a **reversible** neurological emergency because survival is dependent on early administration of its antagonist.
- Differentials include **metabolic encephalopathies, HIE, CO_2 narcosis, cholinergic syndrome, bilateral pontine, and thalamic infarctions**.

- Investigations include **trial of naloxone, CT head** to exclude ICH, and **serum/urine toxicology**. Metabolic screen should be included.
- Treatment consists of **naloxone 2 mg i.v./i.m. every 2–3 minutes** (total of **10–20 mg**). Reversal of coma and respiratory failure less than **10 minutes**. May need **repeated boluses** or **infusion** owing to short half-life.
- Mortality is **approximately 1%** if treated early and **approximately 12%** if unrecognized. Sequelae may occur in **3–7%** of patients, but most recover completely.
- Risk factors for death include **male sex, single marital status, unemployed, chronic use/dependency, i.v. drug use**, and **concomitant use of CNS depressants** (alcohol, benzodiazepines).
- Polysubstance abuse is **common** in opioid abusers (**60–70%**).

PART III

CLINICAL VIGNETTES: GENERAL NEUROLOGY

9

Behavioral Neurology

CASE 1

A 73-year-old woman was brought to the clinic by her daughter. For several months, her daughter noticed that she had become increasingly forgetful, had poor attention to detail, demonstrated a tendency to easily get lost, and had difficulty in grooming herself. Mental status examination revealed impaired short-term memory, calculation, hemispatial neglect, ideomotor apraxia, and anomia with paraphrasic errors. Neurological examination was otherwise normal.

Localization

Memory dysfunction may localize to the bilateral temporal lobes. Inattention may indicate to bilateral frontal lobe dysfunction. Dyscalculia, ideomotor apraxia, and anomia with paraphrasic errors suggest dominant temporal lobe dysfunction. Visuospatial disorientation and hemineglect imply nondominant parietal lobe, whereas ideomotor apraxia suggests dominant parietal lobe dysfunction. In summary, the clinical history and physical examination suggests a disease process with bilateral parietal and temporal lobe dysfunction.

Differential Diagnosis

The most likely diagnosis for a slowly progressive dementia with predominant bilateral parietal and temporal lobe dysfunction is *Alzheimer's disease* (AD). This is the most common degenerative disease of the brain, and accounts for 60% of dementia cases alone, with a further 10% of cases occurring in combination with other disorders. The differential diagnosis for dementia is extensive; the clinical history and examination provide most of the diagnostic clues.

Other considerations include *neurodegenerative* (frontotemporal dementias such as Pick's disease: early, prominent personality and behavioral changes; diffuse Lewy body disease: parkinsonism with visual hallucinations and sensitivity to neuroleptics; corticobasal ganglionic degeneration: usually asymmetrical presentation with alien hand syndrome, parkinsonism, pyramidal signs; progressive

From: *Neurology Oral Boards Review:*
A Concise and Systematic Approach to Clinical Practice
By: E. E. Ubogu © Humana Press Inc., Totowa, NJ

supranuclear palsy: akinetic-rigid state, vertical gaze paresis, axial dystonia; Huntington's disease: behavioral/personality change, chorea), *vascular* (multi-infarct: usually with stepwise pattern of cognitive decline, Biswanger's disease, HIE), *structural/traumatic* (hydrocephalus, posttraumatic, chronic subdural hematomas), *metabolic* (uremia, hepatic encephalopathy, hypercalcemia, Wilson's disease: younger age, "wing-beating" tremor, akinetic-rigid state, Kayser-Fleischer rings in iris), *endocrinopathy* (hypothyroidism, Cushing's syndrome), *nutritional deficiencies* (vitamins B_1, B_{12}, nicotinamide), and *toxin exposure* (chronic CO poisoning, heavy metal intoxication).

Other differentials include *infections* (HIV, neurosyphilis, cryptococcosis, chronic fungal/tuberculous meningitis, Whipple's disease: dementia with ocular palsies and malabsorption, postencephalitis), *prion disease* (Creutzfelt-Jakob disease, Gestmann-Straussler disease), *neoplastic* (brain tumor, meningeal carcinomatosis, limbic encephalitis, postradiation), *connective tissue disease* (SLE, Sjögren's disease, neurosarcoidosis), *disorders of myelin* (MS, Marchiafava-Bignami disease), *epilepsy* (related directly or indirectly to chronic seizures), *pseudodementia of depression, thalamic dementia* ("subcortical dementia" with choreoathetosis: rare), and *inherited* (usually young age of onset: e.g., leukodystrophies, lipid storage disorders, poliodystrophies associated with myoclonic epilepsy, mitochondrial encephalomyopathies).

Investigations

There are no specific tests used in routine clinical practice that reliably diagnose AD. Reversible causes of dementia (~5% of all cases) should be excluded. Laboratory investigations should include CBC with differential, comprehensive metabolic panel, TFT, vitamin B_{12} levels, RPR/FTA-ABS, ANA panel, and urinalysis. CT/MRI of the head should be performed to exclude structural lesions (may show bilateral frontal, parietal and temporal atrophy, sparing pre- and post-central gyri). LP may be needed if CNS infection/inflammation is suspected.

EEG may show nonspecific slowing of background activity. Single-photon emission CT (SPECT)/positron emission tomography (PET) scans may show bilateral parietal and temporal hypoperfusion/metabolism, respectively (not used in routine clinical practice). Other tests should be tailored toward potential diagnoses based on clinical evaluation (e.g., young age of onset, family history, toxin exposure). Neuropsychiatry evaluation may be needed.

Management

Treatment should be tailored to controlling the cognitive and behavioral symptoms. Pharmacological treatment (maintenance doses) of cognitive symptoms consists of acetylcholinesterase (AChE) inhibitors: donepezil 10 mg p.o. at bedtime, galantamine 12 mg p.o. twice a day, rivastigmine 6 mg p.o. twice a day, or *N*-methyl-D-asparate (NMDA) antagonist: memantine 10 mg p.o. twice a day (used as monotherapy or in combination with donepezil in severe cases). These agents modestly slow the rate of cognitive decline with minimal side effects.

Behavioral symptoms, such as depression (~20% of AD patients) require anti-depressants: e.g., SSRIs, agitation/psychosis: atypical or typical neuroleptics, anxiety/insomnia: benzodiazepines, or antihistamines. Nonpharmacological modalities include providing a safe, quiet, and familiar environment, having experienced and trained caregivers to assist with activities of daily living, and emotional support for patients and caregivers.

Prognosis

AD is the fourth leading cause of death in individuals over the age of 65. The mean survival is approximately 8 years from disease onset, with the most common cause of death being bronchopneumonia. Risk factors associated with mortality include male sex, increased severity of cognitive impairment, decreased functional level, history of falls, physical examination findings of frontal release signs, and abnormal gait. The average annual decline in cognitive function is 4–5 points on Mini-Mental Status Examination (MMSE) and 6 points on the Alzheimer's Disease Assessment Scale, usually in a nonlinear fashion.

Counseling

Patients and caregivers should be aware of the irreversibility of AD and the prognostic data. Making families aware of the resources available and clinical expectations is warranted. Referral to patient support groups may be helpful. Sudden cognitive deteriorations should warrant clinical evaluation for a super-imposed medical/surgical condition. The patient will eventually require long-term care at home or in a nursing facility.

SUMMARY

- **AD** is the **most common** cause for dementia and accounts for **approximately 70%** of all cases (alone or with other disorders).
- Differentials include **neurodegenerative, vascular, structural/traumatic, endocrinopathy, nutritional deficiencies, toxin exposures, infections, prion disease, neoplastic, connective tissue disorders, disorders of myelin, epilepsy, depression, thalamic,** and **inherited causes**.
- There are no routinely used diagnostic tests for AD. **Exclude structural lesions** and **reversible causes of dementia**.
- Treatment of cognitive symptoms includes **AChE inhibitors** (e.g., donepezil and/or **NMDA receptor blocker** memantine).
- Behavioral symptoms require both **nonpharmacological** and **pharmacological** intervention.

- AD is the **fourth** leading cause of death in individuals over the age of 65. Mean survival is **approximately 8 years; bronchopneumonia** is the most common cause of death.
- Risk factors are **male sex, increased severity of cognitive impairment, decreased functional level, history of falls, frontal release signs,** and **abnormal gait** on examination.
- The average annual decline in cognitive function is **4–5 points** on MMSE.

CASE 2

A 42-year-old man was brought to the urgent care center by his wife. She was concerned that his attention and concentration had been poor over the previous 48–72 hours. He also seemed more irritable and confused. She was not aware of any illicit drug use. On examination, vital signs were normal. MMSE shows disorientation to place and time, inattention, poor calculation, and reduced recall at 1 and 5 minutes. Neurological examination was otherwise normal.

Localization

Irritability, disorientation, and inattention most likely localize to the frontal hemispheres bilaterally. Poor calculation and recall may localize to the temporal lobes, however, these could occur in association with poor attention/concentration. The clinical manifestations suggest bilateral dysfunction of the cerebral cortex, with predominant frontal and possible temporal lobe involvement.

Differential Diagnosis

The clinical picture is most consistent with an *acute confusional state*. A history of perceptual changes (delusions and hallucinations), emotional disturbances, altered psychomotor activity and disordered sleep-wave cycle would make *delirium* most likely. Delirium is a clinical syndrome with numerous potential causes. The clinical history is vitally important in trying to narrow down etiological factors.

Etiologies for delirium include *drug intoxications* (alcohol, opioids, steroids, anticholinergics, sedatives), *inhalant exposure* (glue, ether, nitrous oxide), *toxin exposure* (heavy metals, organic solvents, CO), *withdrawal syndromes* (alcohol, sedatives, amphetamines), metabolic (hepatic, renal, hypoxia, hypercapnia, hypo/hypercalcemia, hypo/hyperglycemia, hypo/hypernatremia), *endocrinopathies* (hypo/hyperthyroidism, hypopituitarism, hypo/hypercortisolemia), *nutritional* (deficiencies: vitamins B_1, B_6, B_{12}, folate or intoxications: vitamins A and D), *infections* (systemic and CNS), *trauma* (ICH, cerebral contusions, postconcussive), *neoplasms* (primary brain tumors, metastases, paraneoplastic limbic encephalitis), *inflammation* (CNS vasculitis:

primary or secondary), *epilepsy* (post-ictal: after complex partial or generalized seizure, inter-ictal: epileptic delirium, ictal: absence or complex partial SE), *stroke* (usually right MCA, left or bilateral PCA, or thalamic strokes), perioperative (may be multifactorial), *sensory deprivation/overload* and *transient global amnesia* (loss of memory, behavioral change without recollection of events lasting minutes to hours: rare, cause unknown).

Investigations

The history (including drug history: prescribed, OTC, and illicit; toxin/environmental exposures, nutritional history) and physical examination are extremely important to ascertain the etiology for delirium. Laboratory investigations should include CBC with differential, comprehensive metabolic panel, TFT, Mg^{2+}, vitamin B_{12}, folate, RPR/FTA-ABS, ESR/CRP, ANA panel, urinalysis, septic screen (if febrile or afebrile in the elderly): chest X-ray, blood/urine cultures, ABG, and serum/urine toxicology. Head CT should be performed to exclude intracranial pathology (MRI may be needed depending on clinical suspicion). EKG should be included to evaluate for arrhythmias and EEG (if seizures suggested) can also be performed. LP should be considered for CNS infection/inflammation.

Management

The underlying cause for delirium should be identified and treated. Symptomatic therapy should be provided. All potential causative/exacerbating drugs/factors should be eliminated. Electrolyte abnormalities should be corrected. The patient should be kept in a well-lit, quiet room without minimal environmental changes. Moderate sensory stimulation (e.g., radio, television, visitors) should be provided and orientation facilitated by clocks, calendars, family, and personal effects.

Agitated patients may need temporary restraints and neuroleptic/sedative medications. Regulation of sleep–wake cycle can be achieved with hypnotics, such as benzodiazepines (temazepam). A regular sitter may enhance patient safety and compliance. Supportive nursing care (e.g., DVT prophylaxis, regular vitals, nutritional support, bladder/bowel hygiene) is necessary in the acute phases.

Prognosis

Provided the causative factor of the delirium is identified, the prognosis is very good. The average duration is about a few days to 2 weeks, but may extend to 3 months in the elderly. However, recovery back to baseline may not occur in about 5–10%, especially with pre-existing dementia. Risk factors for developing delirium include: age 80 years or more, male sex, underlying brain disorder/dementia, electrolyte/fluid disturbances, malnutrition, multiple medical illnesses, polypharmacy, drug abuse/dependency, infection, sleep disturbance, sensory (visual) impairment, physical trauma, and surgery (cardiac, orthopedic, vascular).

Counseling

Patients and families should be reassured of complete recovery. About 5–40% of hospitalized patients develop delirium, so families and health care workers should be alert to this possibility, especially in patients older than 65 years. Prevention of delirium should be emphasized. Underlying medical and surgical problems should be addressed in the long-term.

SUMMARY

- **Delirium** is a neurobehavioral disorder characterized by **acute mental status changes, inattention,** and **fluctuating course**.
- Etiologies include **drug intoxications, inhalant use, toxin exposures, withdrawal syndromes, endocrinopathies, metabolic, nutritional, infections, trauma, neoplasms, inflammation, epilepsy, stroke, perioperative, sensory changes,** and **transient global amnesia**.
- Clinical history and examination are **critical** in ascertaining etiology. Investigations should be tailored to findings.
- Management should be directed at the **underlying causes** and **symptomatic care**.
- Outcomes are good provided underlying cause is identified and treated. Cognitive recovery expected after a **few days to 2 weeks** if patient is **younger than 65** and **up to 3 months** if patient is **older than 65**. **Approximately 5–10%** of elderly patients do not recover to baseline.
- Delirium occurs in **5–40%** of hospitalized patients.

CASE 3

A 23-year-old woman was knocked unconscious during a collision while playing soccer 2 days ago. She regained consciousness after about 45–60 seconds and felt well enough to go home. She complained of persistent headache, unsteadiness on her feet, poor concentration, and increased irritability. MMSE showed slower than usual thought processing and responses. Further examination, including fundoscopy, was normal.

Localization

Headache is nonlocalizing, and may suggest diffuse meningeal irritation. Poor concentration, irritability, and slowed thought processing may localize to the bilateral frontal and/or temporal hemispheres. Unsteadiness may be secondary to mild bilateral lower extremity weakness (localizes to mesial frontal lobes and their descending corticospinal tracts: bilateral involvement most likely in the brainstem) or truncal/gait ataxia secondary to bilateral midline cerebellar dysfunction (e.g., superior vermis). The most likely localization is the bilateral frontal hemispheres, with diffuse involvement clinically.

Differential Diagnosis

The most likely diagnosis for these nonspecific neurobehavioral complaints following an apparent mild head injury is *postconcussion syndrome* (PCS). The etiology for PCS is unknown: it may reflect early posttraumatic physiological/pathological changes in the brain. Other differentials include *intraparenchymal hemorrhage, subacute subdural hematoma, SAH, cerebral contusions, frontal convexity tumor* (e.g., meningioma: slowly progressive, usually not associated with trauma, unless acute hemorrhage into tumor occurs), *post-ictal state* (there should be history of seizures) and *bilateral ACA ischemia* (would expect evidence of upper motor neuron weakness in the legs).

Investigations

There are no particular tests that diagnose PCS. Plain radiographs should be performed to exclude skull fracture. CT scan of the head should be performed to exclude ICH. MRI of the brain would be required to evaluate for cerebral contusions (may be missed on CT). If history of trauma is unclear, consider screen for common causes of delirium (*see* p. 95). LP is required to exclude SAH if the CT negative. Neuropsychological evaluation may be required in difficult cases.

Management

GCS of 13–14 or 15 or less with radiological abnormalities should warrant admission for close neurological observation. Sudden deterioration warrants emergency evaluation. Cerebral contusions can become edematous and cause herniation, especially transtentorial herniation with temporal lobe contusions. Stable patients should be treated symptomatically. Headaches in PCS are usually responsive to NSAIDs and the neurobehavioral problems treated with SSRIs with good effect. Psychological treatments, including education, reassurance, and cognitive restructuring or reattribution, should be offered as well in an inpatient or outpatient setting within 7 days of mild traumatic head injury.

Prognosis

Substantial/complete recovery is expected in more than 90% of PCS patients. Cognitive recovery is expected between 1 and 3 months after injury, with complete symptom resolution by 3 months in 70–80% of patients. At 1 year postinjury, residual symptoms are present in abut 7–15% of patients.

Risk factors for the development or persistence of PCS include age over 40, female sex, premorbid social or emotional difficulties, co-morbid medical conditions, neurological complication at injury, associated fracture, lower educational level, and intoxication at the time of injury.

Counseling

These patients should be provided with adequate education and reassurance during their initial evaluation. Early psychological treatment (the above measures with cognitive therapy performed less than 5–7 days after injury) could reduce PCS by about 20%. Prognostic data should be shared with patients. Patients and their families should be aware that any neurological deterioration requires immediate medical evaluation.

SUMMARY

- **Postconcussive syndrome** is a neurobehavioral disorder that occurs as a consequence of **mild** traumatic brain injury.
- Differentials include **intraparenchymal hemorrhage, subacute subdural hematoma, SAH, cerebral contusions, frontal convexity tumor, post-ictal state**, and **bilateral ACA ischemia**.
- **CT/MRI of the brain** should be performed to exclude ICH and cerebral contusions.
- Treatment includes **close neurological observation** if **GCS is less than 13–14** or **15 with radiological abnormality**, **NSAIDs** for headache, and **SSRIs** for neurobehavioral symptoms. **Psychological therapy** is useful.
- Complete/substantial recovery is expected in more than **90%** of patients, with residual symptoms in about **7–15% at 1 year**.
- Risk factors for PCS include **age over 40, female sex, socioeconomic, medical**, and **psychological factors**.

10

Cerebrovascular Disorders

CASE 1

A 64-year-old man with CAD and DM was brought to the ER with right-sided weakness, slurred speech, and difficulty expressing himself. He had awoken with these symptoms about 10 hours ago. Vital signs showed a temperature of 37.6°C, HR 88 per minute, BP 145/88 mmHg, and RR 10 per minute. Neurological examination revealed an expressive aphasia, right lower facial palsy, buccal dysarthria, right hemiplegia, and hemisensory loss affecting the face and upper extremity more than the lower extremities. Reflexes were brisk on the right with an extensor plantar response.

Localization

Right-sided hemiplegic and hemisensory deficits indicate left hemispheric dysfunction, involving the frontoparietal cortex, subcortical white matter, internal capsule with thalamic involvement, or brainstem. Lower facial palsy suggests contralateral upper motor neuron dysfunction of the corticobulbar tracts (frontal cortex to upper pons) to CN VII, with resultant buccal dysarthria. However, the expressive (Broca's) aphasia supports frontal lobe involvement. The absence of any cranial nerve deficits makes the brainstem an unlikely localization. The most likely localization is the left frontoparietal cortex supplied by the left MCA vascular territory.

Differential Diagnosis

The differential diagnosis for sudden onset of left frontoparietal cortical dysfunction includes an *acute ischemic stroke, acute ICH* (subarachnoid-aneurysmal and nonaneurysmal/traumatic; intraparenchymal, e.g., secondary to hypertension or amyloid angiopathy, subdural or epidural: may be associated with head trauma, headache, or early alternation in level of consciousness), *post-ictal state following a seizure* (Todd's paralysis: history of preceding partial or complex partial seizure should be obtained), *hemiplegic migraine* (headache may occur hours to days after lateralizing symptoms), *hemorrhage*

From: *Neurology Oral Boards Review:*
A Concise and Systematic Approach to Clinical Practice
By: E. E. Ubogu © Humana Press Inc., Totowa, NJ

into a brain tumor (may have slowly progressive focal signs with sudden exacerbation), or *secondary to toxic-metabolic derangement associated with* a *remote infarct* (diagnosis of exclusion in the acute phase, would expect prior history/residual deficits: MRI-DWI may be negative in the face of acute symptoms). The clinical history does not discriminate between ischemic and hemorrhagic strokes.

Investigations

CT scan of the head without contrast should be performed emergently to exclude an ICH. An intracranial bleed requires neurosurgical consultation, as surgical decompression may be required. If ischemic stroke is suspected, MRI of the brain without gadolinium (with DWI) and MRA (intracranial and extracranial vessels) should be performed as soon as possible. This should confirm the extent of anatomical involvement and assist in deducing the probable etiology for the stroke (large-vessel occlusive, large-vessel thromboembolic, or small-vessel disease). If a high-grade stenosis of the carotid artery is suggested on MRA, cerebral angiography is warranted (gold standard). Carotid USS and TCDs may be useful where MR scans are not readily available.

Routine baseline laboratory investigations (CBC with differential, comprehensive metabolic panel, PT/PTT/INR, Mg^{2+}, PO_4^{3-}) should be performed. Further investigations include EKG, cardiac holter monitor, or telemetry (for cardiac dysrhythmias such as atrial fibrillation), TEE/TTE to assess LV function (<35% associated with stroke) and cardiac sources of emboli, such as mural thrombus, atrial septal defects with patent foramen ovale or valvular vegetations, for example, would be required.

Management

The patient should be admitted to an acute stroke unit or regular nursing floor for further management. Vital signs and neurological assessments every 4–6 hours, bed rest for 24 hours, strict fluid balance with maintenance fluids (i.v. normal saline at 1–2 cc/kg per hour; facilitative hypervolemia and hypertension to keep MAP 90–110 mmHg for 48–72 hours may be required to improve cerebral perfusion), nasogastric feeding and DVT/decubitus prophylaxis, are necessary. Anti-pyretic treatment with acetaminophen is advised if body temperature raises above 37.5°C. Glycemic control with insulin may be required if glucose levels are grater than 150 mg/dL. Electrolyte abnormalities should be corrected.

The use of i.v. unfractionated heparin (15–18 U/kg per hour, keeping PTT between 1.5 and 2.5 × baseline) and oral warfarin (to keep INR 2–3) may be warranted in strokes associated with atrial fibrillation, arterial dissection, and confirmed cardiac sources of embolism. The utility of anticoagulant agents for other stroke etiologies is controversial but widely practiced in the United States and Canada despite lack of supporting data. Antiplatelet agents include aspirin (ASA) 81–325 mg p.o. daily, clopidogrel 75 mg p.o. daily, dipyridamole/ASA 100/25 mg p.o. twice a day or ticlopidine 250 mg p.o. twice a day. Be aware of common side effects (e.g., GI upset with aspirin, headache with dipyramidole/ASA, neutropenia with ticlopidine, etc.).

Carotid endarterectomy may be required for high-grade (70–99%) stenosis. Balloon angioplasty or stenting of the extracranial and/or intracranial arteries are potential alternatives, especially in high-risk surgical patients. Acute rehabilitation (physical, occupational, speech/language therapy within 3 days of stroke) should be initiated to facilitate and maximize functional recovery. Antihypertensives (e.g., ACE inhibitors) should be started about 72 hours after stroke and anti-lipidemic/oral hypoglycemics continued.

Prognosis

In general, 15–20% of acute stroke patients die within the first month post-stroke (heart attacks, cardiac dysrhythmias, pneumonia, cerebral herniation, DVT/PE) with 50% of survivors exhibiting some degree of disability. Severe disability at 1 month despite acute rehabilitation may predict long-term disability. Outcomes depend on the size and severity of stroke on presentation, age, medical co-morbities, and complications of the stroke and its treatments. A hyperdense MCA sign or large volume MCA infarct on CT scan modifies outcomes (*see* p. 17). Studies have not supported improved outcomes of i.v. heparin in acute stroke care. Ischemic stroke recurrence rates are less than 10% per year in patients with symptomatic MCA stenosis, approximately 12% per year in patients with embolic strokes associated with atrial fibrillation and approximately 15% per year in association with symptomatic high-grade carotid stenosis.

Counseling

Counseling should be tailored toward risk-factor modification (e.g., smoking cessation, BP/diabetes control, medication compliance, the use of prophylaxis), treating depression (~25% of all post-stroke patients) and early recognition of symptoms. Prognostic data should be discussed. Stroke patients have a higher risk of all-cause mortality and vascular deaths than their age-matched cohort. If high-grade symptomatic carotid stenosis is present, discussion on carotid endarterectomy should be considered (*see* p. 18). Percutaneous balloon angioplasty and stenting in high-risk patients may result in approximately 5–8% risk of periprocedural or early postprocedural morbidity and mortality with similar rates of stroke prevention but with a 10% risk of re-stenosis at 1 year. Antiplatelet agents reduce risk of stroke recurrence by approximately 10–30% per year, but do not completely eliminate the risk. Warfarin reduces stroke risk by 75% per year in patients with atrial fibrillation.

SUMMARY

- **An MCA stroke syndrome** is caused by either **intrinsic stenosis** or **thromboembolic disease** from the carotid artery or heart.
- Differentials include **acute ICH, post-ictal state, hemiplegic migraine, hemorrhage into brain tumor**, and **toxic-metabolic derangements**.
- **CT scan** should be performed to exclude ICH. **MRI (DWI)/MRA** should be performed to localize and establish etiology for stroke. **TTE/TEE** is required for cardiac causes.
- Treatment includes **supportive care**, facilitative **hypervolemic** and **hypertensive therapy**, and **risk-factor modification**. Heparin use is **controversial** in acute stroke.
- In general, mortality is **approximately 15–20% in first month** post-stroke.
- Stroke recurrence rates are **less than 10% per year** in symptomatic MCA stenosis, **approximately 12% per year** in embolic strokes associated with atrial fibrillation and **approximately 15% per year** in symptomatic high-grade carotid stenosis.
- Antiplatelet drugs reduce risk of stroke recurrence by **approximately 10–30% per year.**
- Warfarin reduces risk of stroke in atrial fibrillation by **75% per year**.
- In medically refractory or patients with high-grade stenoses, **carotid endarterectomy** or **percutaneous balloon angioplasty with stenting** are possible options.

CASE 2

An 81-year-old woman was brought to the ER with an 8-hour history of nausea, vomiting, dizziness, dysphagia, and numbness affecting her face and body that occurred suddenly while she was working in her yard. On examination, temperature was 37.2°C, HR was 88 per minute, BP was 155/75 mmHg, and RR was 16 per minute. Neurological examination revealed a right Horner's syndrome and facial numbness with reduced palatal elevation and gag reflex on the right. Further examination revealed diminished left hemi-body sensation, normal motor strength in all limbs, normal reflexes, and right-sided hemiataxia.

Localization

The presenting symptoms are suggestive of a process that may affect the CN V, VII–X, or XII (or their central connections), as well as the ascending sensory tracts (anterolateral and dorsal columns-medial lemniscal systems), however, the data is nonlocalizing. A right Horner's syndrome (disruption of sympathetic tracts) with right facial numbness (descending spinal nucleus of CN V) could imply right lateral pontine or medullary dysfunction, however, ipsilateral palatal weakness with reduced gag reflex suggest that the right lateral medulla is more likely. Contralateral hemibody sensory loss with ipsilateral hemiataxia (localizes to cerebellum, vestibular nucleus, or their tracts) further supports that the most likely localization is the right lateral medulla.

Differential Diagnosis

The most likely diagnosis is *lateral medullary syndrome* secondary to an ischemic stroke due to *thrombosis of the right verterbral artery* (VA) or *PICA*. Other potential etiological mechanisms for the stroke include VA dissection (could occur with innocuous trauma or spontaneously), *vasculopathy* (primary or second-ary, e.g., drug-induced, connective tissue disorders), *vertebrobasilar dolichoectasia* or *cardioembolic* (more likely to affect anterior circulation). Other differentials include *ICH* (medulla or cerebellum with brainstem compression) or *brainstem tumor* (e.g., glioma: would expect less acute presentation unless there was an acute hemorrhage).

Investigations

For information on investigations, *see* p. 100. MRI neck with dissection protocol should also be performed to evaluate for vertebral dissection. Cerebral angiography would be useful if further invasive interventions were being considered.

Management

The management of a posterior circulation stroke is similar to an anterior circulation stroke, as described on pp. 100–101. Intra-arterial thrombolysis may be attempted in basilar artery thrombosis for up to 12–24 hours after stroke to prevent mortality. Antiplatelet or anticoagulation therapy should be used for secondary prevention of stroke. There are no prospective studies that support the use of anticoagulants over antiplatelet agents in verte-brobasilar thrombotic disease. Transluminal balloon angioplasty and stenting (for stenosis >70%) may be useful in medically refractory patients or patients to whom the use of antiplatelet or anticoagulant drugs is contraindicated. Endarterectomy and extracranial–intracranial bypass are not options for vertebral stenosis.

Prognosis

Symptomatic vertebrobasilar stenosis has a mortality of approximately 25% at 1 year and approximately 55% at 5 years. The risk of recurrent stroke is about 11% per year with basilar artery (BA), approximately 8% per year with VA, and approximately 6% per year with PICA or PCA stenosis.

Vertebrobasilar occlusion confers a mortality of 50–80% within 1 month of presentation with survivors being severely disabled.

Counseling

The principles of patient counseling are similar for most stroke patients, as described on p. 101. Patients should be aware of the prognostic data and higher mortality and morbidity rates associated with vertebrobasilar occlusion. Angioplasty and stenting of the posterior circulation could result in a periprocedural risk of stroke or death of approximately 10–20%, with a mean residual stenosis of 30–40%, less than 10% restenosis rate, and less than 8% recurrent stroke rate per year. This data is based on small case series and not on randomized controlled trials. Whether this procedure confers any benefit above medical therapy has also not been established. Follow-up MRA/contrast angiography is required to confirm recanalization following VA dissection.

SUMMARY

- **Lateral medullary syndrome** is an ischemic stroke in the **PICA distribution**, but is the result of **VA thrombosis** in **approximately 80%**.
- Differential diagnosis includes **brainstem/cerebellar ICH** or **acute hemorrhage into brainstem tumor**.
- Investigations should include **MRI neck (dissection protocol)** to exclude VA dissection. **Cerebral angiography** may be needed.
- Treatment is as described on pp. 100–101. **Intra-arterial thrombolysis** may be considered with basilar artery occlusion. **Angioplasty and stenting** may be required in **medically refractory or contraindicated patients**.
- Symptomatic vertebrobasilar stenosis has a mortality of **approximately 25% at 1 year** and **approximately 55% at 5 years**.
- Recurrent stroke: **approximately 11% per year** with **BA**, **approximately 8% per year** with **VA**, and **approximately 6% per year** with **PICA/PCA** stenosis.
- Vertebrobasilar occlusion has a mortality of **50–80% at 1 month**. Survivors are usually severely disabled.

CASE 3

A 69-year-old man with chronic hypertension and DM presented to the ER with a 12-hour history of right-sided weakness that seemed to fluctuate in severity over this period. On examination, temperature was 37°C, BP was 166/84 mmHg, HR was 72 per minute, and RR was 12 per minute. Neurological examination revealed right lower facial palsy with dysarthria and right hemiplegia with hyperreflexia. Sensory examination was normal.

Localization

Right hemiplegia with hyperreflexia indicates an upper motor neuron process. The absence of sensory findings suggests involvement of the left frontal hemisphere (pre-central gyrus), subcortical white matter, posterior limb of internal capsule, cerebral peduncles (ventral midbrain), ventral pons, or medullary pyramids. The ipsilateral upper motor neuron CN VII palsy points to a lesion rostral to the pons. The absence of aphasia would make a frontal cortex lesion unlikely. The most likely localization is the left posterior limb of the internal capsule.

Differential Diagnosis

The primary differential diagnosis for a pure motor syndrome is an *acute ischemic stroke involving the posterior limb of the internal capsule*, which is secondary to *small-vessel ischemic disease* to perforators from the anterior choroidal artery or lenticulostriate branches of the MCA associated with chronic hypertension and diabetes (in 80–90% of cases). *Thromboembolic* (from ICA), *cardioembolic sources*, or *inflammatory causes* are also possible but less likely. Other differentials for acute right-sided weakness include *ICH* (e.g., putaminal bleed associated with hypertension: would expect more clinical involvement), *post-ictal Todd's paralysis* (history of preceding seizure should be evident), *hemiplegic migraine* (diagnosis of exclusion in the acute phase; associated with headache afterward), *hemorrhage into tumor* (may have prior slowly progressive symptoms), or *toxic-metabolic derangement* associated with old infarct.

Investigations

These should be performed as described on p. 100. An ischemic infarct less than 15 mm diameter defines a lacunar stroke. MRA of the extracranial vessels and TTE/TEE may be negative, but should be considered for risk-factor stratification in the acute stroke patient. Cerebral angiography is rarely warranted unless there is significant ipsilateral carotid stenosis on MRA, as approximately 10–20% of lacunar infarcts are associated with large-vessel atherothrombosis with distal embolization occluding the origin of small-diameter penetrating arteries.

Management

The management of a small-vessel ischemic stroke is similar to large-vessel strokes, as outlined on pp. 100–101. With incomplete deficits on presentation, a stuttering course may be expected despite aggressive therapy and ICH should be excluded if new deficits develop, especially while on antiplatelet agents. There is no defined role for anticoagulant use in lacunar stroke therapy. Hypertension and DM should be controlled pharmacologically.

Prognosis

Small-vessel ischemic strokes confer a better prognosis than large-vessel or cardioembolic strokes, and constitute up to 25% of all ischemic strokes. The average mortality is approximately 2.5% at 30 days and approximately 3% at 1 year. Five-year mean fatality is approximately 27%. Risk factors for death include age, DM, smoking, male sex, non-use of aspirin, and multiple infarcts. Stroke recurrence occurs at approximately 7.5% in the first year, and approximately 22.5% after 5 years. The annual risk after the first year is about 4.5%. Risk factors for stroke recurrence include hypertension, DM, cardioembolic source, and multiple lacunes on CT.

Functional recovery from a lacunar stroke (complete or with minor deficits) occurs in more than 75% of patients at 3 months. Functional independence is approximately 80% at 1 year, approximately 65% at 2 years, and approximately 55% at 3 years. This reduction may be associated with recurrent strokes or effects of co-morbidities such as hypertension, DM, or cardiac disease. Dementia has been reported in about 10% of patients 2–3 years after lacunar strokes and in 15% 9 years afterward.

Counseling

Patients and their families should be aware of prognostic data. The fact that the identified causative stroke is small does not necessarily confer a benign prognosis, as stroke location and severity on presentation could play a role in outcome. Modifiable risk factors (particularly hypertension, smoking, and DM) should be aggressively managed to prevent recurrent strokes and poor outcomes, including the risk of developing multi-infarct dementia. Good general medical follow-up is important. Antiplatelet agents reduce the risk of recurrent stroke but do not completely eliminate that risk. Functionally dependent patients would require assistance with activities of daily living and may need regular nursing care at home or in a skilled nursing facility.

SUMMARY

- **Pure motor syndrome** is a classic lacunar stroke syndrome that localizes to the **posterior limb of internal capsule, subcortical white matter, cerebral peduncles, ventral pons**, or **medullary pyramids**.
- Lacunar stroke account for **up to 25%** of ischemic strokes, and **approximately 55%** of these present as a pure motor syndrome.
- Diagnosis is confirmed by ischemic stroke **less than 15 mm** on CT/MRI.
- Management is similar to large-vessel strokes. Fluctuating course before complete lesion may be expected.

- Mean mortality is **approximately 2.5% at 30 days, approximately 3% at 1 year**, and **approximately 27% at 5 years**. Risk factors for death include **age, DM, smoking, non-use of aspirin**, and **multiple infarcts**.
- Risk of recurrent stroke is **approximately 75% at 1 year** and **22.5% at 5 years**, with a mean annual risk (after first year) **approximately 4.5%**. Risk factors for recurrence include **hypertension, DM, cardioembolic source**, and **multiple lacunes on CT**.
- Good recovery occurs in **more than 75% at 3 months** post-stroke.
- Functional independence occurs in **approximately 80% at 1 year, approximately 65% at 2 years**, and **approximately 55% at 3 years**.
- Risk of dementia occurs in **approximately 10% at 2–3 years** and **approximately 15% at 9 years** post-stroke.

CASE 4

A 61-year-old woman with a 6-week history of fluctuating generalized headaches and mental status changes that lasted a few hours to days, was brought to the ER by her husband. She had complained of transient left-sided weakness that completely resolved, but he was concerned that she was now having problems speaking and moving the right side. On examination, her vital signs were normal. Neurological examination revealed a mild expressive aphasia with right lower facial and upper extremity weakness. Tone and reflexes were increased on the right. Sensory and coordination examinations were normal.

Localization

A generalized headache and mental status changes are nonlocalizing, but may suggest diffuse meningeal irritation. Transient left-sided weakness suggests right cerebral dysfunction (from frontal cortex to the pyramids prior to decussation in the caudal medulla). Expressive aphasia with a right upper motor neuron lesion involving the face and upper extremity localizes to the left frontal cortex. The initial process was diffuse, with subsequent bilateral frontal cortex involvement being most likely.

Differential Diagnosis

The most likely diagnosis is *PACNS*. This is a chronic granulomatous angiitis of small blood vessels in the brain (particularly involving the leptomeninges) of unknown etiology, without systemic involvement. Other differentials include *systemic vasculitides* (e.g., PAN, SLE, or Wegener's granulomatosis: would expect systemic renal, cutaneous, pulmonary symptoms initially with rare subsequent CNS involvement), i.v. *drug abuse* (e.g., sympathomimetics may cause a vasculopathy with resultant stroke in addition to mental status changes or hypersensitivity vasculitis to contaminants), *infection* (may occur in the absence of fever in the elderly, e.g., *viruses*: hemorrhagic meningoencephalitis secondary to HSE: mesial frontal and temporal involvement more likely and clinical course is more acute; VZV-induced CNS vasculitis with stroke weaks to months after ipsilateral cutaneous zoster of CN V_1; HIV, hepatitis B and C; *spirochetes*: syphilis causes chronic meningoencephalitis with focal signs secondary to gumma/granuloma formation or stroke secondary to endarteritis; *Lyme disease*: causes cranial nerve palsies with headache and meningismus; *bacterial meningitis*: e.g., pneumococcus, meningococcus, tuberculosis with associated focal signs secondary to stroke [thrombophlebitis].

Other differentials include *subdural empyema or brain abscess, infective endocarditis with cerebral embolism, fungi with secondary vasculitis* (such as aspergillosis or mucormycosis), *protozoal infections* (e.g., malaria, toxoplasmosis), *neoplasm* (hemorrhagic metastases such as renal cell carcinoma, choriocarcinoma, melanoma, as well as lung and breast cancer causing acute focal signs with carcinomatous meningitis causing mental status changes: would not expect fluctuations, or vasculitis associated with Hodgkin's lymphoma or paraneoplastic vasculitis), *demyelinating disease* (such as MS: headache and mental status changes uncommon) or *hypertensive encephalopathy* (unusual with normal BP).

Investigations

Tests should be tailored to the clinical history, excluding other potential differentials for PACNS. Laboratory tests to consider include CBC with differential, ESR/CRP, ANA panel, RhF, anti-ds-DNA, ANCA, complement levels, cryoglobulins, aPL levels, ACE levels, RPR/FTA-ABS, and serum/urine toxicology. Lyme titers may be performed if history is suggestive. Blood cultures and echocardiogram would be required if endocarditis is suspected. LP should be performed to exclude infection, neoplastic infiltration, and CNS demyelination.

In PACNS, mild pleocytosis, raised protein content, and normal glucose on CSF occurs in 80–90% of cases, but this is nonspecific. CT/MRI of the brain are useful in excluding other diseases and demonstrating the extent of cerebral involvement, and cerebral angiography may show findings consistent with vasculitis in 50–60% of patients (MRA resolution too low for vessel size ~200 μm). Definitive diagnosis requires brain biopsy to include both the parenchyma and leptomeninges (has a perioperative morbidity of ~3% and ~25% false-negative rate).

Management

The management consists of high-dose prednisone (1–1.5 mg/kg per day) in combination with cyclophosphamide (1.5–2.5 mg/kg per day in divided doses) orally or pulsed i.v. cyclophosphamide 500–1000 mg/m^2 every 2 weeks for three doses, then monthly. Risks of cyclophosphamide include bone marrow suppression and hemorrhagic cystitis with increased risk for bladder cancer. Pulsed therapy reduces the risk of adverse effects but may be less efficacious. Intravenous methylprednisolone 1000 mg every 24 hours (in single or divided doses every 6 hours) may be administered for 72 hours prior to starting oral prednisone in more fulminant cases.

Steroid therapy should be tapered over weeks to months once clinical resolution occurs and cyclophosphamide should be continued for 6–12 months before cessation. Precautionary measures, such as DVT prophylaxis, glycemic control, osteoporosis prevention, regular CBC, or urinalysis for microscopic hematuria/ cytology for cancer, are necessary. Other potential steroid-sparing agents include azathioprine and methotrexate.

General supportive care should be provided as described for stroke patients (p. 100). If headache is a persisting problem, adequate analgesia should be provided, avoiding excessive use of NSAIDs owing to potential bleeding risk. Antiplatelet therapy should be added to immunosuppressants to reduce stroke risk. Delirium would require care as described on p. 95. Standard post-operative care would be required following diagnostic biopsy.

Prognosis

Mortality from PACNS is approximately 10%, with full recovery in approximately 80% and approximately 30% relapse rate in a single study with a mean follow-up for 4 years. The use of cyclophosphamide for more than 12 months may be associated with a relapse rate of approximately 10%. A benign variant of PACNS that presents in females acutely (usually with headache), and associated with normal or mildly abnormal CSF and reversible angiographic changes may result in 94% recovery (~30% with mild residual deficits only) with 6% relapse and no deaths with a mean follow-up of 3 years. The use of immunosuppresants has significantly improved the survival rate from CNS vasculitis.

Counseling

Patients should be aware of the significant improvement in prognosis in PACNS with aggressive immunosuppresant therapy; however, such therapy has its own complications that require detailed discussion. The mean duration from symptom onset to histological diagnosis is about 6 months for newly diagnosed cases, so the index of suspicion should be high in cases of unexplained headache, delirium or focal neurological deficits in order to institute therapy early. Patients should be taught to recognize symptoms and advised to seek urgent neurological evaluation promptly.

SUMMARY

- **PACNS** is a vasculitic disorder that affects **small (~200 μm) blood vessels** in the brain without systemic involvement.
- Differential diagnoses include **systemic vasculitides, i.v. drug use, infection** (viral, spirochete, bacterial, fungal, protozoa), **neoplasm, demyelinating disease,** and **hypertensive encephalopathy**.
- Diagnosis is confirmed by **brain biopsy**. Peri-procedural morbidity is **approximately 3%** with false-negative rate of **approximately 25%**.
- Treatment includes **prednisone 1–1.5 mg/kg per day** and **cyclophosphamide 1.5–2.5 mg/kg per day** or **500–1000 mg/m² every 2 weeks for three doses, then every 4 weeks**. The patient should be treated for **6–12 months**.
- Mortality is **approximately 10%**, with **80% recovery** and **approximately 30% relapse rate** over mean follow-up of **4 years**. Treatment for more than 12 months results in **approximately 10% relapse rate**.
- Risks of chronic immunosuppression should be discussed.

11

Pain Syndromes

CASE 1

A 34-year-old woman came to the office complaining of severe, left-sided throbbing headaches that last about 12–24 hours. She has had these headaches once a week for several months. During an episode, she is sensitive to both bright lights and loud sounds and feels nauseous. Sleep seemed to help her headaches. Neurological examination was normal.

Localization

A left-sided headache may suggest meningeal irritation of the left cerebral hemisphere (anterior and middle cranial fossae), or referred dermatomal pain from CN V_1–V_3 (anterolateral cranium) or C2–C3 nerve roots (posterior cranium) on the left. However, headaches could be nonlocalizing. Photophobia and phonophobia may suggest dysfunction in the visual and auditory systems. Nausea could occur because of vestibular (peripheral or central) dysfunction. The normal neurological examination supports the absence of a structural lesion, so the symptoms most likely suggest diffuse functional deficits involving the cerebral cortex and brainstem.

Differential Diagnosis

The most likely diagnosis is *migraine without aura* (*common migraine*). This is a clinical diagnosis. The history should be expanded to ascertain if an aura is present (e.g., scintillating scotomata, parasthesias: would confirm diagnosis of migraine with aura or classic migraine), previous history, aggravating/precipitating factors, family history (~60–90% familial) and prior medication use.

Other causes of headache that should be considered include *IIH* (diffuse headache worse on awakening in obese individuals associated with visual blurring and CN VI palsy), *brain tumor* (usually awakens patient from sleep, may be unilateral or generalized owing to raised intracranial pressure: focal signs expected; systemic signs may occur with malignancy), *ICH* (usually sudden onset with focal signs), *infection* (cranial and intracranial: course is usually

From: *Neurology Oral Boards Review:*
A Concise and Systematic Approach to Clinical Practice
By: E. E. Ubogu © Humana Press Inc., Totowa, NJ

progressive), *vascular malformations* (AVM, aneurysms with sentinel headaches caused by minor bleed) and *giant-cell arteritis* (GCA; usually age over 60, with jaw claudication, temporal tenderness, and visual symptoms; *see* p. 123).

Investigations

No specific investigations are useful to confirm the clinical diagnosis of migraine. CT/MRI of the brain can be performed in atypical or new-onset headaches to exclude intracranial pathology. MRA may be useful if a vascular anomaly is being considered. In patients older than 60 years, CBC, ESR/CRP/fibrinogen should be considered in evaluating for temporal arteritis. LP would be required to investigate IIH.

Treatment

Treatment of migraine consists of abortive and prophylactic regimens. If migraines have lasted several days with minimal or no relief, then the patient is in *status migrainosus* and requires hospital admission. In this scenario, dihydroergotamine (DHE) 0.5 mg i.v. every 8 hours preceded by an i.v. antiemetic such as chlorpromazine or metoclopramide can be administered (can increase DHE to 1.0 mg if more than 50% relief with 0.5 mg dose is not achieved within 1 hour) for 3 days. Vitals should be checked every 4 hours. DHE is contraindicated in patients over age 60, those with uncontrolled hypertension or angina, and those who are pregnant. Electrolyte and fluid imbalances should be corrected. Corticosteroids or i.v. valproic acid (VPA) can also be administered in place of DHE in status migrainosus.

Non-emergent abortive medications include $5\text{-HT}_{1B/1D}$ agonists (triptans), NSAIDs, acetaminophen, ergotamines, combination analgesics with caffeine, antiemetics, and opioid analgesics (in special cases such as pregnancy or CAD). These should be generally administered as early as possible during the development of the migraine attack. Antiemetics should be given if nausea/vomiting exist with the headache. Patients should be advised to rest in a dark, quiet room with an ice pack on the head. Sleep usually results in awakening in a headache-free state.

Prophylactic medications should be considered if the frequency or duration of migraines interferes with the patient's lifestyle. Options include β-blockers, calcium channel antagonists (verapamil is useful in complicated migraine), TCAs, AEDs (e.g., divalproex sodium), methysergide (for intractable migraine only, use for only 6 months at a time owing to potential complication of retroperitoneal, pulmonary, and cardiac fibrosis), NSAIDs (more useful in abortive therapy), and cyproheptadine (nonselective serotonin blocker: useful in children; can cause drowsiness and weight gain).

Prognosis

Migraine attacks tend to recur with varying frequency and duration throughout the patient's life. About 90% of migraineurs develop their attacks by age 40. With increasing age, there is a tendency for the headaches to become milder and less frequent. About 33% of women experience a worsening in migraines around menopause. In uncommon instances, migraine patients may develop associated hemiparesis sporadically or rarely as part of familial hemiplegic migraine. Full recovery after hours or days is expected, unless cerebral infarction occurs.

Counseling

Patients should be encouraged to identify and avoid migraine trigger factors (e.g., alcohol, caffeine, smoking, drugs). Stress reduction (e.g., pharmacological, biofeedback, relaxation therapy) may be needed, but difficult to achieve. Dietary modifications (avoiding foods with nitrites; such as hot dogs and preserved meats, monosodium glutamate and tyramine-containing foods, e.g., red wine, chocolate, ripened cheeses) may be required to control headaches. Regular exercise may improve well-being.

SUMMARY

- **Migraine** is a clinical headache syndrome whose diagnosis is based on its **nature, localization, duration**, and **associative features**.
- Differentials include **IIH, brain tumor, ICH, infection (cranial/intracranial), vascular malformation**, and **GCA (if >60 years)**.
- Diagnosis is based on **history. CT/MRI brain** may be used to exclude intracranial pathology in atypical or new-onset cases.
- Treatment includes **abortive** and **prophylactic regimens**.
- Abortive therapy for status migrainosus includes **DHE 0.5–1.0 mg i.v. every 8 hours** for **3 days**, preceded by an i.v. antiemetic; **corticosteroids** or **VPA**.
- Non-emergency abortive agents include **5-HT$_{1B/1D}$ agonists (triptans), NSAIDs, acetaminophen, ergotamines, combination analgesics with caffeine, antiemetics**, and **opioid analgesics**.
- Patients should rest in a **dark, quiet room** with an **ice pack on the head**.
- Prophylactic agents include β**-blockers, calcium channel antagonists, TCAs, AEDs, methysergide, NSAIDs**, and **cyproheptadine** (in children).
- Patients should identify and avoid trigger factors. **Stress reduction, dietary modification**, and **regular exercise** may be required.

CASE 2

A 41-year-old man came to the ER complaining of severe, pounding right periorbital headaches associated with nasal congestion and rhinorrhea lasting about 45–60 minutes. He had experienced his third episode that night and was unable to fall asleep. He had a similar episode 6 months ago. On examination, temperature was 37.4°C, HR was 96 per minute, BP was 135/85 mmHg, and RR was 16 per minute. He was restless with normal cognition. Neurological examination revealed right conjunctival injection, miosis, and eyelid ptosis.

Localization

Right periorbital headaches with nasal congestion and rhinorrhea may localize to the frontal and maxillary sinuses. Pain associated with conjunctival injection, miosis, and ptosis may imply ipsilateral orbital disease with reduced venous outflow and compromise to the sympathetic fibers innervating the pupillodilator muscles and levator muscles of the eyelid. A partial Horner's syndrome (miosis, ptosis without anhidrosis) implies dysfunction to the sympathetic tracts to the eye distal to the bifurcation of the common carotid artery. However, in many instances, headaches are a nonlocalizing symptom of CNS pathology.

Differential Diagnosis

The most likely diagnosis for a headache syndrome with this constellation of signs and symptoms is *episodic cluster headaches*. Attacks of headaches occur daily for days, weeks, or months before remission. Remission may last for weeks to years before recurrence. *Chronic cluster headaches* occur if these headache attacks last for more than 1 year without remission for more than 2 weeks. The etiology of cluster headaches is unknown. The diagnosis is established clinically and collaborative history about previous attacks essential. Other considerations include headache syndromes such as *short-lasting unilateral neuralgiform headache attacks with conjunctival injection and tearing* (SUNCT syndrome; moderate pain of very short duration, 5–250 seconds and high frequency of attacks), *paroxysmal hemicrania* (excruciating pain with duration 2–45 minutes), *temporal arteritis* (if age >60 years with supportive clinical features), and *atypical migraine headaches*.

Secondary headache causes include *periorbital/facial diseases* (e.g., sinusitis, glaucoma, dental disease, trigeminal neuralgia, posttraumatic/surgical: lack autonomic features and episodic periodicity), *ipsilateral carotid dissection/aneurysm* (causes partial Horner's syndrome: episodic pain and restlessness are not present), *inflammation* (e.g., Tolosa–Hunt syndrome: granulomatous inflammation of superior orbital fissure or cavernous sinus: CN III, IV, V_1, and VI dysfunction; not seen with cluster headaches), *endocrinopathy* (e.g., pheochromocytoma, insulinoma: usually bilateral and ptosis, tearing and nasal stuffiness unlikely),

CN III compression (e.g., by aneurysm: causes mydriasis owing to compression of superficial CN III parasympathetic fibers and partial/complete oculomotor palsy is present), *vascular malformations* (e.g., AVM) and *tumors* (sphenoidal or parasellar meningioma, pituitary adenoma, nasopharyngeal carcinoma).

Investigations

Cluster headaches are diagnosed clinically. CT/MRI of the brain may be performed in atypical episodic cluster or chronic cluster headaches to exclude intracranial pathology. Indirect ophthalmoscopy with pressure evaluation should be considered if glaucoma is suspected. Routine baseline laboratory tests (CBC/basic metabolic profile) should be performed prior to starting pharmacological therapy.

Treatment

Abortive and prophylactic therapies are required. Abortive therapy includes oxygen 100% 8–10 L per minute via loosely applied face mask, intranasal/subcutaneous triptans, DHE, intranasal lidocaine, and olanzapine. These agents aim to reduce the severity and duration of cluster attacks.

Prophylactic agents (to reduce the frequency of attacks) include short-term agents (weeks): corticosteroids, ergotamines, and methysergide and long-term agents (months): lithium (narrow therapeutic window so levels need to be checked; adverse effects include tremor, diabetes insipidus, renal failure, goiter), calcium channel antagonists (e.g., verapamil), methysergide (chest/abdominal CT or MRI to evaluate for retroperitoneal, pulmonary or cardiac fibrosis every 3–6 months with 4-week drug-free periods if used), AEDs (e.g., divalproex sodium, topiramate), indomethacin, chlorpromazine, clonidine, cyproheptadine, and intranasal capcaisin. Combination therapy (e.g., lithium and verapamil) may be required in chronic cluster headaches.

In medically refractory cases, surgery (thermocoagulation of gasserian ganglion, sphenopalatine nerve block, microvascular decompression of CN V, or stereotactic radiosurgery) may be beneficial in some patients, but there is a risk of keratitis and anesthesia dolorosa with any destructive procedure to the CN V.

Prognosis

Cluster headaches are debilitating during the attacks, but confer an overall benign prognosis. About 10% of episodic cluster headaches evolve into chronic cluster headaches that persist into advanced age, with about 50% eventually ceasing. Frequency and severity start to diminish after the age of 50 in general.

Counseling

Triggers (e.g., smoking, alcohol use) should be avoided. Reassurance of the benign nature and absence of intracranial pathology is useful. Educating the patient about stereotypical periodicity and warning symptoms may help reduce anxiety. The severity of attacks may be reduced with appropriate therapy initiated early in the attack. Adverse drug effects should be emphasized, especially in patients taking combination drug therapy for chronic cluster headaches. Surgical options and potential complications should be discussed with medically refractory patients.

SUMMARY

- **Episodic cluster headache** is a headache syndrome diagnosed based on its **nature, localization, duration**, and **associative features**.
- Differentials include headache syndromes: **SUNCT syndrome, paroxysmal hemicrania, temporal arteritis** and **atypical migraine**, and secondary headache causes: **periorbital/facial disease, ipsilateral carotid dissection/ aneurysm, inflammation, endocrinopathy, CN III compression, vascular malformations**, and **tumor**.
- Diagnosis is established **clinically. CT/MRI head** may be performed to exclude intracranial pathology and to reassure patient.
- Abortive treatment includes **100% oxygen, triptans, DHE, intranasal lidocaine**, and **olanzapine**.
- Prophylactic treatment includes **short-term agents** such as **corticosteroids, ergotamines**, and **methysergide**, and common **long-term agents** such as **lithium, calcium channel antagonists, AEDs**, and **methysergide** (used with caution).
- **Surgical options** should be considered in **medically refractory patients**. There is a risk of **keratitis** and **anesthesia dolorosa**.
- Prognosis is **benign. Approximately 10%** of episodic cluster headache become chronic and lifelong. Frequency and severity reduce with **age over 50**.

CASE 3

A 26-year-old woman came to the office complaining of a 3-month history of dull, constant headaches that involved the entire cranium. These headaches were made worse by lying down and coughing. Over the last 2 weeks, she had noticed some blurred vision and diplopia on looking to the left. Neurological examination revealed bilateral papilledema and a partial left CN VI palsy.

Localization

A diffuse headache is nonlocalizing. A partial left CN VI nerve palsy suggests dysfunction of the left CN VI nucleus in the pons or its nerve fibers within its intracranial course to the orbit. However, an isolated CN VI palsy may represent a "false localizing sign" of raised ICP. Bilateral papilledema further supports an elevated ICP.

Differential Diagnosis

The most likely diagnosis for a holocranial headache with a young woman with visual disturbances is *idiopathic intracranial hypertension* (IIH). This is a disorder that most commonly occurs in young, obese females and is believed to be secondary to elevated dural venous sinus pressure. Drugs commonly associated with IIH include *vitamin A analogs* (e.g,. isotretinoin), *tamoxifen, oral contraceptive pills, tetracycline*, and *cimetidine*.

Other differentials include *primary brain tumors* (causing raised ICP: would expect focal signs), *brain abscess, carcinomatous meningitis* (causing diffuse headache and papilledema from optic nerve infiltration), *chronic hydrocephalus* (increased CSF production or reduced CSF drainage), *malignant hypertension, chronic hypercapnia* (from pulmonary diseases or sleep apnea), and *GCA* (if age >60: can cause bilateral anterior ischemic optic neuropathy; associative features should readily distinguish this from IIH).

Investigations

MRI (with MRV) of the brain with contrast should be performed to exclude space-occupying lesions or hydrocephalus. CT is an option if MRI cannot be performed. LP should be performed to measure opening pressure (normal 8–18 cm H_2O, >25 diagnostic) and exclude CNS infection or inflammation. Formal visual fields (perimetry) should be measured to determine any visual deficits, including plotting size of the blind spot. ABG should be considered if there is a history of chronic lung disease or sleep apnea. Baseline electrolytes should be checked prior to therapy. ESR/CRP/fibrinogen should be checked if patient is older than 60 years.

Treatment

The mainstay of treatment for IIH is acetazolamide 250–500 mg p.o. twice a day. Acetazolamide is a carbonic anhydrase inhibitor that lowers CSF production and pressure. The patient should be monitored for metabolic acidosis and distal parasthesias. These are common side effects seen in about 25% of patients. Other options include furosemide, glycerol (0.25–1.0 g/kg per dose two or three times a day) and corticosteroids (short-term therapy in rapidly progressive IIH: may cause weight gain and rebound increase in ICP during taper). Weight reduction in overweight patients often results in resolution of IIH. Medically refractory patients may benefit from serial LPs or lumboperitoneal shunts (with risk of shunt malfunction, infection, etc.).

If visual function is threatened in medically refractory patients, optic nerve sheath fenestration should be performed (about 13% failure rate; complications include pupillary abnormalities, transient visual loss, and extraocular muscle dysfunction, approximately 50% improvement also occurs in nonoperated eye). Standard analgesics may be required for chronic headaches. Close follow-up (including perimetry) may be sufficient for mild cases without papilledema.

Prognosis

The typical course lasts months to years. The major morbidity is papilledema-associated visual loss. Predictors for visual loss include recent weight gain, significant visual loss on presentation, hypertension, high-grade/atrophic papilledema, and subretinal hemorrhages. Severity of headache and CSF opening pressure are not predictors of visual loss. Other causes for loss of visual acuity in IIH include macular edema and exudates, optic disc infarction, chorioretinal folds, and subretinal peripapillary hemorrhage/neovascular membrane. Following medical treatment, about 50–60% of patients improve, approximately 30% remain stable, and 10–20% worsen based on formal perimetry. Symptom recurrence may occur in approximately 10–35% of patients following resolution and may occur years after the initial episode

Counseling

Patients should be aware of the visual sequelae of IIH and the need for medication compliance. Lifelong therapy is usually not warranted, so treatment can be stopped with clinical resolution. Patients should be encouraged to lose weight (may need professional advice/guidance). Worsening despite therapy warrants more invasive therapies. Risks and benefits for surgical approaches should be discussed in detail.

SUMMARY

- **IIH** is a chronic headache syndrome caused by **raised ICP** possibly secondary to **elevated dural venous sinus pressure**.
  Diagnosis is made by excluding other causes of raised ICP, with a CSF opening pressure **of more than 25 cm H$_2$O** on LP.
- Differentials include **primary brain tumor, brain abscess, carcinomatous meningitis, chronic hydrocephalus, malignant hypertension, chronic hypercapnia**, and **GCA**.
- **MRI with MRV** is the neuroimaging modality of choice.
- Treatment includes **acetazolamide, furosemide**, or **glycerol**. **Corticosteroids** can be used short term in "malignant" cases.
- In medically refractory cases, **serial LPs, lumboperitoneal shunt**, or **optic nerve sheath fenestration** (especially with impending visual loss) should be considered.

- **Approximately 10–20%** of patients worsen despite medical therapy. Improvement is expected in **50–60%**; **approximately 30% stabilize**.
- Predictors for visual loss include **recent weight gain, significant visual loss on presentation, hypertension, high-grade atrophic papilledema**, and **subretinal hemorrhages**.
  Opening pressure and **headache severity** are **not** predictors.
- Recurrence may occur in **approximately 10–35%** of patients, usually years after initial episode. Outcomes are similar after recurrence.

CASE 4

A 29-year-old man came to the clinic 8 weeks after a work-related injury to his right foot. There was severe pain after the incident, but the pain subsided over 5–7 days. About 3 weeks ago, he developed deep, burning excruciating pain and noticed intermittent skin color and temperature changes to that foot. On examination, the right foot appeared to fluctuate from pale to reddish-purple and was swollen. Neurological examination revealed reduced range of motion of all movements at the ankles and toes owing to pain. There was subjective allodynia and hyperalgesia to light touch in the foot in a nondermatomal pattern. Reflex examination of the right ankle jerk was deferred.

Localization

Right foot pain may be secondary to neurological or non-neurological causes (i.e., diseases of skin, joints, bone, vascular structures). Focusing on neurological causes, pain with positive phenomena (allodynia, hyperalgesia) may be secondary to nerve root (L4–S1), lumbosacral plexus, or peripheral nerve (sciatic or peroneal, tibial, and plantar) disease. Vasomotor and sudomotor dysfunction localizes to a disorder affecting sympathetic fibers from the intermediolateral cell column in the thoracolumbar spinal cord to the end organs (vascular smooth muscle and sweat glands). The clinical history does not provide any further localizing features, especially with a nondermatomal sensory pattern on exam.

Differential Diagnosis

The most likely diagnosis of a posttraumatic chronic pain syndrome associated with sympathetic skin changes is *complex regional pain syndrome (CRPS)*. The etiology for this syndrome is unclear. The absence of peripheral nerve injury confers a diagnosis of CRPS type I, whereas evidence of such injury confers a diagnosis of CRPS type II.

Other considerations include *malingering* (requires history suggesting secondary gain), *factitious disorder* (in order to assume the "sick role"), intramedullary *lower spinal cord lesion* (e.g., syringomyelia, tumor, vascular malformation:

sympathetic symptoms would be unusual and dissociative sensory loss and bilateral upper motor neuron findings expected), *L4–S1 nerve root compression* (very unlikely based on the history and clinical findings), and *peripheral neuropathy* (asymmetry unusual, and stepwise history of mononeuropathy multiplex absent).

Investigations

There are no studies that definitively diagnose CRPS because this is a clinical diagnosis. Tests should be tailored toward identifying any underlying nerve damage or potential causes for regional pain. Laboratory tests such as CBC with differential, ESR/CRP, and blood cultures are useful in screening for an infective/inflammatory cause of regional pain. Diabetic screen should be considered. Plain radiographs of the foot should be performed to exclude bony injury. Subchondral bone erosion may occur with any condition causing foot disuse. If tolerated, EMG/NCS may help identify and localize any large-fiber peripheral nerve dysfunction, whereas autonomic tests for sudomotor (e.g., thermoregulatory sweat test [TST], quantitative sudomotor axon reflex test [QSART]) and Doppler flowmetry for vasomotor function can be performed (sensitive but not specific for CPRS). In CPRS, investigations are usually normal.

Treatment

The treatment of CPRS requires physical therapy, pharmacotherapy (noninvasive and invasive), and possible surgery for cases associated with nerve injury (CPRS II). Physical therapy (active and passive range of motion, transcutaneous electrical nerve stimulator [TENS], contrast baths, hydrotherapy, and continuous passive motion) is employed to enhance functional recovery and prevent contractures.

Noninvasive pharmacotherapies include NSAIDs, steroids, TCAs, selective serotonin reuptake inhibitors (SSRIs), AEDs (e.g., gabapentin, phenytoin), calcium channel blockers, and α-2 agonists (e.g., clonidine). Invasive measures include epidural sympathetic trunk (intermittent or continuous), i.v. regional anesthesia, and somatic blocks. When there is identifiable nerve injury and failure to respond to medical and physical therapy, neurolysis, neurorrhaphy, neuroma resection, and if necessary, environmental modification of the nerve bed may be required. Sympathectomy (controversial) may be required in severely debilitating, medically refractory cases.

In general, start with the simplest, least expensive, and least invasive modalities first, utilizing more complex and invasive therapies in medically refractory patients. Psychological support and therapy (e.g., biofeedback, relaxation therapy) may help patients cope with CPRS.

Prognosis

Deciphering the true morbidity of CRPS is dependent on how outcomes are defined. Using pain improvement by more than 50% as a measure of good outcome, about 25% of adult patients at 6-month and 35% of patients at 1- and 2-years may report good outcomes with therapy based on a single study. Other studies report improvement in as many as 50–65% of patients. CPRS may result in approximately 25% of patients changing employment and 30% stop working for more than 1 year. However, 70–75% are still able to maintain some full-time employment at 5 years. Active physical therapy may result in good outcomes in children: 88% are symptom free at 2 years with approximately 30% recurrence during therapy, 10% are fully functional with residual pain, and 2% are functionally limited despite therapy. Institution of therapy early may aid in improving outcomes. Failure to improve after 1 year may be a poor prognostic sign.

Counseling

Patients should understand that CRPS is a difficult condition to treat and multiple modalities are usually necessary for symptom control. Pain clinic referral is usually required. Psychological support and continued physical therapy should be encouraged for chronic pain syndromes. Patients with medically refractory pain may consider sympathectomy or chemical ablation with the risk of developing postoperative neuralgia, worsening of CPRS, and abnormal sweating patterns. CPRS II patients may consider surgery to the damaged nerve without guarantee of symptom resolution.

SUMMARY

- **CRPS** is a pain syndrome that consists of **posttraumatic chronic pain, autonomic**, and **dystrophic** changes.
- There is an absence of identifiable nerve damage in **CRPS I** and evidence of nerve damage in **CRPS II**
- Differentials include **malingering, factitious disorder, intramedullary spinal cord lesion, nerve root compression**, and **peripheral neuropathy**.
- Diagnosis is **clinical**. Other potential causes of regional pain should be excluded.
- **Electrodiagnostic studies** are useful in documenting nerve lesions or autonomic dysfunction (**sensitive**, but not specific for CRPS).
- Treatment includes **physical therapy, pharmacotherapy** (noninvasive and invasive), and **possible surgery** in refractory cases. **Psychological support** may be necessary. **Multimodal therapy** is usually required. Treatment should start with **simple, less invasive methods**.
- **Approximately 25%** of patients at 6 months and **about 35–65%** at 1–2 years, have good outcomes following therapy. **Thirty percent** stop working for **more than 1 year**.
- Patients should be aware of **chronicity** and **suboptimal response** to therapy.

CASE 5

A 51-year-old woman complained of several episodes of severe, paroxysmal stabbing pains that affected her right forehead and cheek regions for 3 months. These episodes lasted about 10–30 seconds and were triggered by chewing, washing her face, or brushing her teeth. Her last episode was about 2 days ago. Neurological examination in the clinic was normal.

Localization

Pain affecting the right forehead and cheek could be dermatomal or referred from structures that share similar dermatomal representation. Possible localizing areas include the ophthalmic (V_1) and maxillary (V_2) divisions of the right CN V, right frontal and temporal dura matter (anterior and middle cranial fossae), frontal and maxillary sinuses, nasopharynx, or upper teeth. The clinical history does not suggest pathology that could cause referred pain. In summary, the most likely localization is the right CN V.

Differential Diagnosis

The most likely diagnosis for severe, paroxysmal, stabbing, unilateral facial pain triggered by activities of daily living in a middle-aged woman is *trigeminal neuralgia*. This condition is usually caused by demyelination of the CN V sensory fibers either within the nerve root or the pons (root entry zone). Bilateral symptoms may occur in 3–5%. The most common etiology is *focal nerve root compression* (80–90%). *Vascular compression* via a *dolichoectatic artery or vein* close to the pons accounts for most cases, with compression by a *saccular aneurysm* or *AVM* being less common. Other causes of compression include *neoplasm* (e.g., vestibular schwannoma, meningioma, osteoma, epidermoid cysts) and *skull base deformities* (e.g., osteogenesis imperfecta). Other etiologies for trigeminal neuralgia include *primary demyelinating disorders* (e.g., MS), *infiltration* (carcinoma, amyloidosis), *ischemia/infarction*, and *inherited causes* (familial trigeminal neuralgia: seen in certain hereditary motor and sensory neuropathy (HMSN) kindred in association with glossopharnyngeal neuralgia).

Other differentials for facial pain include *dental disease* (pulpal disease, fractured teeth, periodontal disease), *temporomandibular disorders* (pain is more likely periauricular with radiation to neck and temples, could last hours and may be associated with tenderness of muscles of mastication), *chronic sinusitis, atypical facial pain* (radiates widely beyond trigeminal region and may be associated with stressors/life events, depression, and movements), *postherpetic neuralgia* (continuous dull ache with sharp exacerbations, associated with allodynia and sensory loss usually in the V_1 distribution), *cluster headaches* (*see* pp. 114–116), *chronic paroxysmal* hemicrania (pain usually lasts for several minutes with multiple daily episodes, autonomic features and responsiveness to indomethacin), or *GCA* (or temporal arteritis).

GCA is a chronic inflammatory disorder affecting large and medium-sized arteries in patients older than 60 years; associated with unilateral or bilateral temporal headache, scalp tenderness, jaw claudication, and polymyalgia rheumatica (in 25–50%). Elevated ESR, CRP, or fibrinogen, anemia of chronic disease and thrombocytosis support the diagnosis. Temporal artery biopsy is required for confirmation—at least 20 mm should be obtained to increase diagnostic yield. Complications of GCA include ischemic optic neuropathy, amaurosis fugax, stroke, spinal cord infarction, mononeuropathy multiplex, aortic aneurysms with potential dissection. GCA is treated with high doses of steroids for 3–6 months, with slow taper over 6–12 months with the intention of complete steroid cessation within 2 years depending on clinical response. Prolonged steroid requirements may be needed if fever, weight loss, ESR over 85 mm per hour or anemia were seen on initial presentation.

Investigations

The diagnosis is established clinically. CBC with differential, comprehensive metabolic panel, LFT should be checked before initiating therapy. If GCA is suspected, ESR, CRP, and fibrinogen should be checked as well. MRI (with and without gadolinium with thin cuts through the posterior fossa), MRA or 3D fast-in-flow steady state precession (FISP) sequences can be performed to evaluate for causes of trigeminal neuralgia and exclude other pathologies causing facial pain.

Management

The treatment of trigeminal neuralgia can be divided into medical and surgical modalities. Medical therapy is usually the first option and consists of AEDs such as carbamazepine (first-line agent with ~75% response rates; oxcarbamazepine probably as efficacious), phenytoin, clonazepam, gabapentin, lamotrigine, or topiramate, or TCA (e.g., amitriptyline, desipramine). Mono- or combination therapy could be applied based on patient response.

Surgical therapy is usually reserved for medically refractory patients. Surgical options include *microvascular decompression* (treatment of choice for young, healthy individuals with more than 10 years life expectancy; mortality rate ~0.3%, neurological morbidity ~2% (hematoma, facial palsy) and CN V section ~3.5%; >95% initial home discharge rates with long-term significant or complete pain relief in >90% of patients), *stereotactic radiosurgery* (~75% with initial reduction in pain within 3 months, ~66% with initial reduction in medications, ~50% with long-term cessation of medications, and >80% with improved quality of life. Complete long-term relief occurs in 35–40%, with recurrence of ~25% at 1 year, ~33% at 2 years, and ~40–50% at 3 years: repeat radiosurgery at lower doses can be attempted with similar rates of initial treatment efficacy; most common complication is facial sensory disturbance including anesthesia dorolosa), *percutaneous trigeminal neurolysis* or *angioplasty of Gasserian ganglion, partial sensory trigeminal sectioning*, or *glycerol rhizotomy*. There are no absolute guidelines for choosing between surgical options and treatment efficacy has not been compared by clinical trials within the surgical group or between medical and surgical modalities. Less invasive methods should be considered in older or medically unstable patients in general. If an underlying cause for trigeminal neuralgia is determined, it should be treated appropriately.

Prognosis

Although trigeminal neuralgia is not a life-threatening disorder, the patient's quality of life, including psychosocial well-being can be adversely affected. In medically refractory patients, good postoperative outcomes are predicted by typical presentation and shorter duration of symptoms. In cases associated with vascular compression, arterial compression confers a better outcome following microvascular decompression compared to venous compression.

Counseling

Patients should be advised as to the risks and benefits of medical and surgical therapy for trigeminal neuralgia. Compliance with medication therapy would be important to prevent recurrence. A thorough evaluation for nonvascular compressive causes should be performed and patient should be reassured by negative results. For younger patients (especially women), MS is a diagnostic possibility that warrants full investigation (*see* pp. 181–184) and treatment, if diagnosed.

SUMMARY

- **Trigeminal neuralgia** is a **severe, paroxysmal, stabbing** unilateral facial pain triggered by **activities of daily living** caused by **demyelination of CN V sensory nerve root** or **root entry zone** in the pons.
- Causes include **compression** (vascular, neoplasm, skull base deformities), **primary demyelination, infiltration, ischemia/infarction**, or **inherited**.
- Differentials include **dental disease, temporomandibular disorders, chronic sinusitis, atypical facial pain, post-herpetic neuralgia, cluster headache, chronic paroxysmal hemicrania**, and **GCA**.
- Diagnosis is established **clinically. MR sequences** are useful in determining etiology or excluding other causes of facial pain.
- Treatment can be divided into **medical** and **surgical** modalities. **Carbamazepine** is the first line medical agent with **approximately 75%**

treatment success. Surgery is usually reserved for **medically refractory** patients.

- **Microvascular decompression** is the treatment of choice in **young, healthy patients** with life expectancy **of more than 10 years**.
- **Stereotactic radiosurgery** has an initial treatment response of **75%** within **3 months** and **50%** with complete medication cessation, but with **40–50%** recurrence rates **3 years** postoperatively.
- There are **no** direct comparison clinical trails to ascertain most efficacious treatment for trigeminal neuralgia.
- Trigeminal neuralgia is **not life-threatening**, but can be **significantly disabling**.

12

Neuromuscular Disorders

CASE 1

A 63-year-old woman complained of a tingling sensation involving the index and middle fingers in her right hand for 3 months. These symptoms awaken her from sleep. She also had some neck discomfort without any radiation. She felt that the function in her hand was reduced. On examination, there was subjective sensory loss to pinprick involving the affected digits. Motor examination revealed MRC 4/5 strength in right thumb abduction only. Reflex examination of the upper extremities was normal.

Localization

Parasthesias and reduced sensation in the right index and middle fingers indicates dysfunction in the ipsilateral C6–C7 dermatomes. However, lesions causing these sensory findings could involve the C6–C7 nerve roots, upper and middle trunks or lateral cord of the brachial plexus, or median nerve. Weakness in the right abductor pollicis brevis could indicate disease in AHC, C8–T1 nerve roots, lower trunk, or medial cord of the brachial plexus or median nerve. Although a multilevel radiculopathy (C6–C8) or pan-plexopathy is possible, one would expect more symptoms and signs on clinical evaluation. The most likely localization is the right median nerve.

Differential Diagnosis

The most likely diagnosis is *carpal tunnel syndrome* (CTS), an entrapment neuropathy of the median nerve below the transverse carpal ligament. This is the most common entrapment neuropathy and may be associated with *pregnancy, DM, obesity, hypothyroidism, rheumatoid arthritis, uremia, acromegaly, amyloidosis,* and *inflammation of the bony/ligamentous structures at the wrist.*

Other median nerve entrapment syndromes include *anterior interosseous syndrome* (entrapment by fibrous bands between flexor digitorum superficialis: causes weakness in flexor pollicis longus, pronator quadratus, and flexor digitorum profundus to index and middle fingers without sensory loss), *pronator teres syndrome*

From: *Neurology Oral Boards Review:*
A Concise and Systematic Approach to Clinical Practice
By: E. E. Ubogu © Humana Press Inc., Totowa, NJ

(compression in the lateral forearm between the two heads of pronator teres: would expect weakness in median muscles proximal to the wrist, e.g., flexor carpi radialis, sparing pronator teres itself) and *Ligament of Struthers entrapment* (fibrous band from medial epicondyle to a residual supracondylar spur on the humerus: involves median-innervated muscles above wrist including pronator teres and may cause reduction in radial pulse with fully extended, supinated arm owing to brachial artery compression).

Other causes for median neuropathy include *vasculitis* (systemic or nonsystemic), *trauma, DM, infiltrative* (granulomatous, e.g., sarcoidosis; leukemia, neoplasia), *infective* (e.g., leprosy, HIV), and *demyelinating disorders* (e.g., multifocal motor neuropathy, hereditary neuropathy with liability to pressure palsies). In these cases, median neuropathy may be part of a mononeuropathy multiplex syndrome (*see* p. 131).

Investigations

The clinical history is paramount in establishing the diagnosis of CTS. Laboratory investigations for commonly associated disorders should be tailored based on history. Possible tests include CBC with differential, comprehensive metabolic panel, TFT, fasting glucose or oral glucose tolerance test, ESR/CRP, ANA panel, and RhF. If trauma to the hand, wrist, or arm were of concern, plain radiographs would be useful to exclude bony injury. EMG/NCS would be useful in localizing the median neuropathy to below the wrist and excluding a radiculopathy, plexopathy, or mononeuropathy multiplex in difficult cases. MRI of the hand and forearm may be useful if an infective or infiltrative etiology is highly suggested. In equivocal cases, MRI of the cervical spine could be performed to exclude multilevel C6–C8 radiculopathies.

Management

The treatment of CTS depends on symptom severity. Avoidance of precipitating factors (e.g., reading a newspaper, driving, typing) may be possible, but at many times, impractical. Mild sensory symptoms suggest the use of a neutrally positioned wrist-splint (to be worn at night, during times of activity, or both), NSAIDs, and local corticosteroid injections (e.g., betamethasone with or without lidocaine) into the carpal tunnel. Severe sensory loss and atrophy of thenar muscles would indicate surgical carpal tunnel decompression via sectioning of the volar carpal ligament. This procedure could be performed via open or endoscopic technique. Disorders associated with CTS should be appropriately treated.

Prognosis

In less severe cases, conservative (nonsurgical) measures may result in symptom resolution in approximately 50% of patients. The initial steroid injection into the carpal tunnel may result in about 70% symptom control 2 weeks post-injection and about 50% over 18 months with recurrent injections.

In general, approximately 90–95% of more severely affected CTS patients receive some prompt reduction in hand pain and parasthesias following decompressive surgery. About 70–80% of patients are able to return to work 3 months postoperatively. About 60–75% of CTS patients report being completely or very satisfied with the outcomes of surgery at 6, 18, and 30 months postoperatively. Surgical treatment may decrease the rate of duty modifications, subjective disability ratings, and the likelihood of incurring disability payments compared with nonsurgical treatment in a setting of work-related CTS.

The predictors of less favorable postsurgical outcomes are age over 70, severity of symptoms on presentation, subjective measures of upper extremity functional limitation prior to surgery, mental health status, alcohol use, and the involvement of an attorney or concurrent disability claims (where only ~20% may report being symptom free). Residual motor and sensory symptoms may occur in about 20–40% surgically treated individuals.

Counseling

Patients should be aware of the prognostic data. Work duty or environmental modifications should be advised in work-related CTS. Most of the patients treated conservatively may need surgical decompression in the future despite temporary relief, provided no contraindications exist. Delayed decompression may be associated with poorer postoperative outcomes. Surgical complications (~2–5% of patients) include transient injury to median nerve, incomplete sectioning of the transverse carpal ligament, surgical damage to the palmar cutaneous branch of the median nerve, scarring within the carpal tunnel, and CRPS. Endoscopic techniques appear to offer some advantage over conventional open techniques with regard to the patient's postoperative incision pain, preservation of grip strength, and time to return to work; however, these advantages may be potentially negated by the risk of injury to neurovascular structures and tendons. Surgical failure rate is about 2–5%, and surgical re-exploration may be required.

SUMMARY

- **CTS** is an entrapment neuropathy of the **median nerve within the carpal tunnel**. Other median nerve entrapment syndromes include **anterior interosseous syndrome, pronator teres syndrome**, and **ligament of Struthers entrapment**.
- Other causes of median mononeuropathy include **vasculitis, trauma, DM, infiltrative, infective**, and **demyelinating disorders**.
- Diagnosis requires a **good clinical history** and may be confirmed by **EMG/NCS**. The patient should be evaluated for **associative or causative factors**.
- Treatment consists of **conservative measures** (wrist-splints, NSAIDs, and local steroid injections) and **surgical decompression** (~2–5% failure rate).

- Conservative measures may result in **approximately 50%** improvement (usually short term). Long-term surgical improvement may occur in **up to 75%** of patients. Residual deficits occurs in **approximately 20–40%** of patients.
- **Litigation or disability claims** may adversely reduce subjective assessment of treatment outcomes.

CASE 2

A 59-year-old overweight man complained of a 6-month history of progressive low back pain and weakness in the left foot. He described a dull backache with "electric-shock" radiation down to his leg and a tingling sensation affecting the dorsum and sole of the foot, as well as the lateral ankle. Lifting his foot up while walking was problematic. On examination, there was MRC 3/5 weakness in the left toe and ankle dorsi- and plantarflexors, and 4/5 weakness in the left knee flexors and hip abductors. Sensory examination revealed reduced pinprick sensation affecting the left foot, lateral ankle, and calf. The left ankle jerk was diminished compared to the right.

Localization

Weakness of the toe dorsi- and plantarflexors, as well as hip abductors indicates L5–S1 nerve root involvement. Weakness in the ankle dorsiflexors indicates L4–L5, and ankle plantarflexors/knee flexors suggest S1–S2 nerve root involvement. The diminished left ankle jerk further supports S1 involvement. However, such lower motor neuron weakness may be the result of AHC disease, L5–S1 radiculopathies, lumbosacral plexopathy, or neuropathy (sciatic, peroneal, tibial, and superior gluteal). Sensory loss in a L5–S1 dermatomal distribution excludes AHC disease, and multiple mononeuropathies would be unlikely, especially given the history of radicular back pain. The most likely localization is the left L5 and S1 nerve roots. However, a lumbosacral plexopathy on the left cannot be completely excluded.

Differential Diagnosis

With the history of back pain and overweight body habitus, *lumbar disc degeneration with spondylosis at the L5–S1 and S1–S2 vertebral levels is most likely.* This disorder may cause nerve root impingement via *neuraformaminal or canal stenosis.* Acute disc herniation would be more common in patients younger than 40 years and occurs secondary to trauma. Other potential causes for compressive L5–S1 radiculopathies include *neoplasia* (bony metastases or primary nerve sheath tumor), *infection* (osteomyelitis, discitis, epidural abscess, etc.), *fracture* (e.g., vertebral compression or articular facet), or *spondylolisthesis* (relative movement of vertebral body over another).

Other differential diagnostic considerations for L5–S1 radiculopathies include *lumbosacral plexopathy* or *mononeuropathy multiplex* (asymmetric, stepwise progressive disorder of individual peripheral or cranial nerves secondary to vasculitis, DM, autoimmune disorders, infection, sarcoidosis, or multiple entrapments).

Investigations

Localizing the anatomic site and cause for the radiculopathy is important. Radiographs of the lumbar spine should be performed (if history is suggestive of trauma, infection, or bony neoplasia) as a screening tool. MRI of the lumbar spine without gadolinium is the best test in evaluating for lumbosacral spondylosis and disc degeneration. CT myelography should be used if MRI is not available or is contraindicated. EMG/NCS is useful in differentiating a lumbosacral radiculopathy from plexopathy or neuropathy (sensory nerve action potentials [SNAPs] are preserved in radiculopathies) and may show more widespread muscle involvement than deduced clinically. EMG may further confirm active or chronic nerve root compression.

Management

There are conservative and surgical modalities utilized in the management of patients with lumbosacral radiculopathy. Back-strengthening exercises (performed within limits of patient tolerance through physical therapy), active rehabilitation for muscle weakness, weight reduction, and analgesia (NSAIDs, TCAs, AEDs, or local epidural corticosteroid injections) may be employed initially. Failure to demonstrate adequate radicular pain relief despite conservative therapy for 6–8 weeks, progressive or severe neurological (motor) deficit or traumatic injury, infection, or neoplasia are possible indications for surgery. Lack of objective findings on neurological examination or unidentified nerve root impingement on radiological evaluation should be contraindications for surgery.

Prognosis

Patients with lumbosacral disc degeneration and spondylosis may report improvement in 25–35%, approximately 40% remain unchanged and approximately 30–35% deteriorate despite conservative or surgical measures. In fact, there are no controlled studies supporting the effectiveness of any form of surgical decompression or fusion for degenerative lumbar spondylosis compared with natural history, placebo, or conservative treatment.

With acute disc herniation, neuropathic pain may be relieved surgically in about 80–90% of patients initially, with 1 year outcomes being similar to nonsurgical treatment. In patients with clinical worsening after surgery ("failed back pain syndrome"), possible explanations include surgery at the wrong level, incomplete removal of extruded disc fragments or other compressive material, progression in spinal degeneration, postoperative arachnoiditis, and psychosocial factors that may affect recovery. In cases of lumbosacral radiculopathy associated with other causes, the underlying medical condition could also influence outcomes.

Counseling

Patients should be aware of the outcome data and lack of convincing epidemiological evidence for either conservative or surgical interventions, although particular individuals may respond to different therapeutic modalities. Patients should be encouraged, however, as a multimodal approach may assist with symptomatic relief and enable the patient maintain an adequate functional status. Raising patient expectations, such as promising a potential cure, may be counterproductive. In severely disabled individuals, chronic pain management via specialized services, supportive care, braces, and walking aids may be required.

SUMMARY

- **Degenerative lumbar spondylosis** affects the L4–5 and L5–S1 vertebral levels in **more than 90%** of cases.
- Differential diagnoses for L5–S1 radiculopathies include **lumbosacral plexopathy** and **mononeuropathy multiplex**. Other causes of lumbar nerve root compression include **acute disc herniation, neoplasm, infection, fracture,** or **spondylolisthesis**.
- **Radiographs** are helpful screening tools if **trauma, infection,** or **neoplasms** are suspected. **MRI of the lumbar spine** establishes diagnosis. CT myelograms may be used as a substitute.
- **EMG/NCS** may help exclude plexopathy/neuropathy and provide some evidence for active/chronic/widespread muscle involvement.
- Treatment includes **conservative** (back-strengthening exercises, active rehabilitation for muscle weakness, weight reduction, and analgesia) and **surgical** modalities.
- Indications for surgery include **severe pain** refractory to conservative therapy for 6–8 weeks, **progressive or severe neurological (motor) deficit,** or **traumatic injury, infection, or neoplasia**.
- Contraindications include **lack of objective neurological deficit** clinically or **structural lesion** on radiological evaluation.
- Outcomes are as follow: **25–35%** improve, **approximately 40%** remain stable, and **approximately 30–35%** worsen with conservative/surgical treatments.
- **No scientific evidence** exists supporting the effectiveness of **surgery** for lumbar degenerative spondylosis compared with **natural history, placebo, or conservative treatment**.
- Patients should be aware of outcome data and actively encouraged during therapy.

CASE 3

A 36-year-old woman developed severe pain around the left shoulder and upper arm 5–6 weeks ago. The pain lasted 2 weeks then improved and was described as an intense, sharp pain. For about 3 weeks, the patient complained of progressive difficulty elevating her left arm and lifting objects with relatively preserved grip. On examination, there was weakness and mild atrophy in shoulder abduction, external rotation, and elbow flexion with scapular winging on the left. Sensory examination revealed mild reduction in pinprick affecting the lateral arm and forearm. Reflex examination showed absent left biceps and brachioradialis responses only.

Localization

Pain localized to the left shoulder and upper arm could be secondary to neurological or musculoskeletal disease. The sensory examination supports dysfunction in the C5–C6 dermatomes, which could indicate pathology in the C5–C6 nerve roots, upper trunk, or lateral and posterior cords of brachial plexus or multiple peripheral nerves (axillary, lateral cutaneous nerves of the arm and forearm) on the left. There is also evidence of lower motor neuron weakness in C5–C6 innervated muscles, but this may also implicate AHC, nerve roots, brachial plexus, or multiple nerves (axillary, radial, musculocutaneous, and long thoracic nerve). There is no apparent history of neck pain, so the most likely localization is the upper trunk of the left brachial plexus. However, the absence of neck pain or radicular symptoms does not completely exclude a left C5–C6 radiculopathy.

Differential Diagnosis

The most likely diagnosis is *upper trunk brachial plexopathy.* This is an anatomical diagnosis with several etiologies. Possible etiologies include *idiopathic* (may be *autoimmune* or rarely inherited as a *hereditary neuralgic amyotrophy*: onset usually in first decade, is associated with dysmorphic features and recurrent bouts or hereditary neuropathy with liability to pressure palsies [HNPP]), *traumatic* (direct injury: heavy impact or traction, indirect from bony injury in the neck region or iatrogenic from nerve blocks), *neoplastic* (usually associated with severe pain; primary tumor rare, metastatic disease more common, with predilection for lower brachial plexus), and *radiation-induced* (usually painless, has predilection for upper plexus and could occur months to years after radiation therapy).

With lower trunk brachial plexopathies, *neurogenic thoracic outlet syndrome* (compression of lower trunk, especially T1 fibers, by fibrous band from a rudimentary cervical rib to the scalene tubercle of the first thoracic rib) is another diagnostic consideration. The main differential diagnosis for upper trunk brachial plexopathy is *C5–C6 radiculopathy.*

Investigation

EMG/NCS would be helpful in distinguishing between an upper trunk brachial plexopathy and upper cervical radiculopathy. Preservation of median and radial SNAPs support a radiculopathy. Needle examination may show the extent of motor involvement, and paraspinal muscle involvement is not expected in brachial plexopathy. Myokymic discharges would be expected in radiation-induced plexopathy. If neoplastic plexopathy were considered, CT/MRI of the brachial plexus would be useful in addition to the cancer evaluation, which may include CT-guided biopsy. In traumatic or compressive plexopathy, plain radiographs of the shoulder and neck region would demonstrate bony injury or cervical rib respectively. In hereditary forms, genetic testing could be performed (e.g., deletion in PMP-22 gene on chromosome 17p in HNPP).

Management

Therapy for idiopathic acquired brachial plexopathy consists of pharmacological and nonpharmacological measures. Analgesia is required to control severe pain, and short-term opiate narcotics may be used. There is no concrete evidence that a short course (7–10 days) of corticosteroids influence outcomes, although this may be beneficial in a small number of patients. Nonpharmacological measures include arm immobilization in a sling to minimize pain, physical therapy for muscle weakness, and range of motion exercises to prevent contractures. In severely affected individuals, orthotic devices should be provided to facilitate activities of daily living. For other etiologies, treatment of the underlying cause (i.e., surgical reconstruction in trauma, chemotherapy with neoplasms) is paramount.

Prognosis

Idiopathic brachial plexopathy is usually a monophasic illness that has a benign prognosis. About 60–70% of patients report some degree of improvement within the first month of illness. About 40% of patients report complete recovery by 1 year, approximately 75% by 2 years, and approximately 90% by 3 years. Residual motor and sensory deficits that may not affect daily functioning could persist indefinitely. Predictors of a prolonged course include persistence of severe pain and lack of clinical improvement during the first 3 months of illness. Prognosis for other causes of brachial plexopathy is dependent on the underlying cause, with neoplastic brachial plexopathy being associated with poor outcomes. Supraclavicular traumatic brachial plexopathies are more severe and have a worse prognosis in comparison to infraclavicular lesions. Recovery would be more complete and occur at a faster rate with predominantly compressive (i.e., demyelinating) plexopathies.

SUMMARY

- **Upper trunk brachial plexopathy** may be **idiopathic** (autoimmune or hereditary), secondary to **trauma, neoplasm**, or **radiation-induced**.
- The differential diagnosis is **C5–C6 radiculopathy**.
- Diagnosis is established by **EMG/NCS**. Further studies may be required to decipher potential etiologies.
- Treatment consists of **pharmacological** (analgesia for acute pain) and **nonpharmacological** (physical therapy, immobilization, orthotics) modalities.
- In idiopathic acquired brachial plexopathy, **approximately 60–70%** of patients show improvement within the **first month** of illness, **approximately 40%** recover by **1 year, approximately 75%** by **2 years**, and **approximately 90%** by **3 years** after onset.
- Prolonged course may occur if there is **persistence of severe pain** and **lack of clinical improvement** during the first **3 months** of illness.
- Underlying etiologies influence prognosis of brachial plexopathy: **neoplastic plexopathy** is associated with poor outcomes, and **supraclavicular traumatic plexopathies** are more severe and result in worse prognosis than infraclavicular lesions.
- Compressive plexopathies result in **faster and more complete** recovery.

CASE 4

A 62-year-old man presented to the office complaining of burning pains affecting his feet for several months. He stated that these seemed worse at night and his legs felt numb. More recently, he had noticed some parasthesias in his fingertips and weakness in his toes. On examination, there was a symmetrical distal glove and stocking distribution sensory loss to pinprick, light touch, and vibration sense. Motor examination showed atrophy and mild weakness in the foot intrinsic muscles bilaterally. Ankle jerks were absent bilaterally. There was mild truncal ataxia that was present with eye closure only.

Localization

Symmetrical distal sensory loss to multiple modalities involving the hands and feet suggests bilateral sensory nerve dysfunction (median, radial, and ulnar nerves in the hands, saphenous, superficial and deep peroneal, and sural nerves in the feet) that includes both large, myelinated and small, unmyelinated fibers. Sensory ataxia suggests dysfunction in proprioception. However, bilateral cervical and lumbosacral radiculopathies (C6–C8 and L4–S1) or plexopathies are also possible. Lower motor neuron weakness in the foot intrinsics could also represent peripheral motor nerve dysfunction (medial and lateral plantar, tibial, and peroneal nerves), AHC disease, L5–S1 radiculopathy, lumbosacral plexopathy, distal myopathy, or disorder of neuromuscular transmission (unlikely, usually proximal muscles are involved initially). The most likely localization is peripheral nerve, although bilateral cervical and lumbosacral nerve root or plexus lesions are possible.

Differential Diagnosis

The most likely diagnosis is *sensorimotor polyneuropathy*, which could be predominantly *axonal* or *demyelinating* (early generalized reflex loss and milder atrophy expected). Etiologies include *toxin exposures* (recreational, environmental, nutritional, or heavy metals), *metabolic disorders* (DM, renal/thyroid/liver disease), *nutritional deficiencies* (vitamins B_1, B_6, B_{12}: associated with dorsal column and corticospinal tract dysfunction [*see* pp. 139–141], vitamin E, folate), *medications* (isoniazid, chemotherapeutic drugs: cisplatin, vincristine, phenytoin, colchicine, anti-HIV retroviral drugs), *autoimmune/inflammatory disorders* (chronic inflammatory demyelinating polyradiculoneuropathy [CIDP], vasculitis: primary or secondary, associated with CTDs; sarcoidosis, cryoglobulinemia), *infections* (e.g., leprosy: most common neuropathy worldwide, HIV, HTLV, Lyme disease), and *paraneoplastic disorders* (e.g., sensory neuronopathy with small-cell lung cancer [SCLC]).

Other etiologies include *paraproteinemic/dysproteinemic disorders* (associated with monoclonal proteins that may have anti-myelin-associated glycoprotein [MAG] or anti-sulfonated glucuronyl paragloboside [SGPG] activity, e.g., multiple myeloma), *amyloidosis* (primary, secondary or hereditary), *hereditary disorders* (HMSN, hereditary sensory and autonomic neuropathy [HSAN], porphyria, Fabry's disease, mitochondrial cytopathies: neuropathy, ataxia, and retinitis pigmentosa [NARP], MELAS, myoclonic epilepsy with ragged red fibers [MERRF]; leukodystrophies, e.g., metachromatic leukodystrophy, adrenomyeloneuropathy: would also expect CNS disease as well as neuropathy), and *idiopathic* (may represent ~25% of all neuropathies).

The differential diagnoses for a length-dependent sensorimotor polyneuropathy include *bilateral cervical and lumbosacral radiculopathies* (C6–C8 and L4–S1 nerve roots) and *brachial/lumbosacral plexopathies*.

Investigations

Investigations should be tailored toward potential etiologies based on the clinical history and associated signs. A general screen may include comprehensive metabolic profile, TFT, oral glucose tolerance test, HbA_{1c}, vitamin B_{12} (if 200–350 pg/mL with high clinical suspicion, check methylmalonic acid levels: *see* p. 140), serum/RBC folate, ESR, ANA profile, serum and urine electrophoresis, and immunofixation (paraproteinemia requires further work-up to exclude a myelomatous neoplasm).

Other tests to consider include urine heavy metals and toxicology screen, porphyria screen (urine and blood), cryoglobulins, HIV titers, ACE levels, Lyme IgM and IgG, anti-MAG/SGPG antibodies, anti-Hu (if present, would need to evaluate for SCLC), and genetic tests for hereditary neuropathies, as dictated by clinical history. EMG/NCS would be useful to decipher if the neuropathy is primarily axonal or demyelinating, as well as the pattern of involvement, as these features would guide diagnostic investigations. LP should be performed if CIDP is suspected. If a potentially treatable neuropathy is suspected (e.g., vasculitis, CIDP, leprosy), nerve biopsy (commonly sural) should be performed.

Management

If a potentially treatable neuropathy or specific etiology is defined, appropriate therapy should be instituted (e.g., glucose control in diabetes, immunosuppressants for vasculitis, IVIg/TPE or immunosuppresants for CIDP, antibiotics for Lyme disease/leprosy, vitamin supplementation for deficiencies, cessation of offending drug or toxin exposure). The general principles of care involve symptomatic therapy for neuropathic pain and supportive therapy for the consequences of neuropathy.

Oral analgesics used include TCAs (e.g., amitriptyline, desipramine, nortriptyline), AEDs (e.g., gabapentin, clonazepam, carbamazepine), opiates (in combination with acetaminophen or alone, e.g., oxycodone, MS contin), or antiarrhythmics (e.g., flecainide, mexilitine). Topical agents (e.g., capsaicin, lidocaine) may be used in conjunction with oral agents. Adequate analgesic trial should involve therapeutic dosages and last about 6–8 weeks.

Supportive therapy may include physical therapy to improve or maintain functional status, for gait training, and to prevent contractures, occupational therapy to facilitate self-reliance by maintaining activities of daily living (ADLs), assist devices, ankle-foot orthosis for foot drop, regular foot examination, and the use of properly cushioned shoes to prevent pressure sores. In severely affected patients, ambulation may require the assistance of walking aids or electric wheelchair in nonambulatory patients. In chronic neuropathies (including hereditary neuropathies), orthopedic evaluation and surgery may be required for hammertoes and high-arched foot deformities.

Prognosis

Outcomes are dependent on the underlying cause. In general, peripheral neuropathies are chronically progressive with more proximal involvement and disability expected with time. Symptomatic therapy does not alter the natural history. Treating the underlying cause may slow progression (e.g., diabetic neuropathy), facilitate recovery (e.g., renal transplantation for uremic neuropathy), or have no effect (amyloid neuropathy associated with osteolytic multiple myeloma). Recovery over several months to years is generally expected in adequately treated autoimmune/inflammatory, infectious, or toxic neuropathies, although deficits may persist.

In CIDP, about 70–95% of patients show initial improvement with immunosuppression, with partial or complete remission occurring in about 40–50%, and 50% relapse rate after 4 years of follow-up. Recovery with no or mild-moderate deficits allowing ambulation and employment may be seen in 60–70% of CIDP patients, with approximately 25–30% with severe deficits causing confinement and approximately 10–15% dead due to the disease over mean follow-up of 7.5 years. Anti-MAG neuropathies are usually resistant to immunomodulating therapy.

Counseling

Patients should be aware of the disease chronicity and prognostic data should be tailored toward underlying cause. The fact that 25% of patients with peripheral neuropathy have an unknown cause should be emphasized. An aggressive etiological search for demyelinating neuropathies should be advised because of relatively limited causes and potential for treatment. Genetic counseling should be offered to patients with hereditary neuropathy. Patients should realize that symptomatic and supportive therapies do not alter the natural history of peripheral neuropathies, but may maintain functional status for longer periods of time. Analgesia should be discussed and offered to patients. Patients should be encouraged to undergo an adequate therapeutic trial. In refractory pain patients, referral to a pain specialist for more complex pharmacological and nonpharmacological therapies (biofeedback, relaxation, and hydrotherapy, etc.) would be advisable.

SUMMARY

- **Sensorimotor polyneuropathy** may occur secondary to **toxin exposures, metabolic disorders, nutritional deficiencies, medications, autoimmune/inflammatory, infectious, paraneoplastic, dysproteinemic, amyloid**, and **hereditary disorders** and may be **idiopathic in approximately 25% of patients**.
- Differential diagnosis includes **bilateral cervical and lumbosacral radiculopathies or plexopathies**.
- Laboratory investigations should be tailored toward potential etiologies based on **clinical history, physical signs**, and **EMG/NCS** (axonal or demyelinating) findings.
- Treatment consists of **symptomatic** (analgesic) and **supportive** measures. An adequate analgesic trial should involve **therapeutic drug dosages for about 6–8 weeks**. Supportive measures aid to **maintain or improve functional status** and **limit disability**.
- Prognosis is dependent on the **cause** of the polyneuropathy. Symptomatic and supportive treatments **do not alter** the natural history of the disease.
- Patients should be aware of **disease chronicity**.

CASE 5

A 41-year-old man comes to the clinic complaining of slowly progressive parasthesias that affected his feet, then hands for over 3 months. About 4 weeks ago, he noticed difficulty maintaining his balance, especially with his eyes closed and difficulty walking because of stiffness in his lower extremities. Neurological examination showed MRC 4/5 weakness in hip and knee flexors and ankle dorsiflexion with mild spastic hypertonia bilaterally. Sensory examination demonstrated absent proprioception and vibration in the toes and ankles with reduced pinprick sensation in a stocking and glove distribution bilaterally. Ankle jerks were absent with 3+ reflexes proximally and bilateral extensor plantar responses. Romberg's sign was present.

Localization

Mild weakness affecting the flexor muscles of the lower extremities associated with spastic hypertonia and hyperreflexia is indicative of upper motor neuron lesions affecting the descending corticospinal tracts bilaterally (mesial frontal cortex, cerebral peduncles, basis pontis, medullary pyramids, or ventrolateral spinal cord above L2). Absent proprioception and vibration in the toes and feet (with sensory ataxia demonstrated by Romberg's sign) implies a large fiber sensory neuropathy, lumbosacral plexopathy, dorsal root ganglionopathy, L5–S1 radiculopathy, or dorsal column spinal cord dysfunction at or above the L5–S1 spinal level.

Parasthesias with reduced pinprick in a glove and stocking distribution are most suggestive of a small fiber polyneuropathy, but may localize to bilateral brachial and lumbosacral plexi, sensory neurons (dorsal root ganglions), or bilateral C6–C8 and L5–S1 nerve roots. In summary, the underlying process most likely localizes to the posterior and ventrolateral aspects of the spinal cord above the L2 spinal level, with an associated length-dependent polyneuropathy that predominantly affects sensory nerves.

Differential Diagnosis

The most likely diagnosis for a progressive myeloneuropathy affecting the dorsal columns, corticospinal tracts, and sensory nerves is *vitamin B$_{12}$ deficiency*. This usually due to reduced GI absorption secondary to diminished intrinsic factor production by gastric parietal cells. Dietary insufficiency in strict vegetarians is rare. Pernicious anemia, the hematological manifestation of this disorder, may be absent on neurological presentation.

Other differentials include *vitamin E deficiency (see p. 158), folate deficiency* (rare and clinically indistinguishable from vitamin B$_{12}$ deficiency: would expect low folate, normal methylmalonic acid [MMA] and elevated homocysteine levels), *nitrous oxide intoxication* (occurs ~2–6 weeks after heavy exposure or following general anesthesia in vitamin B$_{12}$-deficient patients), *neurosyphilis (tabes dorsalis)*,

adrenomyeloneuropathy (adult adrenoleukodystrophy [ALD]; *see* pp. 242–246),
HIV/AIDS (vacuolar myelopathy with painful sensory neuropathy), and *hereditary
spastic paraparesis* (HSP; would expect family history; usually AD inheritance, and
can be divided into two forms: *pure form* with only lower extremity spasticity or
complicated form, e.g., optic neuropathy, deafness, ataxia, peripheral neuropathy,
dementia, movement disorder, autoimmune microcytic hemolytic anemia).

Investigations

Laboratory tests should include CBC with differential, comprehensive metabolic panel, fasting glucose, and serum vitamin B_{12}, folate, and vitamin E levels.
Vitamin B_{12} levels less than 200 pg/mL are diagnostic. If levels are between 200
and 350, MMA and homocysteine should be elevated to confirm the diagnosis.
Schilling's test would be useful to confirm GI malabsorption. In equivocal cases,
additional tests such as RPR, FTA-ABS for syphilis, very-long chain fatty acids
[VLCFA] for adult ALD, HIV titers, or genetic tests for spastin in HSP may be
required. EMG/NCS should be considered to demonstrate an axonal sensory or
sensorimotor polyneuropathy. MRI of the cervical and thoracic spine with
gadolinium may show enhancement in the posterior and lateral columns or cord
edema. Symptoms and signs of vitamin B_{12} deficiency may precede MRI signal
changes by 2 weeks. The MRI features are most prominent 3–5 months after disease onset and normalize within 2–3 months of treatment initiation.

Management

Intramuscular injections of vitamin B_{12} are the mainstay of therapy. Replacement therapy provides much more than the daily requirement of 1 μg. Regimens
include 1000 μg i.m. two times a week for 2 weeks, followed by 1000 μg every
month for life or 1000 μg i.m. every day for 1 weeks, then every week for 4 weeks
and then monthly for life. There is no evidence that high doses speed neurological
recovery or cause known adverse effects. Supportive care (e.g., analgesia for neuropathic pain) with antispasticity agents should be provided as needed.

Prognosis

Early recognition and treatment is important because clinical remission is
inversely related to the duration between disease onset and initiation of replacement therapy. With adequate therapy, partial to near complete recovery is expected
within 6–12 months. Myelopathy is most resistant to therapy. A clinical relapse in
vitamin B_{12} deficiency may take 5 years to be recognized following interruption of
replacement therapy because of large body stores in the liver (1–10 mg).

Counseling

Patients should be aware of the potential complications of vitamin B_{12} deficiency:
pernicious anemia, delirium, dementia, psychiatric disturbances, myelopathy, and
peripheral neuropathy. Patients should be encouraged to receive monthly replacement

therapy for life because of the potential reversibility of this disorder and to prevent further neurological or hematological progression.

SUMMARY

- **Vitamin B$_{12}$ deficiency** is a potentially reversible cause of progressive myeloneuropathy. Other causes include **vitamin E deficiency, folate deficiency, nitrous oxide intoxication, neurosyphilis, adult ALD, HIV/AIDS,** and **HSP.**
- Diagnosis is established via reduced serum levels. If levels are 200–350 pg/mL, **MMA** and **homocysteine** levels should be checked. **MRI** may show signal changes (**enhancement/edema**). EMG/NCS shows **axonal neuropathy**.
- Treatment consists of **lifelong i.m. vitamin B$_{12}$ replacement**.
- Prognosis is generally **favorable**, with clinical improvement expected within **6–12 months** of initiating therapy.

CASE 6

A 36-year-old woman noticed sudden weakness of the right side of her face associated with right ear pain. She came to the clinic for evaluation because of progression over the last 48 hours. She also experienced intolerance of loud noises in her right ear and a dry right eye. On examination, there was moderate right facial weakness that was worse in the upper face with less involvement of the lower face and buccal region. The corneal reflex was absent on the right and an upward and outward motion of the eye was seen on attempted right eye closure.

Localization

Right facial weakness without any other cranial nerve findings implies right CN VII dysfunction. Hyperacusis (due to reduced sound dampening by stapedius), reduced lacrimation (reduced parasympathetic supply to lacrimal glands), absent corneal reflex (efferent limb is mediated by CN VII supplying orbicularis oculi), and retroauricular pain (referred otalgia) further support a CN VII lesion. This may localize to the ipsilateral CN VII nucleus in the pons or along its intracranial course (internal auditory canal [IAC] to geniculate ganglion) proximal to or at the branch to stapedius muscle. The absence of ipsilateral CN VI paresis or contralateral hemiparesis makes a pontine lesion less likely. In summary, the underlying process localizes to the right CN VII.

Differential Diagnosis

The most likely diagnosis for an ipsilateral CN VII palsy of sudden onset with maximum deficit within 2–3 days is *Bell's palsy.* This is an idiopathic, infranuclear facial nerve palsy and is the most common cause for an acquired, nontraumatic CN VII lesion. Some authorities believe that this disorder may be secondary to herpes simplex infection (controversial).

Other causes of unilateral CN VII palsy include *trauma* (basilar skull fracture or secondary to sphenoidal electrode placement for video EEG), *infections* (Lyme disease, leprosy, VZV: affects geniculate ganglion causing Ramsay–Hunt syndrome with pain and vesicles in the external auditory canal or soft palate), *ischemia* (hypertension or diabetes, especially in the elderly), *sarcoidosis, neoplasm* (usually slowly progressive; secondary to tumor infiltration into nerve as seen with metastatic disease or leukemia or direct extrinsic compression, e.g., vestibular schwannoma or parotid tumor), and *GBS* (usually facial diplegia is present).

Investigations

Clinical evaluation is the mainstay of diagnosis. CBC with differential and comprehensive metabolic panel should be performed to screen for potential causes. PT/PTT/INR should be checked before LP. LP may be considered as part of the work-up for the first episode, especially if a more systemic illness co-exists, or following the first recurrence. MRI of the head with gadolinium may show contrast enhancement of the affected CN VII. EMG/NCS with blink responses should be performed 2–3 weeks after disease onset to establish the degree of axonal loss. In some clinical studies, transcranial magnetic stimulation has been used to determine early facial nerve integrity following trauma.

Management

Pharmacotherapy for Bell's palsy is controversial. Some authorities advocate 5–7 days therapy with acyclovir (400 mg p.o. five times a day) and oral high-dose corticosteroids (e.g., prednisone 40–60 mg p.o. every day), sighting earlier and increased frequency of recovery when compared to no treatment based on limited retrospective or small randomized controlled studies. Meta-analyses and large population observational studies do not support improved outcomes with medical therapy over nontreatment in Bell's palsy (i.e., its natural history). For secondary causes of unilateral CN VII palsy, the underlying condition should be identified and treated appropriately.

Prognosis

The prognosis is generally favorable in Bell's palsy. Approximately 80–85% of patients completely recover within 3 months of disease onset with severe residual deficits occurring in only about 5%. Prognosis is better if the maximal deficit is partial (~95–100% recovery at 3 months), but worse with Ramsay–Hunt syndrome or severe axonal loss on EMG/NCS (this also increases likelihood of aberrant reinnervation). Complications of CN VII palsy are secondary to aberrant reinnervation: "crocodile tears" (lacrimation while eating), or facial synkinesis (e.g., contraction of orbicularis oculi or frontalis while chewing). Recurrence may occur in 7–10% of patients with Bell's palsy. Predisposing medical conditions include VZV infection, Lyme disease, and sarcoidosis. With increasing number of recurrences, the risk for permanent facial paralysis increases.

Counseling

Prognostic data and information on the patient's chances for complete recovery based on clinical presentation and EMG/NCS findings should be discussed. Patients should also be aware of the controversies surrounding medical treatment of this disorder and allowed to make an informed decision. The risk of recurrence of Bell's palsy should be mentioned, emphasizing that it and may occur many years after the initial episode. Female patients should be informed of an increased incidence of this disorder during pregnancy.

SUMMARY

- **Bell's palsy** is an **idiopathic** infranuclear facial nerve palsy.
- Bell's palsy is the **most common** cause for an acquired, nontraumatic CN VII lesion.
- Other causes include **trauma, infection, ischemia, sarcoidosis, neoplasm**, and **GBS**.
- Diagnosis is made **clinically**. LP and MRI of the head may be performed. EMG/NCS **2–3 weeks** after onset determines severity and aids in prognostication.
- Treatment is **controversial** for Bell's palsy. Options include **acyclovir with corticosteroids** or **no treatment**.
- **Approximately 80–85%** of patients completely recover within **3 months** of disease onset with severe residual deficits occurring in **about 5%**.
- **Partial maximal deficits** predict favorable outcomes, whereas **Ramsay–Hunt syndrome** or **severe axonal loss** on EMG/NCS predict worse outcomes.
- Complications are secondary to **aberrant reinnervation**.
- Recurrences occur in **7–10%** of patients; risks include **VZV infection, Lyme disease**, and **sarcoidosis**.

CASE 7

A 28-year-old woman complained of slowly progressive, difficulty climbing stairs for about 2 months. Over the last 4 weeks, she had also noticed some difficulty lifting her hands above her head, requiring more time for grooming and feeding. On examination, there was MRC 4/5 weakness in shoulder abduction, shoulder and elbow flexion, shoulder and elbow extension, and external rotation of the shoulders bilaterally. Similar weakness was also noticed in the hip flexors, extensors, abductors, and adductors bilaterally. Multimodal sensory examination and reflexes were normal.

Localization

The clinical history and physical examination support bilateral proximal muscle weakness. In general, muscle weakness could be secondary to central (corticospinal tract), AHC, nerve root, plexus, peripheral nerve, and NMJ or muscle disease. Normal reflexes would make central causes unlikely, and a normal sensory examination would make NMJ or muscle disease more likely, although pure motor neuropathies rarely exist. The distribution of muscle involvement includes bilateral C5–C8 myotomes in the upper extremities and L2–S2 myotomes in the lower extremities. However, the pattern of subacute proximal muscle involvement without other clinical features suggests that the pathological process most likely localizes to muscle.

Differential Diagnosis

The most likely diagnosis for a subacute proximal myopathy in this age group would be *inflammatory myopathy*. *Polymyositis* is more likely based on the history. This could be primary or secondary to mixed-connective tissue disease or sarcoidosis. *Dermatomyositis* would have expected characteristic heliotropic or diffuse rash. *Inclusion body myositis* is a neurodegenerative disease more commonly seen in patients over the age of 50 with significant forearm flexor and quadriceps involvement, however, an *hereditary inclusion body myopathy* may occur during early adulthood with relative quadriceps sparing. *Infectious myositis* (e.g., viral: HIV, HTLV, coxsackie, echoviruses, parainfluenza; bacterial: *S. aureus*, or Gram-negative pyomyositis; or parasitic: cysticercosis, trichinosis) is a consideration; a prodromal syndrome and other systemic features would be expected.

Other differentials include *muscular dystrophy* (family history very important: e.g., limb-girdle muscular dystrophy: usually slowly progressive; proximal myotonic myopathy: would require myotonia; oculopharyngeal muscular dystrophy: starts with ocular palsies and ptosis with subsequent dysphagia), *toxic myopathies* (e.g., drug-induced such as from cholesterol-lowering agents, colchicine, steroids, alcohol, chloroquine, azidothymidine [AZT], phencyclidine: history of exposure required), *endocrine myopathies* (e.g., hypo- or hyperthyroidism, Cushing's disease: other features of endocrinopathy expected), *mitochondrial myopathies* (e.g., MELAS, MERRF, Kearns–Sayre syndrome [KSS]: other clinical features, e.g., strokes, seizures, hearing loss, chronic progressive external ophthalmoplegia [CPEO] expected), and *metabolic myopathies* (would expect exercise-induced symptoms and myoglobinuria without fixed weakness, e.g., lipid metabolism: carnitine palmitoyltransferase [CPT]-I and II, carnitine deficiencies; carbohydrate metabolism: myophosphorylase, phosphofructokinase deficiencies).

Further diagnostic considerations include *channelopathies* (e.g., sodium channel: hyperkalemic periodic paralysis, paramyotonia congenita; chloride channel: myotonia congenita; calcium channel: hypokalemic periodic paralysis. Attacks of weakness precipitated by external factors, e.g., cold, dietary intake, exercise; fixed weakness uncommon), *NMJ disorders* (would cause fatigable weakness, e.g., myasthenia gravis: would expect ocular findings, LEMS: would expect dysautonomic features such as dry mouth or blurred vision, for example), *motor neuropathy* (e.g., multifocal motor neuropathy with or without conduction block: would expect distal muscle involvement as well), *polyradiculopathies* (e.g., CIDP: sensory features may be mild, but would expect deficits on examination), and *AHC disease* (e.g., adult SMA, progressive muscular atrophy: lower motor neuron variant of amytrophic lateral sclerosis [ALS]: fasciculations and early muscle atrophy expected).

Investigations

Laboratory investigations should include CK, ESR/CRP, ANA panel, and TFT. Other laboratory tests may include septic screen (CBC, blood cultures, etc., if infectious myopathy is suspected), electrolytes (if endocrine myopathy or channelopathy suspected), serum/urine toxicology, forearm exercise tests (if metabolic myopathy considered), genetic testing for inherited myopathies, anti-AChR and P/Q-type voltage-gated calcium channel [VGCC] antibodies (for MG and LEMS, respectively).

EMG/NCS should be performed to confirm myopathy (irritable, e.g., seen in inflammatory and necrotizing myopathies or nonirritable as seen in muscular dystrophies, endocrine myopathies) and may guide in muscle selection for biopsy. Other neuromuscular disorders can be excluded (e.g., channelopathies, NMJ disorders, polyradiculopathies, AHC disease). Muscle biopsy should be performed to diagnose the underlying process and is particularly useful in inflammatory, toxic, infectious, metabolic, and mitochondrial myopathies and muscular dystrophies.

Management

The mainstay of therapy for inflammatory myopathies is immunosuppresant therapy. Initial therapy involves the administration of corticosteroids, prednisone at 1–2 mg/kg/per day orally (maximum 100 mg per day) until clinical improvement, then slow taper. Steroid-sparing agents (e.g., azathioprine, cyclophosphamide, cyclosporine, or methotrexate) could be added if patients require high-dose steroids for long time courses, patients are steroid-refractory, or they exhibit poor responses, especially during relapse. Prophylactic measures, for example, salt restriction, regular glycemic checks, gastric ulcer, and osteoporosis prevention should be considered for patients requiring corticosteroids; regular CBC and LFT may be required for other immunosuppressants.

For recurrence or refractory cases, monthly IVIg (2 g/kg divided over 2–5 days) may be utilized for short- to medium-term benefit. Physical therapy should be initiated to improve/maintain functional status, for gait training, and to prevent contractures in severely affected individuals. With significant upper extremity involvement, occupational therapy and the use of orthotic devices should be considered.

Prognosis

The survival rate for inflammatory myopathies is approximately 95% at 1 year, approximately 92% at 5 years, and approximately 85–90% at 10 years. Death rate from the disease is highest in the first year and unlikely after about 8 years. Causes of death include cardiac and respiratory failure, intercurrent infection, and complications of therapy. Mortality rates in the pre-steroid era were about 65% at 5 years and 53% at 8 years. Inflammatory myopathies may demonstrate a pattern of early full remission in approximately 15%, monophasic and relapsing-remitting courses in approximately 20%, chronic progressive illness in 35%, with approximately 15% death rate after 20 years follow-up.

With immunosuppressant therapy, complete remission is expected in 40%, with about 43% expected to improve with mild residual deficits and about 17% of patients being refractory with clinical worsening. Predictors of clinical remission include younger age, and short duration of disease before treatment, whereas poor outcomes may be predicted by older age (>60 years), pulmonary/ esophageal involvement, and associated cancer. Drug-induced morbidity may also play a role in long-term outcomes.

Counseling

Patients should be aware that early immunosuppressant therapy improves outcomes, although there are no randomized controlled trials confirming the efficacy of corticosteroids in inflammatory myopathies. Patients should be made aware of the complications or adverse effects of drug therapy. Prognostic data should be discussed in detail. Neoplastic evaluation should be performed in patients older than 60 years with inflammatory myopathy (especially dermatomyositis), and inclusion body myositis should always be considered in this age group, especially in steroid-unresponsive cases. Patients with chronic progressive disease with functional limitations may need ambulatory aids, wheelchairs, or both to facilitate mobility and caregivers may be needed to assist with ADLs.

SUMMARY

- **Inflammatory myopathies** usually present with proximal muscle weakness, and include **polymyositis** and **dermatomyositis**.
- Differential diagnosis includes **infectious myositis, muscular dystrophy, toxic, endocrine, mitochondrial, metabolic myopathies, channelopathies, NMJ disorders, motor neuropathy**, and **AHC disorders**.
- Diagnosis requires **serum CK, EMG/NCS**, and **muscle biopsy**.
- Treatments include **immunosuppressants** such as high-dose **prednisone** with slow taper, **azathioprine, cyclophosphamide, cyclosporine, methotrexate**, and **IVIg every month. Physical** and **occupational therapy** may be required as well.
- **Approximately 95%** 1-year, **approximately 92%** 5-year, and **approximately 85–90%** 10-year survival expected. Causes of death include **cardiac/respiratory failure, intercurrent infection**, and **complications of therapy**.
- Predictors of poor outcomes include **older age, pulmonary/esophageal involvement**, and **cancer**.
- Complete remission expected in **approximately 40%, 43%** improve with mild residual deficits, and **17%** worsen clinically despite therapy.

CASE 8

A 64-year-old male smoker complained of progressive weakness in the lower extremities, dry mouth, blurred vision, and constipation for 4 weeks. He stated that he fatigued easily but felt stronger after brief exercise. On examination, vital signs were normal. There was MRC 4/5 strength in the hip flexors, extensors, and abductors bilaterally. Exercise for 10 seconds improved strength to normal, however, continued exercise for 1 minute caused MRC 3/5 weakness. Sensory examination was normal. Reflex testing showed reduced knee jerks bilaterally that normalized following brief exercise.

Localization

Proximal lower extremity weakness with diminished reflexes could localize to the lumbosacral AHC, L2–S2 nerve roots, lumbar and lumbosacral plexi, multiple peripheral nerves (femoral, inferior and superior gluteal nerves), NMJ, or pelvic girdle muscles. Fatigable weakness is highly suggestive of an NMJ disorder, whereas improvement in strength and reflexes with brief exercise suggests a presynaptic disorder. Pupillary abnormalities, hyposalivation, and constipation suggest parasympathetic nerve dysfunction in the brainstem (CN III, VII, IX, and X) and spinal cord (S2–S4). The most likely localization is a presynaptic disorder affecting the pelvic girdle muscles and parasympathetic nerves.

Differential Diagnosis

The most likely diagnosis is *Lambert–Eaton Myasthenic Syndrome* (LEMS), which is a presynaptic NMJ transmission disorder caused by antibodies against the P/Q-type VGCC. The current smoking history implies that LEMS could be a paraneoplastic disorder associated with SCLC. Paraneoplastic LEMS occurs in 50–70% of cases, whereas autoimmune LEMS may occur in 10–30% of affected patients.

Other differentials include other *NMJ disorders* such as *botulism* (would expect severe dysautonomia and may involve respiratory muscles); *MG* (would expect ocular motor palsies, no improvement with exercise or dysautonomia); *toxic envenomization* (snake, scorpion, spider bites: would expect acute presentation, systemic features, and history of exposure), *primary myopathies* including *inflammatory* (including inclusion body myositis), *toxic, endocrine,* and *infectious myopathies* (dysautonomia unusual), *polyradiculoneuropathies* (e.g., GBS, diphtheria: would expect acute presentation with ascending or descending weakness, sensory findings with hypo- or areflexia), and *AHC disorders* such as progressive muscular atrophy (lower motor neuron [LMN]-ALS), adult-onset SMA, X-linked spinobulbar atrophy (Kennedy's disease: would not expect constipation and pupillary abnormalities, sialorrhea may occur secondary to dysphagia).

Investigations

Antibodies to P/Q-type VGCC should be checked. These may be positive in approximately 75% of patients with paraneoplastic LEMS and approximately 50% of patients without autoimmune LEMS. Other laboratory tests for MG or myopathies (*see* pp. 38 and 145) may be performed in equivocal cases. Diagnosis is confirmed by EMG with RNS: >10% decrement in motor amplitudes on slow RNS at 2–3Hz, with >100% increment on fast RNS at 30–50 Hz or immediately after 10 seconds of maximum exercise (postexercise facilitation). EMG/NCS would also help exclude neuropathic disorders, irritable myopathies, and botulism (fibrillations common due to botulinum toxin-induced chemodenervation).

In paraneoplastic LEMS, cancer evaluation should be performed. Chest X-ray/CT chest may be required every 6–12 months for SCLC (may be diagnosed up to 5 years after LEMS). Bronchoscopy or more frequent CT chest (e.g., every 3 months for the first year) may be required in chronic smokers. Patient should be screened for other autoimmune disorders (e.g., Graves' disease, rheumatoid arthritis, SLE) if autoimmune LEMS suspected.

Management

The management of LEMS includes symptomatic and immunosuppressant therapies. Therapy should be individually tailored based on symptom severity, life expectancy, and underlying cause. Symptomatic therapies include *cholinesterase inhibitors* (pyridostigmine: side effects include diarrhea, increased salivation, nausea/vomiting), *guanidine* (increases ACh release: may cause bone marrow suppression, hepatorenal dysfunction, ataxia, and mood disorder) and *3,4-diamino-pyridine* (3,4-DAP: K^+ channel blocker at motor nerve terminals, causing depolarization and ACh release). 3,4-DAP is not available for general clinical use in the United States, but can be obtained on compassionate basis. It causes transient perioral and digital parasthesias, lightheadedness, and seizures at high doses. These agents may be combined (especially cholinesterase inhibitors and 3,4-DAP), limited by increased risk of side effects.

Immunosuppressant therapy including corticosteroids, azathioprine, and cyclosporine can be used chronically as in MG, but caution required with an underlying neoplasm. Short-term benefit in severe cases may be achieved with IVIg/PE, although responses are less favorable than in MG. Removal of the underlying tumor in paraneoplastic LEMS may be sufficient to facilitate remission. General supportive care for dysautonomia, inlcuding laxatives for constipation, liberal salt diet, mineralocorticoids, supportive stockings for orthostatic hypotension, and saline eye drops for dry eyes should be provided. Physical/occupational therapy is recommended to maintain or improve functional status.

Prognosis

Malignancy adversely affects prognosis in LEMS. In patients with SCLC, median survival is 10 months without LEMS and 17 months with LEMS. In LEMS patients without SCLC, mortality is approximately 15% after mean follow-up of about 10 years. Seventy-eight percent of survivors require chronic immunosuppressant therapy. Death is usually unrelated to LEMS, but complications of therapy may play a role in outcomes. Sustained remission occurs in about 45% of patients, 20% of whom do not require chronic immunosuppression. Transient relapses are associated with reduction in immunosuppressant doses. Remission is expected to occur within 3 years of initiating therapy in responsive patients. About 30% of patients are poorly mobile or nonambulatory despite adequate treatment.

Counseling

Patients should be aware of prognostic data and the need to aggressively search for an underlying neoplasm, especially SCLC. The chances of having paraneoplastic LEMS is reduced if a tumor is not discovered after aggressive evaluation within the first 2 years of symptoms. Drugs that may worsen NMJ muscle weakness (e.g., quinine, *d*-penicillamine, aminoglycoside antibiotics, neuromuscular blocking agents, β-blockers, calcium-channel blockers, Mg^{2+} salts) should be avoided. Systemic/febrile illness or hot environments may cause transient worsening of weakness in LEMS and these should be promptly treated and avoided respectively.

SUMMARY

- **LEMS** is a **presynaptic** disorder of NMJ transmission associated with antibodies to **P/Q-type VGCC**. It could be **paraneoplastic** or **autoimmune** in origin.
- Differentials include **NMJ disorders** (MG, botulism, toxin envenomization), **primary myopathies** (inflammatory, toxic, infectious, endocrine), **polyradiculopathies** (GBS, diphtheria), or **AHC disorders**.
- Diagnosis is via **antibodies to P/Q-type VGCC and EMG with RNS. Neoplastic evaluation** is required.
- Treatment includes **symptomatic, immunosuppressant**, and **supportive measures**. Responders remit **within 3 years** of initiating therapy.
- **Malignancy** (especially SCLC) influences mortality rates in LEMS.
- In non-SCLC patients, mortality is **about 15%**, sustained remission occurs in **45%** and **approximately 30%** have severe deficits despite therapy at **10 years. Approximately 80%** of survivors require chronic immunosuppression.

13

Movement Disorders

CASE 1

A 59-year-old man came to the clinic complaining of a tremor in his right hand for about a year. He stated that this seemed worse at rest. He had also noticed generalized slowness of movements over the last 3 months. On examination, there was a pill-rolling resting tremor on the right, with lead-pipe rigidity and bradykinesia in all extremities, worse on the right. He demonstrated a shuffling gait with a stooped posture and reduced arm swing. Further examination revealed expressionless facies and micrographia.

Localization

The clinical history is classic for parkinsonism, which indicates dysfunction of the substantia nigra in the midbrain or its central dopaminergic connections. The predominant symptoms on the right suggest that the left substantia nigra is more affected. Less often, parkinsonism may be secondary to striatal (caudate and putamen) or globus pallidal dysfunction, maintaining the same contralateral relationship to symptom presentation.

Differential Diagnosis

The most likely diagnosis is *Parkinson's disease* (PD, idiopathic parkinsonism). This is a neurodegenerative disorder affecting the dopaminergic neurons in the zona compacta of the substantia nigra. There are rare familial forms of this disease, inherited mainly in an autosomally dominant fashion. However, secondary causes of parkinsonism should be considered, and a history of drug/toxin exposure, trauma, and vascular disease should be excluded.

Other differentials include *neurodegenerative disorders* such as *diffuse Lewy body disease* (dementia, psychosis including hallucinations, mild parkinsonism with rare tremors, and neuroleptic sensitivity), *multiple systems atrophy* (MSA; parkinsonism with dysautonomia, cerebellar dysfunction, or pyramidal signs), *progressive supranuclear palsy* (PSP; supranuclear gaze palsies, axial dystonia, dysarthria/ dysphagia, tremor rare), *cortical-basal ganglionic degeneration*

From: *Neurology Oral Boards Review:*
A Concise and Systematic Approach to Clinical Practice
By: E. E. Ubogu © Humana Press Inc., Totowa, NJ

(CBGD; alien hand syndrome, pyramidal signs, action/postural tremor, cortical sensory loss, apraxia), *Pick's disease* (frontotemporal dementia, mild parkinsonism and more common in females), *Huntington's disease* (akinetic-rigid variant; classically causes chorea, dementia, and personality/behavioral changes), and *spinocerebellar ataxia* (e.g., Machado Joseph disease [spinocerebellar ataxia {SCA} 3]: earlier age of onset with slowly progressive parkinsonism and ataxia, ophthalmoplegia, muscle weakness, and bulbar dysfunction).

Potential etiologies for parkinsonism include *drugs* (such as dopamine receptor antagonists such as neuroleptics, dopamine depleters, lithium), *toxins* (manganese, methanol, ethanol, 1-methyl-4-phenyl-1,2,3,6-tetrahydropyridine [MPTP]), *vascular* (atherosclerotic: multi-infarct dementia, Biswanger's, hypertensive), *metabolic* (Wilson's disease, acquired hepatocerebral degeneration, lysosomal storage diseases, hypoparathyroidism), *post-anoxia* (low oxygen, carbon monoxide, cyanide exposure), *post-encephalitic* (viral encephalitis, encephalitis lethargica), *prion disease* (Creutzfeldt-Jakob disease [CJD], Gerstmann-Straussler disease [GSD]: early dementia and insomnia, pyramidal signs; seizures, myoclonus, and prominent hallucinations may occur in CJD), *head trauma* (e.g., punch-drunk syndrome in boxers), *neoplasm* (primary brain tumor/metastases), and *hydrocephalus* (acquired with normal or high pressure).

Investigations

The diagnosis is established clinically. There are no laboratory tests that diagnose PD. In atypical cases, laboratory tests may be useful in excluding parkinsonism secondary to identifiable causes. Such tests may include LFT, Ca^{2+}, PO_4^{3-}, and parathyroid hormone (PTH) levels, urine/serum toxicology including heavy metal screen, copper (Cu^{2+}) and ceruloplasmin, and ABG. Neuroimaging (MRI of the brain) would help exclude vascular, post-anoxic, neoplastic, and hydrocephalic etiologies in equivocal cases or if supportive history exists. MRI may also demonstrate patterns of degeneration seen in secondary parkinsonism (e.g., ponto-medullary and cerebellar atrophy in olivo-pontine cerebellar atrophy [OPCA], midbrain/pontine atrophy in PSP, asymmetrical parietal lobe atrophy in CBGD, or frontotemporal atrophy in Pick's disease).

Management

PD treatment is symptomatic and involves pharmacological, surgical, and supportive measures. The decision to treat depends on symptom severity, functional disability, and rate of clinical decline.

Pharmacological therapy includes *levodopa* (with carbidopa to reduce peripheral metabolism: side effects include nausea (most common), orthostasis, dyskinesias, hallucinations, insomnia), *dopamine agonists* (e.g., bromocriptine, pramipexole, ropinirole: cause hallucinations, dyskinesias, nausea/vomiting, and rarely pleuropulmonary or retroperitoneal fibrosis), *anticholinergics* (e.g., trihexyphenidyl, benztropine: more effective for tremor; side effects include decreased memory, confusion, dry mouth, constipation, urinary retention), *catechol-O-methyl transferase (COMT) inhibitors* (e.g., tolcapone, entacapone: used in combination with levodopa/carbidopa: causes hepatotoxicity so requires regular LFT), *MAO$_b$ inhibitors* (e.g., selegiline: side effects include insomnia, dizziness, nausea, dyskinesias, psychosis; neuroprotective role highly controversial), and *NMDA antagonists* (e.g., amantadine: can cause confusion, hallucinations, livedo reticularis, dry mouth). There is no universal consensus on which drug should be used for initial therapy in PD. A general recommendation is starting with a dopamine agonist, then adding levodopa if disability is not adequately controlled in younger patients (age <60) or levodopa if the patient is older than 60 years.

Surgical therapies include *deep brain stimulation* (DBS; thalamus for refractory tremor only; medial globus pallidus for contralateral dyskinesias and tremor; subthalamic nucleus especially for akinesia) and *stereotactic lesioning* (thalamotomy, medial pallidotomy, and unilateral subthalamotomy). These are usually reserved as adjunctive therapy for patients with severe, pharmacologically refractory disease. Subthalamic or medial globus pallidal DBS are the preferable surgical options, but carry an operative risk of approximately 1–2%, 5–8% infection, and about 20–25% hardware failure rate.

Supportive measures include treatment of drug-related effects (dyskinesias, fluctuations, psychiatric disturbances: include altered sleep patterns and rapid eye movement behavior disorder [RBD], and orthostatic hypotension) and other complications of PD (postural instability, depression, dementia, and sexual dysfunction).

Prognosis

In general, PD exhibits a nonuniform pattern of clinical deterioration. Progression in motor disability from symptom-onset to being wheelchair- or bed-bound takes a mean of 20 years in the post-levodopa era. Prior to levodopa availability, the observed progression had a mean of 14 years. The current rate of motor deterioration is about 8–9% per year, with certain subgroups (with tremor dominance) showing a progression of about 3.5% per year. Risk factors for rapid motor progression may include older age at onset, predominant akinetic-rigid state, and dementia. Uncontrolled psychiatric complications (hallucinations, delusions) may increase the risk for nursing home placement. In the post-levodopa era, mortality from PD is about 10% at 5 years, 21% at 10 years, and 38% at 15 years from disease onset. This is a reduction from 33% at 5 years, 61% at 10 years, and 83% at 15 years in the pre-levodopa era.

Counseling

Patients and their families should be aware of disease chronicity and its potential complications, including cognitive, psychiatric, and sleep dysfunction.

Prognostic data should be discussed and interventional options pursued. Patients should be aware of medication side effects (increased with polypharmacy) and complications of therapy. Failure/poor response to levodopa may suggest secondary parkinsonism. Treating postural instability in PD is difficult and patients and caregivers should be aware of the safety implications. Ambulatory aids and supportive devices may be required. Risks and benefits of surgical interventions should be discussed in medically refractory patients.

SUMMARY

- **PD** is an **idiopathic** disorder caused by degeneration of **dopaminergic neurons** in the **substantial nigra pars compacta**.
- Etiologies for parkinsonism include **neurodegenerative disorders, drugs, toxins, vascular, metabolic, post-anoxic, head trauma, post-encephalitic, prion disease, neoplasm,** and **hydrocephalus**.
- Diagnosis is made **clinically**. Other etiologies should be excluded if clinical history is suggestive or atypical features are present.
- Treatment includes **pharmacological, surgical,** and **supportive measures**. Decision to treat depends on **symptom severity, functional disability,** and **rate of clinical progression**.
- Pharmacological treatments include **levodopa/carbidopa, dopamine agonists, anticholinergics, COMT inhibitors, MAO$_b$ inhibitors,** and **NMDA antagonists**.
- Surgical options include **DBS** or **surgical lesioning** of the **subthalamic nucleus, medial globus pallidus,** or **thalamus**.
- Rate of motor progression is about **8–9% per year**. Mean progression to being wheelchair- or bed-bound is **approximately 20 years**.
- Rapid progression may occur with **older age at onset, prominent akinetic-rigid state,** and **early dementia**.
- Mortality is **approximately 10%** at 5 years, **21%** at 10 years, and **38%** at 15 years.
- Patients should be aware of the **complications** of the disease, including non-extrapyramidal features, and PD treatment.

CASE 2

A 42-year-old woman was brought to the clinic by her husband. He had noticed a significant personality change in his wife; she had become more emotionally labile, suspicious, irritable, and compulsive over the last 18 months. About 6 months ago, she developed some jerky, stereotypical movements in her fingers with occasional shoulder shrugging. She was also becoming quite forgetful. On examination, MMSE was 22/30, with deficits in attention and orientation, recall, and calculation. The patient had a tendency to wash her hands every 5 minutes during the evaluation. Motor examination revealed choreoathetotic movements in the fingers and shoulders with normal strength, tone, and reflexes. Sensory examination was also normal. Coordination testing was accurate but interrupted by chorea. Gait was broad-based without truncal ataxia.

Localization

The personality changes and deficits in attention and orientation may imply bilateral diffuse frontal lobe dysfunction. Deficits in recall and calculation could imply bilateral temporal lobe dysfunction. Choreoathetosis may localize to the striatum (caudate nucleus and putamen) or its central connections. A broad-based gait without truncal ataxia may localize to the bilateral mesial frontal lobes or subcortical white matter. In summary, the underlying process localizes diffusely to the bilateral frontotemporal lobes and striatum.

Differential Diagnosis

The most likely diagnosis in this age group would be *Huntington's disease* (HD). This is an autosomally dominant inherited CAG-trinucleotide repeat disorder on chromosome 4 that causes marked striatal (especially caudate) and less severe generalized cortical atrophy. The clinical triad of personality/behavioral changes, chorea, and dementia helps establish the diagnosis. Eliciting a family history would further support the diagnosis clinically.

Other differentials could be divided into *hereditary* and *acquired chorea*. Hereditary forms include other hereditary chorea disorders such as *neuroacanthocytosis* (orofacial dyskinesias, vocal/motor tics, cognitive changes, generalized chorea, parkinsonism, predominantly motor neuropathy, seizures, and >10% RBC acanthocytes in fresh blood smear), *benign hereditary chorea* (usual onset in childhood with static or slowly improving chorea; cognitive deficits mild and psychiatric features rare), *neurodegenerative disorders* (SCA3, dentatorubral pallidoluysian atrophy [DRPLA]: similar to HD with cerebellar ataxia and more common in Japan; Friedreich's ataxia, OPCA, Hallervorden–Spatz disease: late childhood or early adolescent onset with pyramidal and extrapyramidal findings and frozen pained facial expression; and familial basal ganglia calcification), *metabolic disorders* (e.g., porphyria, Wilson's disease, Lesch–Nyhan syndrome, lysosomal storage disorders: earlier age of presentation expected), and *mitochondrial diseases* (e.g., Leigh's disease: subacute necrotizing encephalomyelopathy; chorea with external ophthalmoplegia, respiratory, and swallowing deficits).

Acquired chorea can be classified into *drug-induced* (neuroleptics, antiparkinsonian agents, TCAs, oral contraceptive pills, amphetamines, cocaine), *toxic* (e.g., manganese, carbon monoxide, toluene), *heavy metal-induced* (mercury, thallium), *metabolic* (anoxia, hypo- and hypernatremia, hypo- and hyperglycemia, hypocalcemia, hepatic disease), *endocrine* (hyperthyroidism, hypoparathyroidism, pregnancy), *infectious/postinfectious* (e.g., Syndenham's chorea: post-streptococcal A rheumatic fever in children, slowly progressive with general spontaneous remission: *see* pp. 249–252; encephalitis lethargica or prion diseases), *autoimmune* (e.g., SLE, aPL syndrome), *vascular* (especially in older patients with hemichorea: e.g., ischemic or hemorrhagic infarction, AVMs involving basal ganglia; cognitive and personality changes unexpected), *neoplastic* (primary brain or metastatic), and *traumatic* (ICH with basal ganglia involvement; cortical signs also expected).

Investigations

Genetic testing for the CAG repeat on chromosome 4 should be performed. More than 35 repeats confirms the diagnosis. MRI of the brain may show caudate atrophy with compensatory ventriculomegaly of the frontal horns of the lateral ventricles. PET scans may show striatal glucose hypometabolism early in the disease. If the diagnosis is equivocal or presenting features atypical, laboratory tests for other hereditary or acquired chorea disorders should be considered, for example, genetic tests for hereditary ataxias, comprehensive metabolic profile, peripheral blood smear, TFT, PTH levels, serum/ urine toxicology, urine human chorionic gonadtrophin (hCG), heavy metal screen, ANA profile, and aPL antibodies. Stroke work-up (MRI-DWI, MRA, MRV) is required in hemichorea patients with a sudden onset, especially in elderly patients. "Thrombophilic" screen should be included if the suspected stroke patient is under 45 years of age (*see* pp. 16 and 20).

Management

The treatment of HD is symptomatic and supportive. Chorea should be treated with dopamine antagonists (typical or atypical neuroleptics: haloperidol most effective but has significant side effects, or dopamine depleters such as reserpine or tetrabenazine). Dystonia may benefit from anticholinergic medications (e.g., trihexyphenidyl, benztropine) or medications with significant anticholinergic side effects (e.g., antihistamines, TCAs). These agents could make cognitive deficits worse. Akinetic-rigid states and chorea may be treated with the anti-parkinsonian medication, amantadine. The use of levodopa, dopamine agonists, and inhibitors of dopamine metabolism could make behavioral features and chorea worse. Depression and obsessive-compulsive states can be treated with SSRIs. There are no pharmacological treatments for dementia.

Supportive therapy should include physical and occupational therapy for ambulation and self-care techniques with the provision of aids if required. Behavioral modification therapy is necessary especially for compulsions. Adequate supervision, assistance with ADLs, nutritional, and emotional support are necessary adjuncts.

Prognosis

Despite supportive measures, HD is relentlessly progressive with death expected between 10 and 20 years from symptom onset. The most common cause of death is aspiration pneumonia or asphyxiation secondary to dysphagia. There is a risk of suicide in younger patients. Clinical progression and prognosis are dependent on the age at symptom onset. Juvenile-onset HD ("Westphal variant": predominantly an akinetic-rigid syndrome and paternally inherited) has a worse prognosis with mental retardation (MR) and seizures and faster rate of clinical progression. Late-onset HD has a slower rate of clinical progression and patients may have a normal life expectancy.

Counseling

Patients and their families should be aware of prognostic data and the implications of the disease. Long-term care at home or a specialized facility may be required in the later stages of the disease. Severe dysphagia may warrant placement of a percutaneous endoscopic gastrostomy (PEG) tube. Genetic counseling should be provided for all affected and at-risk families.

The risk of transmission is 50% (incomplete penetrance resulting in <50% risk may occur with CAG repeats 37–42). Paternal inheritance is associated with anticipation and earlier onset of disease. The issue of presymptomatic testing in offspring of affected patients may pose ethical, psychological, and practical social implications (e.g., insurance, employment, marriage) for these individuals. The decision to pursue such testing would depend on the individual's informed choice and understanding the implications of a positive test for an incurable disorder prior to symptom development.

SUMMARY

- **HD** is a neurodegenerative, hereditary choreiform disorder that presents with **behavioral/personality changes, chorea,** and **dementia**. HD is inherited in an **autosomally dominant** pattern.
- HD is caused by a **CAG-trinucleotide repeat** on **chromosome 4**, with **more than 35** repeats being diagnostic.
- Marked **caudate** and diffuse **cortical** atrophy may be seen in MRI.
- Differential diagnosis can be divided into **hereditary** and **acquired** chorea.
- Hereditary forms include **neuroacanthocytosis, benign hereditary chorea, neurodegenerative, metabolic,** and **mitochondrial** causes.
- Acquired forms include **drug-induced, toxic, heavy metal-induced, metabolic, endocrine, infectious/postinfectious, autoimmune, vascular, neoplastic,** and **traumatic**.
- In **atypical cases,** laboratory and radiological tests may be required to exclude other etiologies for chorea.

- Treatment consists of **symptomatic** and **supportive** measures. **Dopamine antagonists** are most effective for chorea.
- HD is relentlessly progressive, with death expected **10–20 years** after symptom onset. Cause of death is usually **aspiration pneumonia** or **asphyxiation** secondary to dysphagia. **Suicide** may occur in young patients.
- Outcomes and clinical progression depend on **age of onset**.
- Patients should be made aware of prognostic data. **Genetic counseling** should be provided to affected and at-risk families.

CASE 3

A 52-year-old man has had problems with his gait for more than 9 months. His colleagues at work had noticed a worsening tendency to stumble and head nodding. On examination, cranial nerves were normal. Motor examination revealed normal strength, bulk, and reflexes. Sensory examination revealed mild distal stocking distribution sensory loss to vibration and pinprick. Coordination testing showed titubation, severe truncal ataxia with an inability to perform heel-to-toe tandem walking, and mild bilateral appendicular ataxia that was worse in the lower extremities. Gait testing revealed a broad-based gait and Romberg's sign was absent.

Localization

Titubation, truncal ataxia, and a broad-based gait suggest midline cerebellar dysfunction. Bilateral appendicular ataxia suggests bilateral dysfunction of the lateral cerebellum. Distal sensory loss suggests a peripheral neuropathy or bilateral lumbosacral plexopathies or L4–S1 radiculopathies. An absent Romberg's sign provides further evidence that the truncal ataxia is not caused by distal sensory loss. The most likely localization is the midline cerebellum with some involvement of the lateral cerebellar hemispheres, in association with a mild sensory peripheral neuropathy.

Differential Diagnosis

The most likely diagnosis for chronic, predominantly midline, cerebellar dysfunction associated with a mild sensory neuropathy is *alcoholic cerebellar degeneration*. This may be the most common cause of acquired cerebellar dysfunction and is seen in chronic alcoholics who are more likely to be malnourished. This may occur either as a result of *chronic thiamine deficiency* or *alcohol toxicity*.

Other diagnostic considerations could be divided into *acquired* and *inherited* etiologies. Acquired etiologies include *vitamin E deficiency* (progressive gait and appendicular ataxia, large-fiber sensory neuropathy, areflexia, retinopathy, ophthalmoparesis and dysarthria: may be caused by intestinal malabsorption or liver disease), *paraneoplastic cerebellar syndrome* (associated with ovarian and other gynecologic and breast cancers, associated with downbeat nystagmus, opsoclonus, and anti-Purkinje cell antibodies, e.g., anti-Yo, Ri, Ma, Tr, CV2: precedes diagnosis of malignancy in ~60–70%), *drugs* (e.g., phenytoin, lithium, 5-fluorouracil), *toxins* (e.g., toluene, carbon tetrachloride), heavy metals (e.g., methyl mercury, thallium), *metabolic/endocrine* (hepatic disease, myelinolysis related to hyponatremia, hypothyroidism), *structural* (causes of hydrocephalus: communicating and noncommunicating, or foramen magnum compression, including brain tumors), and *infections* (prion: CJD, GSD, kuru: progressive cerebellar signs may occur before other features such as myoclonus or dementia; bacteria, e.g., CNS tuberculosis, bacterial abscess; parasites, e.g., cysticercosis).

Hereditary etiologies include *spinocerebellar ataxias* (e.g., predominantly cerebellar forms, with autosomally dominant inheritance such as SCA 5, 6, or 11), *idiopathic late-onset degenerative ataxias* (e.g., MSA, late cortical and cerebellar atrophy of Marie–Foix–Alajouanine: resembles alcoholic cerebellar degeneration, Ramsay–Hunt syndrome of dyssynergia cerebellaris progressiva), *DRPLA* (more common in Japan: choreoathetosis and parkinsonism present) and *mitochondrial disorders* (e.g., KSS, MELAS, MERRF, NARP).

Investigations

The clinical history and physical findings are most useful in establishing the diagnosis. There are no laboratory tests to confirm the diagnosis, although other potential causes of progressive cerebellar dysfunction could be excluded in clinically equivocal cases. Such tests may include serum electrolytes, TFT, serum/urine toxicology including heavy metal screen, vitamin E levels, anti-Purkinje cell antibodies (positive test would require further evaluation for an occult malignancy), genetic tests for hereditary ataxia, LP for CSF examination to exclude infections, EMG/NCS (to evaluate for associated neuropathy or myopathy), lactate/pyruvate levels, and muscle biopsy for mitochondrial encephalomyopathy, and postmortem brain examination for prion diseases. CT/MRI of the brain is useful in excluding structural causes, and may show anterior and superior vermal (in alcoholic cerebellar degeneration) or nonspecific cerebellar atrophy.

Management

The management of alcoholic cerebellar degeneration involves alcohol cessation and chronic thiamine replacement. Nutritional support should be provided for malnourished patients. Patients may require physical and occupational therapy to help cope with their functional limitations. For patient safety, ambulatory devices should be used to improve gait stability. Other complications of chronic alcoholism commonly co-exist, so these should be addressed and adequately treated.

Prognosis

Some improvement may occur in milder cases of alcoholic cerebellar degeneration treated early, however, response to therapy is limited if patients are already nonambulatory or wheelchair-confined. Gait/truncal ataxia is relatively resistant to treatment. Residual deficits are common even in patients with some treatment response. Prognosis would be modified by concomitant neurological and systemic complications of chronic alcoholism.

Counseling

Chronic alcoholics should be aware that this complication may occur in approximately 10–15% and is commonly associated with cognitive deficits and Wernicke–Korsakoff syndrome (*see* pp. 79–82). Patients should be aware of other complications of alcohol use. Chronic alcoholism should be addressed through medical counseling and supportive groups (e.g., Alcoholics Anonymous). Chronic vitamin supplements may be needed.

SUMMARY

- **Alcoholic cerebellar degeneration** may occur in **approximately 10–15%** of chronic alcoholics because of **degeneration of the anterior/superior vermis**.
- Differentials can be divided into **acquired** and **hereditary**.
- Acquired chronic ataxias include **vitamin E deficiency, paraneoplastic, drugs, toxins, heavy metals, metabolic/endocrine, structural**, and **infectious** etiologies.
- Hereditary chronic late-onset ataxias include **spinocerebellar ataxia syndromes, idiopathic late-onset degenerative, DRPLA**, and **mitochondrial disorders**.
- Diagnosis is established **clinically. Brain CT/MRI** may show **vermal atrophy**. Other causes should be excluded in equivocal cases.
- Treatment involves **alcohol cessation, chronic thiamine supplementation**, and **supportive** measures.
- **Residual deficits** are expected despite treatment.

CASE 4

A 37-year-old woman had noticed progressive difficulty using her right hand for about 1 year. Her fingers and hand became tight when she attempted to write or paint but were normal otherwise. She did not complain of similar symptoms elsewhere. Neurological examination was normal. On attempting to write, there was dystonic posturing of the right wrist and metacarpophalangeal joints in a hyperflexed position, with hyperextension of the thumb and index fingers, resulting in illegible script.

Localization

Focal dystonia of the right hand and fingers suggests hyperexcitation of the agonist and antagonist muscles of the right hand and fingers or reduced inhibition of those muscle groups. Hyperexcitation could localize to the contralateral (left) frontal cerebral cortex, whereas reduced inhibition may localize to the contralateral basal ganglia and its central connections (including the thalamus) or ipsilateral cervical spinal cord interneurons (C6–T1). The otherwise normal neurological examination makes a focal lesion in the cerebral cortex, thalamus, or spinal cord unlikely. The most likely localization is the left basal ganglia (putamen, globus pallidus, or caudate nucleus).

Differential Diagnosis

The most likely diagnosis is *focal hand dystonia*, an occupational dystonia (includes writer's cramp). This is a primary, idiopathic focal or segmental dystonia that commonly starts in the second to fourth decades of life. Other differentials include *idiopathic torsional dystonia* (a primary generalized idiopathic dystonia: may initially present in older individuals as a focal dystonia; more common in children between 6 and 12 years old) and *secondary dystonias.*

Secondary dystonias may be the result of *neurodegenerative disorders* (e.g., PD, CBGD, PSP, MSA, SCA 6, and HD), *neurometabolic disorders* (e.g., Wilson's disease, adult-onset GM_1/GM_2 gangliosidoses, metachromatic leukodystrophy), *drugs* (e.g., L-Dopa, dopamine agonists, neuroleptics), *toxins* (e.g., manganese), *trauma* (head injury, limb trauma with CRPS, postsurgical e.g., thalamotomy), *vascular* (*post-stroke*: ischemic or hemorrhagic involving the putamen, thalamus, globus pallidus, or caudate: may cause hemidystonia weeks after acute insult; *post-anoxia*: may occur years or decades after perinatal injury; *vascular anomalies*, e.g., AVMs, cavernous angioma), *infections* (encephalitis, cerebral abscess), neoplasia (primary brain tumor or metastatic disease), *mitochondrial disease* (e.g., Leigh's disease, Leber's hereditary optic neuropathy with dystonia, MELAS), or *psychogenic* (should be a diagnosis of exclusion) causes.

Investigations

The clinical history and examination are paramount in diagnosing an occupational dystonia. Laboratory investigations can be modified to exclude possible differentials, but should be guided by the clinical history. Such tests include CBC with differential, comprehensive metabolic panel, LFTs, serum copper/ceruloplasmin, serum lysosomal enzymes, lactate/pyruvate, and genetic tests for hereditary dystonias and certain neurodegenerative or neurometabolic disorders.

MRI of the brain may be useful in hemidystonia to exclude focal brain lesions, as well as exclude other potential causes of generalized dystonia,

EMG/NCS may exclude associated peripheral neuropathy or myopathy. EEG may be useful to exclude frontal lobe seizures in atypical cases, especially in paroxysmal nocturnal dystonia and electroretinogram may be useful in evaluating for Leber's hereditary optic neuropathy.

Management

Focal hand dystonia could be difficult to treat. EMG-guided injections of botulinum toxin may be administered periodically (every 6–12 months) into selected muscles (efficacy of ~85% for focal hand dystonias at 6–8 weeks; adverse effects include transient weakness in injected or surrounding muscles). This may be considered first-line treatment owing to the poor response to oral medications, such as anticholinergics, baclofen, and benzodiazepines.

Supportive therapies can be utilized in less severe cases or as an adjunct to botulinum toxin therapy. These methods include splinting/immobilization, ergonomic alternatives in writing or instrument handling or equipment modification, sensory motor retuning with or without biofeedback, training the contralateral side, and orthosis. Stereotactic nucleus ventrooralis thalamotomy may be useful in medically refractory patients, but this has not been proven in large series or randomized controlled trials.

Prognosis

The natural history of focal hand dystonia is progression for 6–12 months, then plateau without major fluctuations or remissions for several years. Less commonly, evolution to a generalized dystonia may occur. In writer's cramp, long-term periodic botulinum toxin injections may result in normal writing in approximately 45% of patients, with efficacy lasting about 6 months after 3–9 year follow-up. About 10% received partial benefit and 20–45% may experience suboptimal results or treatment failure. Poor outcomes were associated with secondary dystonia, tremulous variants, progressive cases (>12 months), and long duration from onset before treatment. In focal hand dystonia in musicians playing string instruments, about 40% maintain professional abilities, approximately 40% were capable of playing nonprofessionally at leisure, and about 20% had to completely stop playing instruments after appropriate pharmacological/supportive measures.

Counseling

Patients should be aware of the idiopathic etiology for most focal hand dystonias, the chronic nature of the disease, and the suboptimal response to therapy. Patients should be made aware of the prognostic data, and other etiologies (including family history, which may be present in ~20% of patients with writer's cramp) should be thoroughly investigated for in equivocal or atypical cases.

SUMMARY

- **Focal hand dystonia** is an **occupational dystonia** of unknown etiology (primary, idiopathic focal dystonia).
- Differentials include **idiopathic torsional dystonia, drugs, toxins, neurodegenerative, neurometabolic, traumatic, vascular, infectious, neoplastic, mitochondrial,** and **psychogenic etiologies.**
- Diagnosis is established by **clinical history** and **examination**. Other potential etiologies should b excluded in equivocal or atypical cases.
- Treatment of focal hand dystonia is challenging.
- Options include **periodic botulinum toxin injections, anticholinergics, baclofen, benzodiazepines, physical, occupational** or **psychological** therapies, **orthoses,** and **ergonomic alterations.**
- Most untreated cases progress for **6–12 months**, then plateau.
- Initial response to botulinum toxin injections could be as high as **85%** at **6–8 weeks**. Efficacy lasts about **6 months**.
- Long-term benefit in writer's cramp: **approximately 45%** normal writing, **approximately 10%** partial, and **approximately 20–45%** with suboptimal or treatment failure after **3–9 years. Secondary dystonia, tremulous variant, progression of more than 12 months,** and **long duration from onset to treatment** are poor prognostic factors.
- **Approximately 40%** of professional musicians with focal hand dystonia are still capable of playing professionally with adequate treatment.
- Patients should be aware of the **idiopathic etiology, chronic nature of the disease,** and the **suboptimal response** to therapy in focal hand dystonias.

CASE 5

A 23-year-old man was brought to the ER by his roommate. He observed that his friend had become more irritable and impulsive over the last month. The patient felt he was being followed by green monsters and heard voices constantly telling him that the police wanted him. On examination, resting tremor with bradykinesia and mild lead-pipe rigidity, worse on the left, were present. Jaundiced sclerae were also observed.

Localization

Irritability and impulsive behavior could imply bilateral anterior frontal or limbic cortex dysfunction. Formed visual and auditory hallucinations may localize to the dominant or bilateral temporo-occipital and superior temporal lobes, respectively. Bilateral parkinsonism localizes to the substantia nigra in the midbrain (or its central connections via the nigrostriatal or pallidonigral tracts), worse on the right. Jaundiced sclerae imply hepatocellular dysfunction in conjugated bilirubin metabolism. In summary, the underlying disorder involves the bilateral anterior frontal or limbic, temporal and occipital cortices with bilateral (right>left) substantia nigral and associated hepatic dysfunction.

Differential Diagnosis

Psychosis, parkinsonism, and liver disease in a young adult most likely implies an inherited hepatocerebral disorder. The most likely diagnosis for such a disorder is *Wilson's disease*. This is an autosomal recessive (AR)-inherited defect in the gene producing a Cu^{2+}-transporting P-type ATPase (ATP7B) on chromosome 13. This protein is required for the efficient excretion of Cu^{2+} into bile. Approximately 45% of patients present with liver disease, 35% with neurological disease, 10% with psychiatric disease, and 10% with cardiological, endocrine, orthopedic, hematological, or ophthalmologic disorders. Kayser–Fleischer rings (greenish discoloration of Descemet's membrane of the iris) are present in 95% of patients with neurological involvement, 50–60% without neurological involvement, and 10% of asymptomatic patients.

Differentials include *chronic acquired hepatocerebral degeneration* (neuropsychiatric disorder associated with chronic liver failure, secondary to associated manganese or ammonium toxicity), *schizophrenia with neuroleptic-induced parkinsonism* (drug history would help exclude this), *parkinsonism with psychosis* (e.g., PD, DLBD: *see* pp. 151–154, older age of onset would be expected), HD (*see* pp. 154–158), *rheumatic (Syndenham's) chorea* (*see* pp. 249–252), *Hallervorden–Spatz syndrome* (more likely to present in late childhood or early adolescence, *see* p. 155), *adult-onset leukodystrophies* (e.g., metachromatic, ALD: *see* pp. 242–246), *post-ictal psychosis* (history of ictal event and absence of parkinsonism expected), *vitamin B_{12} deficiency* (parkinsonism unexpected, but psychosis may be the presenting feature; *see* pp. 139–141), or *toxin exposures* (e.g., methanol, cyanide, ethylene glycol, or carbon monoxide: encephalopathy with parkinsonism).

Investigation

Kayser–Fleischer rings and low ceruloplasmin levels (<20 mg/dL) in a patient with a suggestive history are diagnostic of Wilson's disease. Other supportive tests include serum Cu^{2+} (<100 μg/dL) and 24-hour urinary Cu^{2+} (>100 μg). In equivocal cases, liver biopsy can be performed. This may show elevated hepatic Cu^{2+} (>250 μg/g dry weight) and evidence of fatty liver, micronodular cirrhosis, chronic active hepatitis, or fibrosis. Genetic testing can be used to confirm the diagnosis, but its usefulness is limited by the large number of known mutations (the most common mutation in Europe and North America is only seen in ~45% of affected patients).

Additional tests include CBC with differential and Coomb's test (for hemolytic anemia), comprehensive metabolic panel, PT/PTT/INR (before biopsy), LFT, ammonia level, TFT, PTH (hypothyroidism and hypoparathyroidism are less common complications), vitamin B_{12} levels and serum/urine toxicology screen. MRI of the brain may show signal changes in the basal ganglia or subcortical white matter or generalized atrophy. In rare equivocal cases, evaluation for other inherited disorders (e.g., leukodystrophy, HD) would be necessary.

Management

Any suicidal or homicidal ideation warrants admission to a secured psychiatric unit. Symptomatic therapy (e.g., antipsychotics, L-Dopa) may be required in the early phases of treatment. The management of Wilson's disease can be divided into medical and surgical modalities.

Medical therapy includes *dietary measures:* avoidance of Cu^{2+} (liver, shellfish, legumes, chocolate, nuts, or water with concentrations >1 ppm or 0.1 µg/L) and *inhibition of GI Cu^{2+} absorption by zinc salts* (zinc acetate or zinc sulfate), and *chelation therapy* (d-penicillamine—most commonly used initial agent; ADRs include vitamin B_6 deficiency, skin lesions, bone marrow suppression, nephritic syndrome, and MG; trientine or tetrathiomolybdate). In general, 60–85% of medically treated patients respond. About 20–50% of patients treated with d-penicillamine alone may discontinue therapy owing to side effects.

Surgical treatment via liver *transplantation* (orthotopic or living-related donor) is usually reserved for patients with fulminant or advanced liver failure or patients refractory to medical therapy, apart from those with severe refractory neuropsychiatric disease (with significant irreversible neurodegeneration). Wilson disease accounts for about 10% of patients with fulminant liver failure referred for emergency liver transplantation. Liver transplantation, if successful, dramatically improves neurological function within 3–4 months with restoration of normal Cu^{2+} homeostasis within 6 months.

Prognosis

Early recognition and institution of therapy are important to prevent irreversible hepatocerebral degeneration. If untreated, Wilson's disease is universally fatal, with death secondary to hepatic failure. Life expectancy is normal in treated patients that respond to medical therapy. In patients requiring liver transplantation, 1-year survival is about 85% posttransplantation, with early deaths commonly attributed to complications from immunosuppressant use. In the last decade, 5-year survival (including graft survival) rate is greater than 80%.

Counseling

Patients and their families should be encouraged by the excellent prognosis in treatment-responsive patients. Medical compliance should be emphasized and frequent (every 1–3 months) 24-hour urinary Cu^{2+} levels can be checked to monitor compliance and drug efficacy (not useful in patients treated with zinc salts alone). For patients requiring liver transplantation, the perioperative risks and risks of chronic immunosuppression need to be weighed against the potential reversal of the clinical manifestations of this disorder. Presymptomatic screening (physical, metabolic, and genetic) should be made available to all siblings (25% risk of Wilson's disease) and first-degree relatives (0.5% risk). Medical therapy should be offered to individuals diagnosed with Wilson's disease.

SUMMARY

- **Wilson's disease** is an inherited disorder due to gene defects in a **Cu^{2+} transporting P-type ATPase** (ATP7B) on **chromosome 13**.
- Clinical presentation commonly involves **hepatic, neurological**, or **psychiatric** features.
- Differential diagnosis includes **chronic acquired hepatocerebral degeneration, schizophrenia with neuroleptic-induced parkinsonism, parkinsonism with psychosis, HD, rheumatic chorea, Hallervorden–Spatz syndrome, adult leukodystrophy, post-ictal psychosis, vitamin B$_{12}$ deficiency**, and **toxin exposures**.
- Diagnosis is confirmed by **low serum ceruloplasmin, low serum Cu^{2+}**, or **elevated 24-hours urinary Cu^{2+}. Liver biopsy** and **genetic testing** are also useful in certain cases.
- Treatment includes **medical** (dietary and chelation therapy) and **surgical** (liver transplantation) modalities.
- Indications for liver transplantation include **fulminant or advanced liver failure** or patients **refractory to medical therapy**.
- If untreated, the disease is **uniformly fatal**: cause of death is **liver failure**. Life expectancy is **normal** in medically treated patients.
- One-year survival rates of patients undergoing liver transplantation is **approximately 85%** with 5-year survival rates **greater than 80%** over the last decade.

14

Epilepsy

CASE 1

A 43-year-old man was brought to the clinic by his spouse. He has had three to four episodes of "fits" that lasted 2–3 minutes. On further questioning, she stated that he developed generalized stiffness with upward eye deviation lasting about 5–10 seconds. Following that, he developed generalized rhythmic contraction of all his extremities with urinary or fecal incontinence. During these episodes, he was unresponsive and it took about 30 to 60 minutes for him to fully recover to normal. Neurological examination was normal.

Localization

Generalized hypertonia and rhythmic contractions (clonus) of all extremities without other signs would suggest diffuse hyperexcitability in either the cerebral motor cortex or subacute to chronic lesions affecting the descending motor pathways (cerebral cortex, subcortical white matter, posterior limb internal capsule, cerebral peduncles, basis pontis, pyramidal tracts, or lateral spinal cord [above or at the level of C5]) bilaterally. However, unresponsiveness after an episode (suggestive of global cerebral dysfunction) and a normal neurological examination infer that the most likely localization is the bilateral cerebral motor cortex (predominantly frontal lobes).

Differential Diagnosis

The most likely diagnosis is *GTC seizures*. These could either be *primary generalized* (more common in children) or *complex partial seizures with secondary generalization*. An aura or some focal signs are usually present in secondary generalized seizures.

Other diagnostic considerations include *syncope* (cardiac, cerebrovascular, hypotensive, vasovagal, hypovolemic, metabolic), *drop attacks* (cerebrovascular, paroxysmal hydrocephalus, third ventricular and posterior fossa tumors, vestibular disorders), *myoclonus* (multifocal or generalized; loss of consciousness and tonic phase unlikely and jerks are usually asynchronous: etiologies

From: *Neurology Oral Boards Review:*
A Concise and Systematic Approach to Clinical Practice
By: E. E. Ubogu © Humana Press Inc., Totowa, NJ

include *epileptic disorders, neurodegeneration, infections* [viral], *metabolic, toxins/drugs, post-hypoxia,* and *hereditary), psychogenic* (pseudoseizures: *see* pp. 173–176; rage attacks, panic attacks: intense fear/discomfort with symptoms, such as palpitations, diaphoresis, dyspnea, nausea, dizziness/lightheadedness, loss of control or fear of death or parasthesias that suddenly develop and peak within 10 minutes), and *paroxysmal choreoathetosis* (kinesigenic or nonkinesigenic: change in level of consciousness and synchrony of limb movements unexpected).

Etiologies for GTC seizures in this age group include *idiopathic epilepsy* (no apparent cause identified), *metabolic derangements* (e.g., hypo- or hypernatremia, hypo- or hyperglycemia, hypocalcemia, hypomagnesemia, uremia, hepatic failure, hypoxia), *drug intoxication* (amphetamines, cocaine, TCAs, bupropion), *drug withdrawal* (alcohol, GABAergic agents, AEDs), *toxins* (heavy metals such as mercury, lead), *infection* (causes of meningoencephalitis: bacterial, viral, fungal), and *neoplasia* (focal lesions are more likely to present with secondary generalization, but mesial frontal lesions could primarily generalize).

Investigations

Epilepsy is a clinical diagnosis, so further history for exacerbating/ precipitating factors, family history, prior history, toxin/drug exposure, and prior head injury/CNS infections would be required. Laboratory tests should be tailored toward potential etiologies: CBC with differential, comprehensive metabolic panel, Mg^{2+}, PO_4^{3-}, ABG, serum/urine toxicology, urinalysis, and venereal disease reference laboratory (VDRL) / FTA-ABS. LP should be performed if CNS infection is suspected. EKG may help exclude cardiac arrhythmia, which could cause syncope or occur secondary to seizure.

MRI brain (with and without contrast; seizure protocol with thin cuts through the temporal lobes) is the radiological assessment of choice for seizure patients to exclude cerebral pathology that could cause epilepsy. EEG can be performed as a guide to clinical diagnosis (only ~30–50% of GTC seizure patients have interictal abnormalities on EEG).

Management

The decision to treat recurrent seizures (i.e., epilepsy) is dependent on its frequency, effect on patient lifestyle, safety and tolerability of AEDs, and the underlying cause. If a reversible underlying cause was identified (e.g., metabolic derangement), long-term AED therapy would not be required.

AED options for GTCs (primary or secondarily generalized) include *VPA* (drug of choice for primary generalized GTC; ADRs: tremor, nausea, hepatic toxicity, hirsutism, weight gain), *phenytoin* (ADRs: ataxia, hirsutism, gingival hyperplasia, rash, sedation), *carbamazepine/oxcarbamazepine* (ADRs: ataxia, hepatic dysfunction, hyponatremia: less common with oxcarbamazepine), *phenobarbital* (ADRs: sedation, irritability), *lamotrigine* (ADRs: rash including fatal

Stevens-Johnson syndrome, ataxia, headache, dizziness), *topiramate* (ADRs: cognitive slowing, confusion, renal stones, parasthesias, somnolence) and *gabapentin* (ADRs: ataxia, dizziness, fatigue).

Levetiracetam (ADRs: somnolence, tremor, irritability, thrombocytopenia), and *zonisamide* (ADRs: headache, somnolence, rhinitis, nausea, rash) can be used as adjunctive therapy in refractory cases. Phenytoin, carbamazepine, and phenobarbital are more efficacious in secondarily generalized seizures, whereas data supporting the use of the newer AEDs includes both partial and generalized epilepsy patients. Monotherapy is the target because of cumulative adverse effects and the risk of noncompliance with polytherapy.

In medically refractory patients (therapeutic dose administration of more than three AEDs for 6 months to 2 years), *vagal nerve stimulation* (side effects: dyspnea, hoarseness, cough, and parasthesias) or *epilepsy surgery* (more efficacious for partial seizures with secondary generalization, especially of temporal onset, e.g., anterior temporal lobectomy, lesion excision, amygdalohippocampectomy, multiple subpial transactions, corpus callosotomy) may be considered in carefully selected patients.

Prognosis

With GTC seizures, risk of recurrence is about 30–50% within 5 years, with approximately 80–90% lifetime risk depending on the etiology. Precipitating factors can be identified in about 40% of patients, and commonly include sleep deprivation with or without alcohol abuse and AED noncompliance. The risk of recurrent seizures is approximately 1 seizure per year in untreated and approximately 0.2 seizures per year in treated patients after about 10 years mean follow-up.

About 60–70% of adult patients with primary idiopathic generalized epilepsies (including myoclonic epilepsies) experience excellent seizure control with AEDs over a 5-year period, with more than 90% maintaining adequate employment. Prognosis is also modified by the underlying cause, with outcomes being better with metabolic etiologies. A seizure-free period of more than 2 years, and a normal neurological examination, intelligence, and EEG are favorable factors for stopping AEDs in patients requiring long-term therapy. Prognosis is less favorable in patients with localization-related epilepsies with secondary GTC seizures.

Counseling

Patients should be aware of the importance of AED compliance and their adverse effects. The risks of SE and its prognosis (*see* pp. 33–36) should be highlighted. Regular AED levels may be required as a guide during initial drug titration and should be checked if a seizure occurs. Other routine blood tests (CBC, basic metabolic profile, LFT, or urinalysis) may be required to monitor for AED adverse effects. Patients should be counseled on avoidance of known precipitants (especially sleep deprivation and alcohol) and should obtain a medical alert bracelet.

The use of AEDs in pregnancy should be discussed with women of childbearing age, and folic acid should be prescribed. Slow AED weaning should be considered in patients with good prognostic indicators. In refractory cases, video EEG or intracranial monitoring may be required for focus localization prior to surgery.

SUMMARY

- **GTC seizures** could be **primary** or **secondary** to a partial seizure.
- Differentials include **syncope, drop attacks, pseudoseizures, myoclonus, paroxysmal choreoathetosis**, or **psychogenic** causes.
- Etiologies for adult GTC include **idiopathic, metabolic, drug intoxication/withdrawal, toxins, infection**, and **neoplasia**.
- Laboratory evaluation should be tailored toward potential etiologies. **MRI** is the diagnostic test of choice in evaluating for cerebral lesions.
- Treatments include **VPA** (drug of choice in primary generalized GTC), **phenytoin, carbamazepine**, and **phenobarbital**.
- In secondarily generalized GTC, AEDs such as **lamotrigine, topiramate, oxcarbamazepine**, and **gabapentin** can also be used as initial monotherapy. Adjunctive AEDs include **levetiracetam** and **zonisamide**.
- **Vagal nerve stimulation** and **epilepsy surgery** should be considered in medically refractory cases.
- Primary GTC have a good prognosis if treated, with **approximately 60–70%** with excellent control and **more than 90%** maintaining employment over **5 years** follow-up and **about 0.2 seizures per year** recurrence over **10 years** follow-up.
- **Metabolic** and **idiopathic** causes are more favorable than **localization-related** etiologies.
- **Counseling** is important in reducing morbidity and mortality related to seizures.

CASE 2

A 56-year-old woman was brought to the ER. Her son stated that she complained of nausea, perceived pungent smells and a feeling of unfamiliarity with her surroundings about an hour ago. About 30 seconds later, she became very quiet, then developed forced head and eye deviation to the left, continuous lip smacking, and right facial and arm twitching lasting about 2 minutes. She had been sleepy ever since. On examination, she was oriented to person only and exhibited global deficits on MMSE. Motor examination showed mild right lower facial droop and MRC 4/5 weakness in the right upper extremity. There was symmetrical withdrawal to noxious stimulation. Reflexes were generally brisk with bilateral extensor plantar responses.

Localization

Nausea (epigastric fullness), perception of pungent smells, *jamais vu*, and oral automatisms are highly suggestive of an irritative lesion of mesial temporal lobe. Forced head and eye deviation to the left could suggest left temporal or right frontal lobe hyperactivity or left frontal hypofunction (tonic eye deviation to the left that cannot be overcome by oculocephalic maneuvers suggests a right pontine lesion). Right lower facial and arm twitching (with subsequent palsies) suggests involvement of the left frontal cortex. The most likely localization is the left mesial temporal cortex with spread to the ipsilateral frontal cortex. There is also evidence for global cerebral dysfunction (somnolence, cognitive deficits, and generalized hyperreflexia).

Differential Diagnosis

The most likely diagnosis for a sudden paroxysmal event with evolution over seconds to minutes with this localization is *temporal lobe seizures*. This is a complex partial seizure of temporal lobe onset and accounts for about 70% of all complex partial seizures. Alternation of consciousness is not expected in simple partial seizures.

Etiologies include *mesial temporal sclerosis, trauma, congenital malformations* (including subclinical heterotopias), *infections* (viral: especially HSE; bacterial, fungal, and parasitic: causing abscesses or cysts such as cysticercosis: most common cause of epilepsy in central America), *cerebral infarction* (ICH, SAH, or ischemia: chronic or acute), *neoplasms* (primary: e.g., astrocytoma, pleomorphic xanthoastrocytoma, meningioma, oligodendroglioma, neuronal cell tumors, etc., or secondary metastases), and *idiopathic*. Metabolic etiologies tend to cause GTC seizures.

Other differential diagnoses to consider include *atypical hemiplegic migraine* (aura is atypical, as well as convulsions), *acute left ICA, anterior choroidal, or inferior MCA stroke/transient ischemic attack* (TIA; positive symptoms are unusual and neurological deficit expected at onset), *transient global amnesia* (TGA; positive symptoms unlikely), and *pseudoseizures* (most unlikely with the clinical presentation and physical signs). *Focal/segmental myoclonus* is possible, but behavioral changes unexpected. *Syncope* and *drop attacks* are less likely to present with focally, and should not demonstrate focal signs unless associated with previous encephalomalacia or subsequent head injury.

Investigations

These are similar to those described on p. 168, with more emphasis on assessing for structural causes. As for all possible seizure disorders, a comprehensive history is required to help establish the diagnosis. Interictal EEG may be abnormal in about 50–70% of patients.

Management

A single complex partial seizure does not require AED therapy, unless a structural cause is identified, as this increases the risk of recurrent episodes (epilepsy). In patients with temporal lobe epilepsy, AEDs should be administered (*see* pp. 168–169). Carbamazepine and phenytoin are the usual first-line agents, but therapy should to tailored toward the patient achieving seizure-free control with monotherapy. In refractory patients, vagal nerve stimulation (~50% reduction in seizures without reduction in AEDs) or epilepsy surgery (~65–70% seizure free, 20–25% improvement, with negligible perioperative mortality, ~4% minor, and ~1% major complication rates) should be offered in adequately selected patients (*see* p. 169), especially if the seizure focus or a focal lesion is identified.

Prognosis

In general, the risk of seizure recurrence after an unexplained seizure is about 25–80%, depending on the seizure type (partial more likely than generalized), presence of pre-existing neurological disease, or epileptiform discharges on EEG. The risk of recurrence is highest within the first 6 months, and is >80% after the second seizure.

In temporal lobe epilepsy, 1-year seizure-free status is expected in approximately 60% of treated patients; when associated with mesial temporal sclerosis, approximately 15–45% of patients may be seizure free at 1 year. Temporal lobe seizures are less likely to become secondarily generalized in comparison to extra-temporal complex partial seizures. Intractable seizures become more likely if adequate seizure control is not achieved with time. Patients with chronic epilepsy have psychological morbidities such as depression and anxiety (10–25%), as well as behavioral, cognitive, and memory deficits. In general, patients with complex partial seizures are more likely to require lifelong AED therapy than GTC seizures, especially if identifiable brain lesions are present.

Counseling

Patients with a single seizure should be aware that they might never have another episode. Epileptic patients should be aware of prognostic data and the potential role of epilepsy surgery in medically refractory individuals. Prognostic data for epilepsy surgery (risk–benefit assessment) should be discussed with adequately selected medically refractory patients. Outcomes are better for temporal over extra-temporal epilepsy, including GTC seizures. The neurological sequelae of temporal lobe surgery should also be discussed. The general principles of epilepsy counseling apply as outlined on pp. 169–170.

SUMMARY

- **Temporal lobe epilepsy** is a **localization-related**, **partial** seizure disorder that could be **simple** or **complex**, depending on alterations in level of consciousness. It accounts for **approximately 70%** of complex partial seizures.
- Causes of temporal lobe epilepsy include **mesial temporal sclerosis**, **trauma**, **congenital malformations**, **infections**, **cerebral infarction**, **neoplasms**, and **idiopathic**.
- Differentials include **atypical hemiplegic migraine, stroke/TIA, TGA, pseudoseizures, atypical syncope/drop attacks**, and **focal/segmental myoclonus.**
- Investigations should include **MRI of the brain** to assess for structural causes.
- Treatment **may not be necessary** for a single complex partial seizure.
- First-line AED options include **carbamazepine** and **phenytoin**. Newer AEDs (**oxcarbamazepine, lamotrigine, topiramate**, and **gabapentin**) have demonstrated efficacy as **monotherapy** in partial seizures.
- Medically refractory cases should be considered for **vagal nerve stimulation** or **epilepsy surgery**. Of adequately selected patients, **80–90%** experience benefit from temporal lobe surgery.
- Seizure-free rate at 1 year is **about 60%** with treated temporal lobe epilepsy, **approximately 15–45%** if associated with **mesial temporal sclerosis**. Chronic AED use is more likely to be required than in generalized epilepsies.
- **Psychological** morbidities are relatively common in chronic epileptics. **Behavioral**, **cognitive**, and **memory** deficits may also occur.

CASE 3

A 23-year-old woman was brought to the ER by her friends. She was reported to have had a convulsion after an argument with her boyfriend. She was observed to scream, then fall to the ground with all her limbs shaking violently in an uncoordinated manner for about 5 minutes, during which she asked that no one touch her or put anything in her mouth. Neither tongue biting nor urinary incontinence occurred. Neurological examination was normal. Following clinical evaluation, she had another episode, with irregular contractions of her left upper and lower extremities with head nodding.

Localization

An abrupt fall to the ground may suggest sudden loss of lower extremity muscle tone caused by upper motor neuron pathology in the mesial frontal lobes or their descending tracts (subcortical white matter, posterior limb of internal capsule, cerebral peduncles, basis pontis, pyramids, or spinal cord) or LMN disease involving the AHC, nerve roots (L2–S2), lumbosacral plexus, multiple peripheral nerves, NMJ, or multiple muscles. Bilateral upper and lower extremity muscular activity suggests activation of bi-hemispheric motor (predominantly frontal) cortices; however, normal mentation during the event makes volitional muscle activation more likely. The subsequent episode suggests volitional activation of the right frontal hemisphere (for left-sided movements) with some bilateral activation causing head nodding. The normal neurological examination makes true pathology less likely. The process is most likely nonphysiological, with volitional activation of the frontal lobes bilaterally.

Differential Diagnosis

The most likely diagnosis is *pseudoseizures*. These are nonepileptic spells that may superficially resemble GTC seizures and more commonly occur in females. There is usually a history of psychological disturbance or secondary gain (e.g., to play the sick role: factitious disorder, or overt benefit: malingering). However, approximately 10–40% of patients with pseudoseizures may have a seizure disorder, so that should be thoroughly investigated for.

Differential diagnoses include *simple partial frontal lobe seizures* (may be fast, frequent, and bizarre with normal level of consciousness and normal interictal EEG), *syncope* (especially vasovagal), or *drop attacks* (*see* p. 167: convulsions may occur as a result of transient cerebral hypoxia and recovery is usually rapid), *narcolepsy* (cataplexy: sudden loss of muscle tone associated with emotion, consciousness retained but increased muscle activity unexpected), *multifocal/generalized myoclonus*, or *panic attacks* (*see* p. 168).

Investigations

An elaborate collaborative clinical history or witnessing an event helps establish the diagnosis. Serum prolactin levels are invariably normal in pseudoseizures, but could also be normal in frontal lobe seizures. Interictal or ictal EEG recordings can be performed, however, normal results do not completely exclude a seizure disorder. Video or long-term ambulatory EEG monitoring would correlate the episodic behavioral spells with cerebral dysrhythmias; so negative testing further supports the diagnosis. Any other medical problems (e.g., drug intoxication, trauma) in addition to pseudoseizures should be adequately investigated.

Management

Patients with pseudoseizures should be informed that their spells are nonepileptic and should be referred to a psychiatrist for therapeutic intervention. AEDs have no role in treating pseudoseizures. Treatments include psychotherapy (supportive, psychodynamic), behavioral (biofeedback, relaxation), hypnosis or drugs for co-existing anxiety or depression. Neurologists should provide supportive care and continued reassurance to patients with pseudoseizures.

Prognosis

Complete cessation of pseudoseizures may occur in about 30% at 6 months after diagnosis, with cessation in approximately 35–50% at 1–6 years mean follow-up. About 50% of patients previously taking AEDs for misdiagnosis of seizure disorder will cease taking these medications over 5 years. About 10% of patients develop new somatic complaints within 6 months of diagnosis.

Factors highly predictive of recurrent pseudoseizures despite adequate counseling and treatment include duration of pseudoseizures before diagnosis, history of affective disorder, recurrent major depressive episodes, dissociative disorder, somatoform disorder, personality disorder (borderline, histrionic), denial of stressors or psychosocial problems, chronic abuse (physical, emotional, sexual, or mixed), and noncompliance with treatment options. Morbidity could also occur as a consequence of chronic AED use or therapeutic interventions (e.g., intubation, pharmacological coma for pseudo-SE).

Counseling

Counseling is an integral part of the therapeutic approach in pseudoseizures. This should be done in a nonconfrontational way that is not condescending in order to acquire and maintain patient trust. Psychiatric co-morbidities are relatively common in this disorder, and may occur in more than 80% of patients. These problems should be professionally managed. Patients should be made aware that early therapeutic intervention and adequate treatment of psychiatric co-morbidities improve outcomes. Patients should be weaned off AEDs slowly and should have the option of whether to continue neurological follow-up.

SUMMARY

- **Pseudoseizures** (or nonepileptic seizures) superficially resemble GTC seizures and are associated with **psychological illness** or **secondary gain**.
- **Approximately 10–40%** of patients with pseudo seizures have a seizure disorder.
- Differentials include **simple partial frontal lobe seizures, syncope, drop attacks, narcolepsy, multifocal/generalized myoclonus**, and **panic attacks.**
- Normal **video** or long-term **ambulatory EEG** establishes diagnosis in clinically suspected cases. Serum **prolactin** levels may be useful.
- Treatment includes **counseling, psychotherapy, behavioral therapy, hypnosis,** and **drugs** (antidepressants and anxiolytics).

- **Approximately 10%** of patients develop new somatic symptoms within 6 months of initial diagnosis.
- **Approximately 30%** of patients have complete cessation at **6 months**, with **approximately 35–50%** cessation rates at **1–6 years** mean follow-up.
- Predictors of recurrent episodes include **pseudo seizure duration**, history of **affective disorder**, recurrent **major depressive episodes, dissociative, somatoform or personality disorders, denial of stressors** or **psychosocial problems, chronic abuse**, and **noncompliance** with treatment options.
- Referral should be made to a **psychiatrist** for management, but the **supportive role** of the neurologist is also essential.
- **Early treatment** improves outcomes.

CASE 4

A 59-year-old man came to the office complaining of "fainting spells" for 3 months. He stated that he developed lightheadedness that occurred with positional change, followed by nausea, blurred vision, and generalized weakness resulting in passing out and falls. His wife had noticed that he remained unconscious for about 30 seconds and she had observed convulsions after a fall. These episodes were occurring approximately once a week and he seemed to make a rapid recovery from them. On examination, vital signs, including orthostatic BP and HR evaluations were normal. Neurological examination was also normal.

Localization

Lightheadedness is a nonspecific complaint. True vertigo (illusion of rotation) would imply vestibular dysfunction. Nausea may be secondary to medullary disease, whereas blurred vision could imply disease affecting the anterior visual pathways bilaterally. Generalized weakness suggests bilateral upper motor neuron (motor cortex, subcortical white matter, posterior limb of internal capsule, cerebral peduncles, basis pontis, pyramids, or spinal cord) or LMN disease (AHC, nerve roots, lumbosacral plexi, multiple peripheral nerves, NMJ, or multiple muscles).

Loss of consciousness implies bilateral cerebral cortex dysfunction or dysfunction of the reticular-activating system in the brainstem (pons, medulla), and subsequent convulsions could be secondary to loss of descending cortical inhibition of the brainstem. Motor cortex hyperexcitability would be unusual in this setting. In summary, the underlying process diffusely localizes to the cerebral cortex, anterior visual pathways, and brainstem bilaterally.

Differential Diagnosis

The most likely diagnosis is *syncope*: a symptom complex associated with transient hypoperfusion or hypoxia to the brain with loss of consciousness, loss of postural tone, and absence of neurological sequelae. Tonic-clonic movements may occur (convulsive syncope) and these may be rarely prolonged with severe cerebral anoxia following cardiac arrest. The sensation of an impending syncopal attack is called presyncope.

Differential diagnoses include *seizures* (e.g., atonic, GTC, or complex partial seizures: usually have longer ictal and postictal phases with distinct stereotypical motor phenomena that result in falls), *drop attacks* (secondary to cerebrovascular disease—vertebrobasilar and ACA: would expect further localizing signs; paroxysmal hydrocephalus with third ventricular and posterior fossa tumors), *cataplexy* (as part of narcolepsy: loss of tone associated with emotion, hypnagogic hallucinations, and sleep paralysis; loss of consciousness and convulsions unexpected), *vestibular disorders* (otolithic crises in Ménière's disease), *cerebellar disorders* (with truncal ataxia: presentation usually progressive), and *metabolic encephalopathies* (e.g., hepatic failure, uremia).

Etiologies for syncope include *cardiovascular disease* (secondary to reduced cardiac output or dysrhythmias), *cerebrovascular disease* (bilateral arterial occlusive disease in carotid arteries or vertebrobasilar system, vasculopathy: vasculitis or vasospasm from multiple causes), *hypotension* (*orthostatic* in dysautonomia: *primary autonomic failure* e.g., Riley–Day syndrome, MSA, or *secondary to peripheral neuropathies*: DM, alcohol, amyloidosis, porphyria, or GBS; *drug-induced* e.g., antihypertensives, neuroleptics, TCAs, or cholinergic agents or vasovagal: may be associated with change in emotional state), *hypovolemia* (e.g., following blood loss, burns, or sepsis), *metabolic* (e.g., hypoxia, hyperventilation-induced alkalosis: usually psychogenic in origin; or hypoglycemia), *situational* (usually associated with certain events e.g., micturition, defecation, and tussive syncopes), or *idiopathic* (~20% of all cases).

Investigations

Investigations should be individualized toward particular etiologies suspected during clinical evaluation and need to exclude other disorders. CBC with differential, basic metabolic panel, chest X-ray, and EKG should be considered in all patients. Prolonged Holter monitoring (>24 hours) or telemetry evaluation should be performed if cardiac dysrhythmias are suspected. Further possible investigations include Doppler ultrasonography (including TCD), MRI brain and MRA intra- and extracranial vessels, echocardiography, exercise/stress testing, and neurophysiology (peripheral: EMG/NCS and autonomic testing and/or central: EEG, polysomnography with multiple sleep latency test).

Management

The treatment of syncope should be tailored to the underlying cause, as well as general supportive measures. Admission to the hospital for evaluation and care depends on the severity of the clinical suspicion for etiology. In patients with cardiac dysrhythmias, referral to cardiology for evaluation and permanent pacemakers is required. With dysautonomia associated with orthostasis, options include liberal salt diet, increased fluid intake, compression stockings, drugs (e.g., midodrine, mineralocorticoids), moderate exercise, and tilt-table training: unproven in randomized controlled trials. In cases associated with hypovolemia, fluid replacement should be instituted. Metabolic causes should be reversed, if possible. Offending drugs and toxins should be stopped. Supportive measures include advice about maneuvers that may prevent loss of consciousness, to assume a supine position when presyncopal, and to avoid activities that may lead to serious injury. Syncopal triggers, such as heat, alcohol, prolonged standing, lack of sleep, large meals, fasting, and dehydration, should be avoided to prevent precipitating attacks.

Prognosis

Prognosis is dependent on the underlying etiology, however, cardiac disease adversely affects prognosis of patients with syncope. Syncopal patients with cardiac disease may have a 1-year mortality of approximately 20–35% secondary to underlying cardiovascular disease rather than cardiogenic syncope. Patients with known causes of syncope without cardiac disease have a mortality rate of about 10% at 1 year, with about 6% death rate in idiopathic cases over the same time period. Possible predictors of poor outcomes (life-threatening cardiac arrhythmias or death) at 1 year in syncope patients include age 45 or older, a history of heart failure, a history of ventricular arrhythmias, and an abnormal ECG. There is an approximately 5% risk of developing poor outcomes with none of these predictive factors, whereas the presence of three or four of these confers a risk of 60–80%.

Counseling

Patients should be aware that syncope with cardiovascular disease might result in poor outcomes modifiable by early permanent pacemaker insertion and aggressive treatment of the underlying disease. Permanent pacemakers may reduce likelihood of recurrent syncope by 80–90% in patients with bradycardia on tilt-table testing over follow-up of 2–4 years. Patients should be aware that approximately 20% of patients with syncope do not have a demonstrable cause, emphasizing the importance of supportive care in this group. Education on protective measures and avoidance of triggers should take place in an attempt to prevent injury and reduce the frequency of attacks.

SUMMARY

- **Syncope** is a symptom complex associated with **transient hypoperfusion** or **hypoxia** to the brain with **loss of consciousness, loss of postural tone**, and **absence of neurological sequelae.**

- Differentials include **seizures, drop attacks, cataplexy, vestibular, cerebellar**, and **metabolic** disorders.
- Treatments include addressing the **underlying cause** and providing **supportive care**: protective advice and avoidance of triggers.
- Prognosis depends on etiology. Co-existence of cardiac disease in syncopal patients results in 1-year mortality of **approximately 20–35%**.
- In non-idiopathic syncope without cardiac disease, mortality rate is **about 10%** at 1 year, with idiopathic syncope, **approximately 6%**.
- Possible predictors of poor outcomes at 1 year in syncope patients include **age 45 or older, history of heart failure, history of ventricular arrhythmias**, and **an abnormal EKG. Three to four predictors** confer **60–80%** risk, whereas **no factors** confers **approximately 5%** risk.
- **Permanent pacemakers** may reduce likelihood of recurrent syncope by **80–90%** in patients with bradycardia on tilt-table testing over follow-up of **2–4 years**.
- Etiologies include **cardiovascular, cerebrovascular, hypotensive** (including **dysautonomia**: primary or secondary to peripheral neuropathy, drugs, or vasovagal disease), **hypovolemic, metabolic, situational**, and **idiopathic** (~**20%** of all cases).
- Investigations should include **CBC with differential, basic metabolic profile, chest X-ray**, and **EKG**. Further tests should be tailored toward potential causes and differentials based on history.

15

Neuroimmunology

CASE 1

A 39-year-old woman came to the ER complaining of progressive left-sided weakness for 3 days. A few days prior, she had gradually developed right-sided sensory loss that lasted 48 hours with complete resolution. On further questioning, she stated that she experienced partial left visual loss 10 weeks ago that seemed to have recovered completely over 2 months and noticed double vision on looking to the left. Neurological examination revealed a left afferent pupillary defect, right adduction paresis with left abduction nystagmus, mild left lower facial droop, MRC 4/5 strength in the left upper and lower extremities, mild right hemisensory loss to pinprick and light touch, and left-sided hypertonia and hyperreflexia with an extensor plantar response.

Localization

Left hemiplegia secondary to an upper motor neuron lesion localizes to the right cerebrum (motor cortex: frontal lobes), subcortical white matter, posterior limb of the internal capsule, cerebral peduncles or pons above the level of the facial nucleus. Right hemisensory loss localizes to the left parietal cortex, subcortical white matter, thalamus (ventral posterior lateral [VPL] and ventral posterior medial [VPM] nuclei) or upper midbrain. A left afferent pupillary defect implies left optic nerve disease, whereas the right internuclear ophthalmoplegia localizes to the right medial longitudinal fasciculus (from midbrain to medulla). In summary, the underlying process is multifocal, with possible involvement of the right frontal and left parietal cortices, left optic nerve, and right brainstem.

Differential Diagnosis

The most likely diagnosis for a subacute presentation of focal neurological deficits disseminated in time and space in this age group is *multiple sclerosis* (MS). MS is primarily an inflammatory demyelinating disease of the CNS. Clinical course may be relapsing-remitting, primary or secondary progressive, or progressive-relapsing. The differential diagnoses for MS are limited in a

From: *Neurology Oral Boards Review:*
A Concise and Systematic Approach to Clinical Practice
By: E. E. Ubogu © Humana Press Inc., Totowa, NJ

relapsing-remitting course, however, these may be more extensive for the initial or an acute episode or a primary progressive course.

Diagnostic considerations include *inflammatory diseases* (e.g., ADEM: monophasic illness following vaccination or viral infection), *collagen vascular diseases* (primary: PACNS or secondary: SLE, PAN, Wegener's granulomatosis [WG], rheumatic arthritis [RhA], Sjögren's syndrome, Behçet's disease), *granulomatous disease* (e.g., sarcoidosis), *infections* (HIV, HTLV-1, JC virus: causes progressive multifocal leukoencephalopathy [PML], neurosyphilis, Lyme disease), *neoplasia* (e.g., lymphoma, paraneoplastic encephalomyelopathy), *toxic/metabolic* (vitamin B_{12} deficiency: peripheral neuropathy present; Marchiava–Bignami disease, central pontine myelinolysis, carbon monoxide poisoning), *mitochondrial disorders* (e.g., Leigh's disease: subacute necrotizing encephalomyelopathy), and *adult-onset leukodystrophies* (e.g., adrenomyeloneuropathy).

Investigations

MRI of the CNS with and without gadolinium is the radiological modality of choice as a diagnostic aid in MS for both acute and chronic lesions. Further diagnostic aids include CSF examination for oligoclonal bands, elevated IgG synthesis rate (>3.0) or IgG index (>0.7), as well as excluding CNS infection. Evoked potentials (visual, somatosensory, or brainstem) may be utilized, but are not as sensitive as MRI (abnormal in 75–85% of definite MS cases in comparison to ~95% with MRI).

If atypical features are present, further diagnostic work-up should be tailored toward excluding other diseases based on the clinical evaluation. Such tests may include ANA panel, ds-DNA, RhF, SSA/SSB, anti-neutrophil cytoplasmic antibody [ANCA], HIV titers, HTLV-1, Lyme titers, VRDL/FTA-ABS, vitamin B_{12} levels, and lactate/pyruvate. Brain biopsy may be required for tumor-like MS presentations to exclude CNS tumor, as well as to exclude PACNS if clinically suspected.

Management

The treatment of MS includes treating acute attacks to limit sequelae, prophylactic medications to prevent or reduce rate of progression, and symptomatic/ supportive therapy. Acute attacks or relapse are treated with high-dose corticosteroids, i.v. methylprednisolone 500–1000 mg　every day divided every 6 or 12 hours for 3–7 days, with or without short-course prednisone taper over 7–10 days. Prophylactic medications include the disease-modifying drugs interferon β-1b, interferon β-1a and glatiramer acetate. These agents may reduce the rate of relapse or clinical progression by 20–30% over 2–5 years. Side effects include local infection-site reactions, flu-like symptoms, myalgias, fatigue, depression, and anxiety. Regular CBC, LFT, and electrolyte checks (every 3–6 months) may be required for interferon-β therapy, especially during the first 1–2 years of therapy.

For progressive disease, immunomodulatory drugs such as methotrexate, cyclosporine, cyclophosphamide, azathioprine, total lymphoid irradiation, mitoxantrone (risk of cardiotoxicity), mycophenolate mofetil, or interferon-β may be employed to treat this difficult and moderately refractory MS phase.

Symptomatic therapies include antidepressants (SSRIs, TCAs, etc.) for depression (as many as 50% of MS patients are affected by depression), anticholinergics for hyperreflexic bladder, α-blockers, or cholinergics/catherization for flaccid bladder, amantadine/pemoline for fatigue, antispasticity drugs (baclofen, tinzanidine, dantrolene, benzodiazepines) for muscle spasticity, AEDs for tremor, clonus, and pain, and sildenafil for sexual dysfunction. More invasive methods, for example, botulinum toxin injections for focal spasticity or bladder augmentation for spastic bladder may be required in more severe cases.

Supportive care includes physical/occupational therapy to improve with functional capabilities, coping strategies or lifestyle modifications to facilitate ADLs, cognitive-behavioral therapy, and emotional support. In more severe cases, ambulatory aids or wheelchairs and other home-assist devices and caregiver support may be necessary.

Prognosis

Patients with optic neuritis have a 50–70% chance of developing MS if initially associated with brain lesions on MRI and approximately 10–20% chance if no MRI lesions are present, over 5 years. Presentation with ATM confers a 60–90% risk of developing MS over 3–5 years in patients with MRI lesions and 10–30% in patients without lesions. Mortality from MS is difficult to ascertain because of co-existing diseases of aging, but MS may reduce life expectancy by 10–15 years. Benign and malignant/fulminant variants exist. Early disability and death are more common with fulminant variants such as Devic's disease (neuromyelitis optica), or Marburg's disease.

MS relapse rate is approximately 0.8–1.2 per year in untreated patients and about 0.4–0.6 per year in treated cohorts. About 15% of clinically diagnosed MS patients never have a second attack. Patients with mild disease 5 years after diagnosis have approximately 7.5% and approximately 10% risk of developing severe disease at 10 and 15 years, respectively. Prognostic indicators include gender (males are worse), age at onset (later ages less favorable), initial presenting feature (optic neuritis has better prognosis than brainstem/cerebellar disease), and initial disease course (relapsing form has better prognosis than progressive forms).

Counseling

Patients should be aware of the potential chronicity and complications of MS. Prognostic data should be discussed in detail. There are no longer term studies on the efficacy and risks of disease-modifying drugs and patients should be aware of the risks for developing MS after an initial attack. Neutralizing antibodies may develop in 25–50% of patients receiving interferon-β for longer than 6 months, and this may result in loss of efficacy. The treatment resistance of progressive forms of MS may result in trials of different immunomodulating agents with varying side effects. Supportive care from family and friends should be encouraged.

SUMMARY

- **MS** is a primarily **demyelinating inflammatory** disease of the CNS with lesions disseminated in **time** and **space**.
- Differentials include **ADEM, collagen vascular diseases, sarcoidosis, infections, neoplasia, toxic/metabolic, mitochondrial disorders**, and **adult-onset leukodystrophy**.
- Diagnosis is **clinical**, aided by **MRI with and without gadolinium**, **CSF** examination for **oligoclonal bands, IgG synthesis rate** and **IgG index**, and **evoked potentials**.
- Treatments include **corticosteroids** for acute attacks, **disease-modifying drugs** for relapsing-remitting disease, **immunomodulators** for progressive disease, as well as **symptomatic** and **supportive** measures.
- Presentation with optic neuritis confers **approximately 50–70%** 5-year risk of MS if initial MRI brain lesion present, and **approximately 10–30%** without.
- MS relapse rate is **approximately 0.8–1.2 per year** in untreated patients and **about 0.4–0.6 per year** if treated.
- Patients with mild disease at 5 years have **approximately 7.5%** and **approximately 10%** chance of severe disease at **10** and **15 years**, respectively.
- Prognostic indicators for poor outcomes include **male gender, older age at onset, brainstem/cerebellar presentation**, and **initial progressive course**.

CASE 2

A 49-year-old man presented to the ER with sudden onset of bilateral lower extremity weakness. About 1 week prior, he complained of low-grade fever, generalized malaise, and myalgias. Two days afterward, he developed sudden left-sided sensory loss followed by right facial weakness and double vision on looking to the right that worsened over 2 days. On examination, he was afebrile and without nuchal rigidity. Cranial nerve examination revealed limitation of right eye abduction and right facial weakness. Motor examination revealed paraparesis (MRC 3/5) with reduced tone. Sensory examination reveals astereognosis and agraphesthesia on the left. Reflexes were normal in the upper extremities and reduced in the lower extremities.

Localization

The left-sided astereognosis and agraphesthesia suggest a right parietal cortex lesion. The right CN VI and VII nerve palsies most likely localize to the right pons. Paraparesis may localize to the bilateral mesial frontal cortex, subcortical white matter, cerebral peduncles, basis pontis, pyramidal tracts or corticospinal tracts of the spinal cord, or PNS (lumbosacral AHC, nerve roots, plexi, multiple nerves, NMJ, or muscle). Reduced tone and reflexes in the lower extremities implies PNS disease, but the sudden onset is more consistent with CNS dysfunction. This is most likely in the spinal cord with associated "spinal shock." In summary, the underlying process is multifocal, localizing to the right parietal cortex, right pons, and bilateral ventral spinal cord.

Differential Diagnosis

The most likely diagnosis for a multifocal disorder that occurs suddenly with subsequent progression days after a viral prodrome that affects the brain and spinal cord is *acute disseminated encephalomyelitis* (ADEM). This is a monophasic disorder that may occur following systemic viral infection or postvaccination, and is characterized pathologically by perivascular inflammation, edema, and demyelination in the CNS. Possible etiological agents for postinfectious ADEM include *rubella, mumps, herpes simplex, influenza, EBV, CMV, coxsackievirus, mycoplasma, Lyme disease*, and *malaria*. Vaccines implicated in the past include *rabies, smallpox, pertussis, diphtheria, rubella*, and *measles*.

Other differentials include *MS* (recovery is less rapid), *CNS vasculitis* (PACNS or secondary to systemic vasculitis), *multiple cerebral embolic infarcts* (e.g., infective endocarditis, ulcerated plaque), *chronic meningitis* (such as fungal or TB: multiple cranial neuropathies common and spinal cord disease less likely), *multiple brain abscesses, sarcoidosis, brain metastases* (symptoms usually present less acutely), and *mitochondrial encephalopathy* (e.g., Leigh's disease: presents more subacutely).

Investigations

MRI of the brain and spinal cord with and without gadolinium is the diagnostic test of choice in demonstrating the lesions of ADEM. These findings are somewhat indistinguishable from MS. CSF examination may reveal cell count less than $100/\mu L$ in 85–100% of cases, with modest increase in protein in 40–60% of patients. CSF IgG synthesis is normal and oligoclonal bands are usually absent. Gram stain and cultures would exclude chronic meningitides. In atypical cases, blood tests for systemic vasculitides (ANA panel, ds-DNA, RhF, SSA/SSB, ANCA), lactate/pyruvate, serum ACE levels, and serial blood cultures may be required to exclude other differentials. MRA/TEE may be required if embolic etiology highly considered. In equivocal cases, brain biopsy may be required to exclude PACNS, brain metastases, or sarcoidosis.

Management

The mainstay of therapy is corticosteroids, although this is not supported by controlled trials. Therapeutic options include high-dose methylprednisolone (500–1000 mg i.v. every 24 hours) for 5 days only or with slow steroid taper over 4–6 weeks in patients with improvement but moderate to severe deficits after initial therapy; i.v. cyclophosphamide (1000 mg for 5 days), plasmapheresis or IVIg (0.4 g/kg per day for 5 days) may be used in steroid-unresponsive cases. Supportive care, such as adequate nutrition and hydration, regular nursing checks, DVT/GI prophylaxis, capillary glucose (while on i.v. steroids), speech, physical, and occupational therapy should be instituted. Eye patches should be considered to reduce diplopia.

Prognosis

Mortality occurs in about 10–20% of cases, and is associated with more severe and fulminant initial clinical presentations. Recovery may take days, but usually occurs over weeks to months. Complete recovery is expected in approximately 50%, with minor residual deficits occurring in about 30–35% of patients and moderate deficits in approximately 10–15%. About 20–30% of patients initially diagnosed with ADEM may develop clinical MS. The second episode of neurological deficit usually occurs within 1 year of the initial episode. Factors most predictive of ADEM over MS clinically include older age of onset, preceding infection, early brainstem involvement, infratentorial lesions, and elevated CSF albumin fraction, although these features are not exclusive to ADEM.

Counseling

Patients should be aware of the monophasic nature of this disease and risk of actually having MS. Recurrences have been described in ADEM, but these may represent relapsing-remitting MS. Prognostic data, including likelihood of complete recovery should be discussed.

SUMMARY

- **ADEM** is an acute **monophasic** demyelinating disorder of the CNS that may be **postinfectious** or **postvaccination**.
- Postinfectious etiologies include **viruses, bacteria, spirochetes**, and **parasites**.
- Postvaccination etiologies include **rabies, smallpox, pertussis, diphtheria, rubella**, and **measles**.
- Differentials include **MS, CNS vasculitis, multiple cerebral infarcts, chronic meningitis, multiple cerebral abscesses, sarcoidosis, brain metastases**, and **mitochondrial disease**.

- Investigations include **MRI** and **CSF** examination. Other differentials should be excluded in atypical cases.
- Mainstay of treatment is **high-dose corticosteroids**. Other treatments include **cyclophosphamide, plasmapheresis**, and **IVIg**.
- Mortality is **approximately 10–20%**. Complete recovery occurs in **about 50%** of patients. Mild residual deficits occur in **approximately 30–35%** and moderate deficits in **approximately 10–15%**.
- About **20–30%** initially diagnosed with ADEM develop clinical MS, with second episode occurring within the **first year** of initial presenting symptoms.

16

Sleep Disorders

CASE 1

A 25-year-old woman complained of an 8-month history of excessive day-time somnolence. She stated that she had to take multiple naps during the day and had vivid dreams on falling asleep. Her friend had witnessed loss of muscle control in her legs following a significant change in emotional state such as anger or laughter. She had also experienced episodes of being paralyzed on awakening. Neurological examination was normal.

Localization

Excessive daytime somnolence (EDS) implies poor nocturnal sleep, which could be secondary to difficulty initiating or maintaining sleep. Dysfunctional sleep is nonlocalizing, and may implicate dysfunction in sleep or alerting centers in the hypothalamus, thalamus, or brainstem. Vivid dreams could be normal or represent visual hallucinations. Visual hallucinations may localize to the bilateral occipital cortex (elementary figures) or temporo-occipital junction (well-formed figures). Sudden lower extremity atonia may localize to the bilateral mesial frontal lobes, subcortical white matter, cerebral peduncles, basis pontis, pyramidal tracts, or corticospinal tracts in the spinal cord. Transient quadriparesis suggests bilateral upper or LMN dysfunction. There are no features in the history that suggest one over the other. In summary, the underlying process most likely involves the bilateral cerebral cortex, diencephalon, and brainstem.

Differential Diagnosis

The most likely diagnosis for a sleep disorder with EDS, hypnagogic hallucinations, cataplexy, and sleep paralysis is *narcolepsy*. This is rapid eye movement (REM)-sleep disorder associated with dysfunction in orexin (hypocretin)-secreting cells in the hypothalamus, and may be linked to human leukocyte antigen (HLA) DQB1*0602 on chromosome 6 in all ethnic groups. In 60–100% of cases, cataplexy occurs with EDS only. Sleep paralysis may

From: *Neurology Oral Boards Review:*
A Concise and Systematic Approach to Clinical Practice
By: E. E. Ubogu © Humana Press Inc., Totowa, NJ

occur in 25–50% of cases and the classic tetrad (as in this case) occurs in approximately 10% of patients. Other differentials that should be considered could be divided based on symptoms.

Differentials for EDS include *obstructive sleep apnea* (OSA), *sleep deprivation, drug-induced hypersomnolence* (alcohol, sedative-hypnotics, antihistamines, etc.), *medical causes* (chronic obstructive pulmonary disease [COPD], CHF, peptic ulcer disease, sleeping sickness), *neurological causes* (stroke, headache, painful peripheral neuropathies, fatal familial insomnia, AD, brain tumors: diencephalic or midbrain), *psychiatric illness* (psychoses, anxiety/panic disorders, bipolar disorder: these may cause nocturnal insomnia with subsequent EDS), *circadian rhythm disturbances*, and *idiopathic hypersomnia* (excessive sleepiness associated with normal or prolonged non-REM sleep episodes: sleep is unrefreshing despite duration and cataplexy not expected).

Differentials for hypnagogic hallucinations include *psychoses* and *lesions of temporo-occipital cortex* (tumor, stroke, hemorrhage, abscess, etc). Differentials for cataplexy include *drop attacks, syncope* (*see* pp. 167, 176–179), and seizures (atonic, complex partial, or absence). Sleep paralysis may occur as an *isolated and physiological response*, as part of familial sleep paralysis or could be mistaken for an *upper brainstem stroke* ("top of the basilar syndrome" secondary to basilar artery thrombosis: transient symptoms unexpected) or *hyperkalemic* or *hypokalemic periodic paralysis* (Na^+ and Ca^{2+} channelopathies respectively; associated with changes in serum K^+).

Investigations

The diagnostic tests of choice include overnight polysomnography and multiple sleep latency test. Polysomnography may show short sleep latency, excessive sleep disruption with frequent arousals, reduced total sleep time, reduced slow-wave sleep, and sleep-onset REM. Multiple sleep latency test may show a mean sleep latency of less than 8 minutes, or more than two sleep-onset REM (out of four to five recordings), or both. In equivocal cases, neuroimaging (CT/MRI of the brain), EEG, electrodiagnostic tests, pulmonary function tests, cardiological evaluation, and serum/urine toxicology may be required to exclude other etiologies.

Management

The mainstay of treatment for narcolepsy is pharmacological. Treatments can be divided into drugs to control EDS (sleep attacks) and drugs to control cataplexy and the other manifestations of the disorder. EDS may be controlled with amphetamines such as methylphenidate, pemoline, dextroamphetamine, adderall, or modafinil (side effects include headache, nervousness, with or without nausea). The treatment of cataplexy and the other manifestations of narcolepsy include TCAs (e.g., imipramine, clomipramine) and SSRIs (e.g., fluoxetine, paroxetine). Nonpharmacological measures include general improvement in sleep hygiene and short, scheduled daytime naps. Lifestyle and job modifications may be necessary to ensure a safe environment. Involvement in a narcolepsy support group and regular exercise could also be useful.

Prognosis

Narcolepsy is a chronic, nonprogressive lifelong disease. Its natural history is poorly defined, but patients with narcolepsy have worse functional ratings and higher disability scores than age-matched controls with time. Narcoleptics may also develop OSA, periodic leg movements of sleep (PLMS), or RBD that require additional treatment. Pharmacological treatment for narcolepsy may result in more than 70–80% improvement in symptoms, with approximately 50–60% of patients reporting significant symptomatic relief. Prognosis is also influenced by the risk of chronically taking these medications.

Counseling

Patients should be aware that narcolepsy is a lifelong disease that can be debilitating. Pharmacological options should be discussed with the patient and a risk–benefit analysis needs to be performed individually. Patients with narcolepsy may develop anxiety, depression, sexual dysfunction, morning headaches, or memory dysfunction, so patients should be counseled to seek medical intervention if these arise. Driving and operating heavy machinery should be avoided and involvement in a narcolepsy support group may help with coping with the disease.

SUMMARY

- **Narcolepsy** is a **REM-sleep disorder** associated with dysfunction of **orexin (hypocretin)**-secreting cells in the **hypothalamus**.
- The classic tetrad consists of **EDS** (sleep attacks), **hypnagogic hallucinations, cataplexy,** and **sleep paralysis**.
- Differential considerations for EDS: **OSA, sleep deprivation, drug-induced hypersomnolence, medical causes, neurological causes, psychiatric illness, circadian rhythm disturbances,** and **idiopathic hypersomnia**.
- Differential considerations for hypnagogic hallucinations include **psychoses** and **lesions of temporo-occipital cortex,** for cataplexy include **drop attacks, syncope,** and **seizures** and for sleep paralysis include **normal** physiological response, **familial sleep paralysis, upper brainstem stroke,** or **periodic paralysis**.

- Diagnostic tests of choice are **overnight polysomnography** and **multiple sleep latency test**.
- Pharmacological treatments include **amphetamines** and **modafinil** for EDS, **TCAs** and **SSRIs** for cataplexy and other symptoms.
- Nonpharmacological treatments include **general improvement in sleep hygiene**, **short**, **scheduled daytime naps**, **lifestyle** and **job modifications**, involvement in a **narcolepsy support group**, and **regular exercise**.
- **Long-term disability** expected with chronic narcolepsy.
- **Risk–benefit ratio** needs to be considered in narcoleptics on long-term pharmacotherapy.

CASE 2

A 67-year-old man came to the clinic with his wife. She was concerned that over the past 4 months, he had been having "violent dreams" resulting in aggressive behavior in bed. During the past week, she had been struck several times on the face and chest and he had kicked the bedside lamp over. He denied any recollection of any of these events. Neurological examination was normal.

Localization

Aggressive violent behavior may indicate dysfunction of the limbic cortex (bilateral mesial frontal and temporal lobes, especially the amygdala). Aggressive behavior may also occur with global cerebral dysfunction (delirium or dementia) without any particular localizing features. The occurrence of these episodes during sleep may also implicate dysfunction in sleep-modulating centers in the hypothalamus, thalamus, or brainstem (midbrain and pons). In summary, the clinical presentation is nonlocalizing, with possible involvement of the bilateral cerebral cortex, diencephalon, and brainstem.

Differential Diagnosis

The most likely diagnosis for violent aggressive behavior during REM sleep in an elderly main is *REM sleep behavior disorder* (RBD). This is an idiopathic disorder in 50–60% of patients. In the remainder, causal associations that have been described include *neurodegenerative disorders* (e.g., PD, MSA, DLBD, CBGD, PSP), *sleep disorders* (e.g., narcolepsy), *toxins* (e.g., alcohol), *drugs* (e.g., sedative-hypnotics, TCAs, anticholinergics), or *thalamic/brainstem lesions*. Differentials include *nocturnal complex partial seizures* (temporal or frontal foci), *psychiatric disorders* (e.g., pain attack, psychosis), *delirium* (*see* pp. 94–96), or *sleep disorders* (e.g., night terrors, nightmares, sleep walking, confusional arousals).

Investigations

The diagnostic test of choice for RBD is nocturnal polysomnography. This shows REM sleep without muscle hypotonia/atonia. In atypical cases, standard 16-channel EEG may be performed to exclude complex partial seizures. Laboratory investigations may include serum/urine toxicology screens if there is a history of drug/toxin exposure. MRI brain may be useful in establishing secondary causes for RBD if suggested by the clinical evaluation.

Management

Any underlying conditions should be identified and appropriately treated if possible. Pharmacological treatment for RBD consists of low-dose medium- to long-acting benzodiazepines, such as clonazepam. There is an approximately 90% response rate to this medication that occurs early in the treatment course. Patients may need to sleep alone with the removal of any potentially dangerous objects in proximity to the bed until symptoms are controlled. Supportive care and reassurance should be offered to bed partners.

Prognosis

RBD is a life-long, chronic sleep disorder that is usually adequately controlled with benzodiazepines. Cessation of medication usually results in symptom recurrence. Prognosis would also be modified by any underlying secondary causes.

Counseling

Patients should be aware of the excellent response to benzodiazepines and the risks and benefit of chronic use should be discussed fully. Bed partners should be provided with reassurance and emotional support. Alcohol and other drugs that may induce RBD should be avoided.

SUMMARY

- **RBD** usually presents with **aggressive behavior** during **REM sleep** and is more common in **elderly men**.
- Etiologies include **idiopathic** (50–60%), **neurodegenerative disorders, sleep disorders, toxins, drugs,** or **thalamic/brainstem lesions**.
- Differentials include **nocturnal complex partial seizures, psychiatric disorders, delirium**, or **sleep disorders** such as night terrors, nightmares, sleep walking, and confusional arousals.
- **Absence of REM sleep hypotonia/atonia** on **nocturnal polysomnography** establishes the diagnosis. Secondary causes should be evaluated for if clinically indicated.
- Treatment of choice is **medium- to long-acting benzodiazepines** (e.g., **clonazepam**), with **approximately 90%** response rate.

- **Supportive care, emotional support**, and **injury precautions** are necessary adjuncts to pharmacotherapy.
- **Cessation of drug therapy** results in **symptom recurrence**.
- RBD is a **chronic disorder** and prognosis may be modified by identifiable underlying causes.

CASE 3

A 48-year-old woman complained of progressively worsening urge to move her legs while lying down in bed for about 3 months, especially before falling asleep. She experienced a creepy, unpleasant sensation in her legs before the urge to move. These symptoms were readily relieved by walking around her bedroom but returned once she got back into bed. Her spouse had also noticed intermittent repetitive stereotypical lower extremity movements when she was asleep. Dramatization showed that she flexes her hip and knee, dorsiflexes the ankle, and extends the great toe. Neurological examination was normal.

Localization

Abnormal sensory perception in the lower extremities may be secondary to peripheral nerve dysfunction (sensory nerves, lumbosacral plexi, lumbar and sacral nerve roots, or dorsal root ganglia) or central dysfunction (e.g., lumbar and sacral spinal cord, periaqueductal gray of the midbrain, thalamus). Abnormal stereotypical motor activity may suggest hyperexcitation of the frontal cortex or lack of cortical inhibition of brainstem (e.g., red nucleus in midbrain, vestibular nucleus at the pontomedullary junction) and spinal cord AHC that influence motor activity. The normal examination does not provide any further localizing clues. In summary, the underlying process most likely affects central or peripheral sensorimotor pathways or both.

Differential Diagnosis

The most likely diagnosis for a non-REM sleep disorder characterized by irresistible urges to move the legs in association with creeping sensations that is relieved by walking, and associated with *periodic leg movements of sleep* (PLMS) is *restless legs syndrome* (RLS). RLS is a complex sensorimotor sleep disorder of unknown etiology that predominantly affects the legs. PLMS may occur in approximately 80% of patients with RLS.

In a few patients, RLS is caused by *neurological disorders*: *central causes* include MS, hyperexplexia, PD, myelopathy; *peripheral causes* include poliomyelitis, lumbosacral radiculopathy, polyneuropathy, Isaac's syndrome (neuromyotonia) or *mixed* (ALS); *medical causes* include iron-deficiency anemia, uremia, DM, hypothyroidism, peripheral vascular disease, and cancer;

drug etiologies include as Ca^{2+} channel antagonists, antiemetics, lithium, TCAs, SSRIs, alcohol, caffeine, sedative-hypnotic drug withdrawal; or *pregnancy.*

Differentials include *akathisia* (motor restlessness commonly associated with neuroleptics, present mostly during the day with an inability to stand or sit still), *myokymia* (undulating muscle movements associated with nerve demyelination), *painful nocturnal leg cramps, essential myoclonus* (benign myoclonic jerks of unknown etiology), *hypnic jerks* (sudden brief myoclonic jerks of limbs or entire body lasting for a few seconds at sleep onset and triggered by stress, fatigue, or sleep deprivation), *cramp-fasciculation syndrome* (a syndrome of peripheral nerve hyperexcitability), *complex regional pain syndrome,* and *anxiety/depression.*

Investigations

RLS is a clinical diagnosis, so a detailed clinical history is paramount. If PLMS is suggested clinically, overnight polysomnography should be performed. Sleep disturbance (with arousals) and more than five PLMS per hour of sleep is diagnostic of PLMS. Secondary causes for RLS should be investigated for. Laboratory tests may include CBC with differential, electrolytes, iron studies including ferritin and transferrin, vitamin B_{12} levels, folate, fasting glucose or oral glucose tolerance test, TFT and serum/urine toxicology. EMG/NCS should be performed to exclude lower motor neuron and peripheral sensory causes for RLS, as well as to exclude conditions that resemble idiopathic RLS.

Management

In general, any underlying conditions or exacerbating factors should be eliminated in treating secondary RLS. Drugs should be started at the lowest therapeutic dose and slowly increased to maximum effect. Pharmacological treatment includes *dopaminergic agents* such as *carbidopa/levodopa* (ADRs: nausea/vomiting, headache), pergolide (ADRs: hypotension, nasal stuffiness), *pramipexole* and *ropinirole* (ADRs: nausea, sleepiness, peripheral edema); *AEDs* such as *gabapentin* (ADRs: somnolence, ataxia, fatigue at higher doses), *carbamazepine* (ADRs: ataxia, hepatic dysfunction, hyponatremia); *benzodiazepines* such as *clonazepam, temazepam* (ADRs: daytime somnolence, confusion, respiratory and cardiac depression at high doses, tolerance/dependence); *opioids* such as codeine, oxycodone, tramadol, methadone (ADRs: constipation, urinary retention, tolerance/dependence); *adrenergic agents* such as *propranolol* (β-blocker) or the central α_2 agonist, *clonidine,* and *baclofen.* In mild cases of RLS-PLMS, one may start with gabapentin, whereas moderate to severe cases may be treated with dopamine agonists pramipexole or ropinirole initially. Polypharmacy may be required in refractory cases.

Prognosis

RLS is not a life-threatening disorder, but if untreated, may cause significant reduction in the quality of life and functional capabilities of patients. There is an approximately 80% good response rate to drug therapy in RLS at a mean follow-up of 16 months. Outcomes may be better in patients with RLS without PLMS. For secondary RLS, prognosis would also be modified by the underlying cause.

Counseling

RLS is a relatively common sleep disorder, affecting about 5–20% of the general population. Patients and their bed partners should be reassured that the condition is not life-threatening. Pharmacotherapy should be offered to patients with symptoms significant enough to affect their quality of life and functional status. They should be aware of the potentially good response rates, as well as the adverse effects of these drugs. Secondary causes should be treated meticulously and specialist help may be required for medical causes of RLS.

SUMMARY

- **RLS** is a **non-REM sleep disorder** characterized by **irresistible urges** to move the **legs** in association with **creeping sensations** that are relieved by **walking**.
- **PLMS** occur in about **80%** of RLS patients.
- Causes include **idiopathic** and **secondary** etiologies such as **neurological disorders, medical disease, drugs/toxins**, and **pregnancy**.
- Differentials include **akathisia, myokymia, painful nocturnal leg cramps, essential myoclonus, hypnic jerks, cramp-fasciculation syndrome, complex regional pain syndrome**, or **anxiety/depression**.
- Diagnosis is established **clinically**. If PLMS is suggested, nocturnal polysomnography showing **more than five PLMS per hour of sleep with arousals** is diagnostic.
- Treat any **underlying conditions** and remove **exacerbating** or **causative** agents.
- Pharmacotherapy of RLS includes **dopamine agonists, AEDs, benzodiazepines, opioids, adrenergic agents**, and **baclofen**.
- **Approximately 80%** of patients demonstrate good responses after mean follow-up of **16 months**. Better outcomes may occur if **PLMS is absent**.
- RLS-PLMS is not a life-threatening disease, but may significantly **reduce quality of life** and **functional capabilities** if untreated. Prognosis may be modified by underlying causes.
- Patients should be aware of prognostic data and **reassurance** should be provided to patients and their bed partners.

CASE 4

A 57-year-old overweight man complained of excessive daytime fatigue, forgetfulness, and increased irritability for about 6 months. He stated that he frequently woke up at night with choking spells, resulting in poor sleep. His wife said that he has had spells of breathing cessation during sleep that concern her. Clinical examination was nonrevealing.

Localization

Forgetfulness and irritability could localize to the bilateral temporal or frontal lobes. EDS implies poor nocturnal sleep (insomnia), and is nonlocalizing. Choking and intermittent apneic spells could indicate upper airway obstruction or dysfunction of respiratory centers in the medulla. In summary, the underlying process localizes diffusely to the cerebral cortex, with brainstem involvement or airway disease.

Differential Diagnosis

The most likely diagnosis for a chronic sleep disorder characterized by EDS with poor nocturnal sleep associated with choking and apneic spells in an overweight man is *obstructive sleep apnea-hypopnea syndrome* (OSAHS). This is a syndrome that occurs mainly in men over the age of 40 (~85% of cases) or postmenopausal women and associated with obesity in approximately 70% of patients. Other causes of sleep apnea include *central* (dysfunction of medullary respiratory centers causing cessation of airflow without respiratory effort) or *mixed* (central and upper airway obstruction) etiologies. In some patients, OSAHS is associated with hypertension, cardiac arrhythmias, or CHF.

Differentials for sleep-disordered breathing include *upper airway resistance syndrome* (subtle airflow limitations due to resistance of airways, resulting in frequent nocturnal arousals without apnea/hypopnea), *Cheyne-Stokes breathing* (central apnea interspersed between crescendo–decrescendo respiratory sequence in a cyclical pattern), *dysrhythmic/ataxic breathing* (nonrhythmic respiratory pattern with irregular amplitude and rhythm, associated with brainstem dysfunction), *apneustic breathing* (prolonged inspiratory phase associated with pontine lesions), and *alveolar hypoventilation* (associated with neuromuscular disorders such as MG, GBS, or myotonic dystrophy causing a restrictive lung deficit).

Investigations

Nocturnal polysomnography should be performed to establish the diagnosis of OSAHS. Findings include apnea-hypopnea index (AHI: number of apneic or hypopneic episodes per hour of sleep) >5 (mild: 5–19, moderate: 20–49 and severe: >50), arousal index (AI) >15 (10–15: borderline, <10: normal), reduced oxygen saturations (<90%), and reduced stage III, IV non-REM and REM sleep. Other causes of sleep-disordered breathing can be deduced with polysomnography. Pulmonary function tests should be considered to exclude intrinsic bronchopulmonary disease in OSAHS or restrictive respiratory deficits as seen in neuromuscular disorders. Cardiac evaluation (such as EKG, Holter monitor, telemetry, or echocardiogram) may be required if there is clinical evidence of heart disease.

Management

Therapy for OSAHS can be divided into general or direct modalities. General measures include weight reduction, treating any associated diseases, and avoidance of alcohol or sedative-hypnotics. Direct therapy can be divided into pharmacological, mechanical, and surgical options. Medications have very limited role in treating OSAHS; partial success in mild OSAHS has been described with protriptyline. Mild central apnea syndrome may respond to acetazolamide at high altitudes.

Mechanical devices include nasal continuous positive airway pressure (CPAP; option of choice), bivalve positive airway pressure (BiPAP), and dental and tongue-retaining devices. Surgical therapy should be considered for severe cases refractory to nasal CPAP: uvulopalatopharyngoplasty (UPPP: ~50% of patients significantly improve but many still require CPAP for residual apneas), tonsillectomy, adenoidectomy, maxillofacial reconstructions, or in rare cases, tracheostomy. Diaphragmatic pacing or electrophrenic respiration may be used in patients with central apnea syndrome.

Prognosis

Data on the natural history of OSAHS is limited by the lack of prospective studies. OSAHS may be a progressive disorder with worsening apneic/hypopneic spells if left untreated. Poor quality of life usually results in patients seeking medical attention. Morbidities associated with OSAHS include hypertension, cardiac arrhythmias, angina, MI, and stroke. These medical complications may occur in about 20–45% of patients over a mean follow-up of 17 months. Mortality is increased in comparison to matched controls and is associated with the increased risk of cardiovascular disease. Treatment (nasal CPAP, UPPP) has been shown to improve outcomes in moderate to severe cases (AHI >35) in comparison with patients who refused therapy.

Counseling

Patients should be aware of the prognostic data and potential benefit of treatment. Compliance with CPAP/BiPAP should be encouraged and measures should be undertaken to maximize patient comfort (such as humidified air, mask modifications). Complications should be aggressively treated and specialist cardiological consultation should be sought. Weight reduction and cessation of alcohol and sedative use should be advised.

SUMMARY

- **OSAHS** is a **chronic, progressive** sleep disorder most common in **obese men over the age of 40**.
- Etiologies for sleep apnea include **upper airway obstruction, central** (medullary) or **mixed (both)**.
- Differentials for sleep-disordered breathing include **upper airway resistance syndrome, Cheyne-Stokes, dysrhythmic/ataxic** or **apneustic breathing**, or **alveolar hypoventilation**.
- Diagnostic test for OSAHS is **nocturnal polysomnography. AHI >5, AI >15, reduced oxygen saturations (<90%)** and **reduced stage III, IV non-REM and REM sleep** are diagnostic variables.
- Treatment includes **general measures** and **direct therapy**. Direct therapy includes **medications** (limited use, in mild cases only), **mechanical** (especially CPAP), and **surgical** (especially UPPP) options.
- Complications of OSAHS are **cardiac, neurological**, and **social**.
- Mortality is **increased** in OSAHS secondary to **cardiovascular disease** and treatment has been shown to improve outcomes.

17

Infectious Diseases

CASE 1

A 29-year-old woman was seen in the ER complaining of a left-sided headache for several weeks. She had noticed progressive weakness and lack of sensation affecting the right face and arm for about 3 weeks. She now felt nauseous and febrile. On examination, she had a temperature of 38.6°C, HR 112 per minute, BP 114/68 mmHg, and RR 16 per minute. She had poor oral hygiene. Neurological examination revealed right spastic hemiparesis, hemisensory loss, and inferior quadrantanopsia. There was right-sided hyperreflexia with an ipsilateral spastic gait.

Localization

The left-sided headache may suggest to the meningeal irritation over the left cerebral cortex or referred from mucosal membranes of ipsilateral extracranial tissues such as the sinuses, or inner ear. However, this complaint could also be nonspecific. Right spastic hemiparesis indicates an upper motor neuron dysfunction of the left frontal cortex, subcortical white matter, posterior limb of the internal capsule, cerebral peduncles or pons above the level of the facial nucleus. Right hemisensory loss may localize to left parietal cortex, subcortical white matter tracts, thalamus or midbrain above the level of the mesencephalic nucleus of CN V. Right inferior quadrantanopsia localizes to the left parietal cortex. In summary, the underlying process most likely localizes to the left fronto-parietal cortex.

Differential Diagnosis

The most likely diagnosis for a slowly progressive left frontoparietal lesion in a febrile patient with a headache and poor oral hygiene is *cerebral abscess*. This is a focal suppurative disease of brain parenchyma that most frequently occurs due to spread from a contiguous cranial site of infection such as teeth, sinuses, or ear. Other sources of infection include *direct implantation* (open-head injury, neurosurgery, craniofacial osteomyelitis), *hematogenous spread* (congenital heart

From: *Neurology Oral Boards Review:*
A Concise and Systematic Approach to Clinical Practice
By: E. E. Ubogu © Humana Press Inc., Totowa, NJ

disease with left-to-right shunts, bronchiectasis, lung abscess), or *unknown* (~10–20% of cases).

Brain abscesses usually contain mixed organisms (~30–60%). In immunocompetent individuals, such organisms may include streptococci, *Enterobacteriaceae*, *S. aureus*, anerobes (e.g., bacteroides) and Gram-negative bacteria (e.g., *Actinobacillus, Proteus, E. coli*). In the immunocompromised, organisms may include *Listeria, Mycobacterium, Toxoplasma, Cryptococcus* or fungi such as *Aspergillus, Mucor* (especially in DM) or *Candida*. In tropical countries, tuberculosis, helminths, and parasites are common causes of cerebral abscesses.

Differentials include *subdural empyema, cranial epidural abscess, meningitis* (viral and other aseptic causes, bacterial), *embolism from infective endocarditis, rupture of mycotic aneurysm, neoplasm* (primary brain or metastatic), or *tumor-like demyelinating lesions* (e.g., MS).

Investigations

Neuroimaging (CT/MRI) of the brain is the diagnostic modality of choice for cerebral abscess and used for posttreatment follow-up. Ring-enhancing lesion(s) with surrounding edema is the expected finding. Intraparenchymal air without open head injury or neurosurgery is suggestive. LP is contraindicated in suspected or proven cases due to the risk of precipitating rupture or inducing herniation. CBC with differential may reveal peripheral leukocytosis, and blood cultures may be useful if hematogenous spread is suspected as a cause. Diagnostic brain biopsy may be required to evaluate for neoplasm if there is no response to antibiotic therapy.

Management

The source of the infection should be sought after and adequately treated. Antibiotic therapy is empirical and based on the localization of the abscess and inferred infection source. The following antibiotic therapies are recommended for specific lesion types:

- Frontal lesions: metronidazole and third-generation cephalosporin or penicillin.
- Temporal or cerebellar lesions: metronidazole, penicillin, and ceftazidime.
- Multiple abscesses: metronidazole, nafcillin, and cefotaxime.
- Penetrating wounds: nafcillin and cefotaxime.
- Postneurosurgical: ceftazidime and vancomycin.

Duration of treatment is also empirical: intravenous therapy can be given for 6–8 weeks, with oral therapy for 2–3 months. Surgical treatment (total excision or stereotactic CT-guided aspiration) should be considered as this may reduce time course of i.v. therapy by 1–2 weeks and may be required as a life-saving measure in cerebral herniation. Contraindications include multiple or deep abscesses,

abscesses less than 2.5–3 cm diameter, dominant hemisphere lesions, early shrinkage with antibiotic therapy or an associated meningitis or ependymitis. If mass effect or raised ICP is present, additional therapy (corticosteroids, hyperosmolar agents, cautious hyperventilation, etc.) may be required. AEDs are usually administered symptomatically or prophylactically after surgical treatment.

Prognosis

The mortality rate from cerebral abscess is less than 10%. This is attributed to improved neuroimaging techniques that facilitate early recognition and antibiotics and neurosurgical techniques to treat and enhance recovery. Death is most likely associated with cerebral herniation as a result of mass effect, suppurative ventriculitis from abscess rupture (confers mortality of >80%) or septicemia. Rapid disease progression prior to hospitalization and poor level of consciousness on admission are poor prognostic signs. Approximately 50% of survivors are neurologically normal with no deficits after aggressive antibiotic and surgical intervention. About 25–50% of patients develop seizures during the early phases of the disease and this may contribute to morbidity and mortality (e.g., SE). Recurrence may occur in about 15% of patients, with the risk increased about threefold for multiloculated in comparison to uniloculated lesions. Persistence of MRI gadolinium enhancement after 6 months may predict recurrence in approximately 20% of cases.

Counseling

Patients should be aware of prognostic data and need to complete a course of antibiotics and undergo surgical treatment if indicated. Patients should be educated on the signs of abscess recurrence and should seek immediate medical care. Symptomatic AEDs can be discontinued after 12 months of therapy provided the patient is seizure-free, and prophylactic AEDs can be stopped after a minimum of 3 months postoperatively. Underlying causes of infection should be eliminated and specialist consultation (e.g., dental, otolaryngological, cardiac, etc.) may be required.

SUMMARY

- **Cerebral abscess** is a **focal suppurative** disease of brain parenchyma.
- This may occur secondary to microbial spread from **contiguous cranial sites, direct implantation, hematogenous**, or **unknown** sites.
- Cerebral abscesses usually contain **mixed organisms** (Gram-positive, Gram-negative, and anerobes), or **fungi, parasites**, and **helminths**.
- Differentials include **subdural empyema, cranial epidural abscess, meningitis, embolism from infective endocarditis, mycotic aneurysm rupture, neoplasms**, or **tumor-like demyelinating lesions**.

- **CT/MRI brain** is the diagnostic test of choice.
- Treatment should be targeted toward the **underlying source**. **Antibiotic therapy** should be instituted and empirical regimens depend on **cerebral location** and **infection source**.
- **Surgery** reduces need for i.v. antibiotic therapy by **1–2 weeks**.
- Additional therapy would be required for complications such as **cerebral edema/herniation**, **ventriculitis**, or **seizures**.
- Mortality is **less than 10%**, with **rapid disease progression** prior to hospitalization and **poor level of consciousness** on admission being poor prognostic signs.
- Recurrence rate is **approximately 15%**; higher risk with **multiloculated** lesions.
- **Approximately 50%** of patients become neurologically normal after treatment.

CASE 2

A 41-year-old man with a chronic cough and weight loss for 3 months came to the clinic complaining of headache, neck stiffness, and increasing lethargy with malaise for about 6 weeks. About 1 week ago, he developed a right facial droop and difficulty chewing. On examination, temperature was 38.1°C, HR 88 per minute, BP 144/68 mmHg, and RR 18 per minute. Neurological examination revealed positive Brudzinski sign, normal MMSE with slow and deliberate responses, right-sided facial palsy, localization of sound to the left ear with Weber's test using a 256 Hz tuning fork, and a normal Rinne's test.

Localization

Headache in association with neck stiffness and a positive Brudzinski sign suggests meningeal inflammation. Slow, deliberate responses with a normal MMSE may suggest mild, diffuse dysfunction of the cerebral cortex. Right-sided facial palsy indicates a CN VII lesion from its origin in the pons or its peripheral course through the internal auditory canal, geniculate ganglion, and stylomastoid foramen to the muscles of facial expression. Right-sided sensorineural hearing loss supports dysfunction of the cochlear division of CN VIII (also runs through internal auditory canal), cochlear nuclei, spiral ganglion (organ of Corti), or central pathways (less likely to cause unilateral hearing loss owing to extensive bilateral connections). In summary, the underlying process localizes diffusely to the cerebral cortex and its surrounding meninges and the right CN VII and VIII.

Differential Diagnosis

Subacute meningitis with basal skull involvement resulting in unilateral CN VII and VIII nerve palsies in association with a chronic cough and weight loss is suggestive of *tuberculous meningitis* secondary to infection with *Mycobacterium tuberculosis* (TB). Neurological TB may affect approximately 1% of patients with pulmonary TB, and CNS infection may occur either during the primary infection or secondary to subsequent immunosuppression. The meninges are the primary site of infection and the incidence of CNS TB has increased with the HIV/AIDS epidemic worldwide. Other differentials include *granulomatous infectious meningitis* (e.g., neurosyphilis, Lyme disease, brucellosis, fungal meningitis, toxoplasmosis), *untreated/partially treated bacterial meningitis, connective tissue disorders* (e.g., SLE, Behçet's disease, PACNS, sarcoidosis), or *neoplastic meningitis* (e.g., carcinoma, lymphoma, or leukemia).

Investigation

Where available, rapid testing for TB in sputum (amplifies and detects RNA or DNA with specificity of >95% and sensitivities of 40–80% in AFB-negative sputum and >95% in AFB-positive sputum; results within 24 hours) may be performed. LP should be performed for AFB smear (diagnostic in ~10–30% of patients) and culture (may take 6–8 weeks and is diagnostic in ~50–70% of patients) if TB meningitis is suspected. PCR (~70–80% sensitivity) should be considered for more rapid diagnosis and may be required in negative CSF culture cases. Cell count usually shows lymphocytic pleocytosis; CSF protein is usually elevated with low CSF glucose. In atypical cases, CSF cytology, Gram-stain, and ACE levels may be warranted. Other tests may include chest radiography, CT/MRI of the brain with and without contrast for basal meningeal enhancement), PPD testing, ANA panel, serum electrolytes, sputum/blood cultures, and HIV serology. In equivocal cases refractory to therapy, meningeal biopsy may be warranted to establish the diagnosis.

Management

The mainstay of treatment for TB meningitis is combination antimicrobial therapy. Empirical treatment should be instituted once suspected clinically, as CSF cultures take weeks and there is about a 25–30% false-negative rate. Such a regimen may include *isoniazid* (10 mg/kg per day p.o., ADRs: peripheral neuropathy: prevented by pyridoxine 25–50 mg p.o. daily, hepatoxicity), *rifampin* (10 mg/kg per day p.o., ADRs: hepatoxicity, drug interactions with cytochrome P450 induction), *pyrazinamide* (35 mg/kg per day p.o., ADR: hepatotoxicity) and *ethambutol* (25 mg/kg per day p.o. ADR: toxic optic neuropathy), or *streptomycin* (10 mg/kg per day i.m. ADR: vestibular toxicity).

These agents are administered once a day. This regimen should be continued for 2 months, and if there is clinical improvement, this can be reduced to two drugs (usually isoniazid and rifampin) for 10 months. If there is concurrent HIV infection or potential for drug-resistant disease, five to seven drugs should be initiated before drug susceptibility is known. Other agents include ethionamide, cycloserine, kanamycin, clofazimine, rifabutin, fluoroquinolones, and para-aminosalicylic acid.

Corticosteroid therapy (e.g., dexamethasone or prednisone) as adjunctive therapy for 1–2 months may improve neurological outcomes, especially if there is evidence of brain edema, hydrocephalus, complicated meningitis, vasculitis, arachnoiditis, visual loss, adrenal insufficiency, or severe infection with multi-drug-resistant strains.

Repeat CSF examination and neuroimaging every 3–6 months during therapy is useful in monitoring treatment efficacy. Monthly visual (including color perception) and hearing evaluations are required if treating with ethambutol or streptomycin respectively. Regular LFTs should be performed because of potential for hepatoxicity with several drugs. Complications of TB meningitis (*see* below) should be aggressively treated (e.g., shunting for hydrocephalus, fluid restriction for SIADH).

Prognosis

TB meningitis is potentially a life-threatening disease, especially when untreated. In untreated cases, mortality is greater than 90%, with death within 6 weeks of clinical onset. In treated cases, mortality is approximately 10–20% in immunocompetent and about 30–35% in immunosuppressed patients. Hydrocephalus, brain infarction, or coma on presentation may predict poor outcomes. Complications may occur in varying degrees in as many as 50–60% of patients, and include progressive hydrocephalus, brain edema associated with tuberculomas, blindness, vasculitis and stroke, seizures, SIADH (normovolemic hyponatremia), and arachnoiditis.

Counseling

Patients should be advised to complete course of therapy to facilitate recovery and comply with routine follow-up care to reduce irreversible sequalae adverse drug effects. Patients should be aware that this disease may cause recurrent meningitis if inadequately treated. Complications are more common when treatment is suboptimal or initiated late. Prognostic data should be discussed with all patients. Close personal contacts should be evaluated with PPD skin testing for possible exposure and prophylaxis instituted with isoniazid in positive cases.

SUMMARY

- **TB meningitis** is a **subacute-chronic** infectious disease of the CNS that has a predilection for the **meninges**.
- Neurological TB may affect **approximately 1%** of patients with pulmonary TB.
- Differentials include **granulomatous infectious meningitis, untreated/ partially treated bacterial meningitis, connective tissue disorders**, or **neoplastic meningitis**.
- Rapid diagnosis may be facilitated via **RNA/DNA amplification and detection tests in sputum** (~95% specific) or **PCR in CSF** (70–80% sensitive). **CSF cultures** are positive in about 50–70%.
- Treatment involves combination therapy: **isoniazid, rifampin, ethambutol**, and **pyrazinamide** for **2 months**, then **isoniazid** and **rifampin** for **10** months. Close follow-up is necessary. **Corticosteroids** are of benefit in certain situations and improve outcomes.
- Complications may occur in **50–60%** of affected patients.
- Mortality is **approximately 10–20%** in immunocompetent and **about 30–35%** in immunosuppressed treated patients. If untreated, mortality is **greater than 90%**, with death occuring within **6 weeks** of clinical presentation.

CASE 3

A 33-year-old woman complained of a diffuse, intermittent headache with mild neck stiffness, generalized malaise, and lethargy for 6 months. Over the preceding 3 weeks, she developed progressive left-sided weakness and sensory loss noticed by her close friend. On examination, vital signs showed temperature 37.9°C, HR 72 per minute, BP 114/78 mmHg, and RR 14 per minute. There was generalized lymphadenopathy and MMSE shows poor attention and orientation. Further neurological examination revealed left spastic hemiparesis with hyperreflexia, hemisensory loss, and hemispatial neglect to visual and tactile stimuli.

Localization

A chronic diffuse headache with a low-grade fever and neck stiffness suggests meningitis. Poor attention and orientation may suggest global cerebral dysfunction (mainly frontal and temporal lobes). Generalized malaise, lethargy, and lymphadenopathy may indicate a systemic illness. Left hemiparesis (UMN type) could localize to the right frontal, subcortical white matter, posterior limb of internal capsule, cerebral peduncles, or upper pons above facial nucleus. Left hemisensory loss with visual/tactile hemineglect localizes to the right parietal lobe. In summary, the underlying process is most likely a chronic systemic illness associated with chronic meningitis, mild diffuse cerebral dysfunction, and a subacute right frontoparietal lesion.

Differential Diagnosis

The most likely diagnosis for a chronic systemic illness with diffuse lymphadenopathy associated with focal and generalized neurological deficits is *HIV/AIDS*. Meningitis may be a sign of HIV-seroconversion or occur with CD4 counts <500/mm^3. Focal deficits could be secondary to *cerebral toxoplasmosis* (an opportunistic infection seen in ~5–15% of AIDS patients, usually with CD4+ counts <200/mm^3), *primary CNS lymphoma* (B-cell type; seen in 2–5% of AIDS patients, with CD4+ counts <200/mm^3), or *PML* (CNS demyelination caused by reactivated infection with JC virus in oligodendrocytes, seen in ~5% of AIDS patients, usually with CD4+ counts <200/mm^3). *Toxoplasmosis* seems most likely.

Other causes of focal cerebral lesions include *cerebral abscess* (bacterial or fungal), *subdural empyema, cranial epidural abscess, embolism from infective endocarditis, rupture of mycotic aneurysm, metastatic brain lesions,* or *tumor-like demyelinating lesions* (e.g., MS, VZV). Other potential differentials for chronic meningitis include *untreated/partially treated bacterial meningitis* (e.g., *Salmonella, Listeria, M. tuberculosis, pneumococcus), aseptic (or viral) meningoencephalitis* (e.g., CMV: course can be acute and fulminant), *granulomatous infectious meningitis* (e.g., neurosyphilis, Lyme disease, brucellosis, *Cryptococcus, Candida, Histoplasma), connective tissue disorders* (unrelated to HIV infection, e.g., SLE, Behçet's disease, PACNS, sarcoidosis), *neoplastic meningitis* (e.g., lymphoma, leukemia, carcinoma), or *drug-induced* (e.g., NSAIDs, trimethoprim-sulfamethoxazole, isoniazid, ciprofloxacin, sulfonamides).

Investigations

CT/MRI of the brain with and without contrast should be performed to diagnose CNS toxoplasmosis (ring-enhancing lesion; multiple in ~70%). Primary CNS lymphoma is more likely to be a solitary lesion with homogenous enhancement, less cerebral edema, and more likely to cross the midline. Neuroimaging can also exclude other causes of focal cerebral disease. An adequate trial of anti-toxoplasmosis antibiotics also helps establish the diagnosis. *Toxoplasma* IgG antibodies are usually, but not invariably positive. HIV titers should be performed. CBC with differential, including CD4+ count is important to check if HIV positive. In equivocal cases, blood cultures, ANA profile, and stereotactic brain biopsy may be required to establish a diagnosis.

Management

First-line antibiotic therapy for CNS toxoplasmosis includes pyrimethamine (may cause renal insufficiency or rash), sulfadiazine, and folinic acid (to prevent hematological toxicity from pyrimethamine) for 3–6 weeks or trimethoprim-sulfamethoxazole for 30 days. Second-line agents are similar to above but clindamycin replaces sulfadiazine. Macrolides such as azithromycin, clartithromycin, and atovaquone are third-line agents. Initial treatment requires 10–14 days to establish clinical/radiological efficacy. Early use of corticosteroids should be limited, as this drug may shrink primary CNS lymphoma and one cannot ascertain whether the antibiotics or steroids resulted in clinical and radiological improvement. Antimicrobial therapy (first-line drugs) should be continued as secondary prophylaxis against CNS toxoplasmosis recurrence and may be discontinued if CD4 count is greater than 200/mm^3 for 3 months.

Highly active antiretroviral therapy (HAART) should be started if the patient is symptomatic of HIV infection or asymptomatic if CD4+ count is less than 200/mm^3 or viral load is greater than 10^5 copies/mL. HAART drugs include *nucleotide* (e.g., tenofovir) or *nucleoside reverse transcriptase inhibitors* (e.g., zidovudine, lamivudine, didanosine, stavudine), *non-nucleoside reverse transcriptase inhibitors* (e.g., efavirenz, nevirapine, delavirdine), *protease inhibitors* (saquinavir, indinavir, ritonavir, etc.), or *fusion inhibitors* (e.g., enfuvirtide). Initial preferred regimens for chronic untreated HIV infection include zidovudine plus lamivudine plus efavirenz, tenofovir plus lamivudine plus efavirenz, or zidovudine plus lamivudine plus ritonavir/lopinavir. In general, these drugs commonly cause nausea, vomiting, diarrhea, headache, and rash.

Specific ADRs include *peripheral neuropathy* with didanosine and zalcitabine, *pancreatitis* with stavudine and didanosine, *nephrolithiasis* with indinavir, *bone marrow suppression*, and *myopathy* with zidovudine. Other complications of HIV (neurological and non-neurological; *see* below) should be thoroughly identified and adequately treated with medical subspecialty assistance as required.

Prognosis

With early identification and treatment, CNS toxoplasmosis is not a life-threatening disease. If treatment is inadequate or delayed, or CNS toxoplasmosis is a late complication of HIV infection (especially with CD4+ counts <100/ mm^3), approximately 40–50% mortality may occur at 6 months after symptom onset. In general, the median survival of HIV-infected patients diagnosed with an AIDS-defining opportunistic infection is about 46 months (11 months pre-HAART). Mortality is about 20% at 24 months and about 33% at 36 months after diagnosis.

HIV-infected individuals have a mortality rate of approximately 9% per year, with a shift in cause of mortality from opportunistic infections, end-stage AIDS (wasting syndrome), and malignancy to end-organ failure with the routine use of HAART drugs. About 11% of patients currently living with HIV infection are older than 50 years old, so other causes of mortality and morbidity in an aging population are more likely to contribute to prognosis with increasing HIV survival.

Complications of HIV infection can be divided into *neurological* and *non-neurological diseases*. Neurological complications, apart from those listed on p. 208 include *HIV-associated dementia* (seen in 10–75% of patients), *cryptococcal meningitis, CMV encephalitis, vacuolar myelopathy, CMV polyradiculitis, shingles, GBS* (associated with CSF pleocytosis), *CIDP, mononeuropathy multiplex, distal symmetrical polyneuropathy*, and *myopathies*. Non-neurological complications include *Pneumocystis carinii pneumonia, oral candidiasis, Kaposi's sarcoma*, and *non-Hodgkin's lymphoma (NHL)*.

Counseling

Patients should be counseled prior to HIV testing on the implications of a positive result. Combination HAART regimens cost between $1100 and $1600 per month (2003 average wholesale price). HAART drugs should be initiated as discussed here and compliance with close follow-up is required. Adverse effects of HAART drugs should be managed aggressively and regular testing for drug resistance undertaken. HIV transmission preventative measures should be taught to patients and cessation of high-risk behaviors advised. Prophylaxis against opportunistic infections should be provided. Complications of HIV infection should be discussed and patients should be educated on the early recognition of these diseases. Support groups for patients and their families, as well as educational resources, should be made available to patients. Emotional support may be required in dealing with the social, physical and psychological consequences of HIV/AIDS.

SUMMARY

- **HIV/AIDS** is a worldwide epidemic that usually presents nonspecifically as a **generalized systemic illness** with subsequent **neurological complications** in more advanced disease.
- **Toxoplasmosis** is an opportunistic infection and a common cause of **focal CNS deficit** in HIV patients and **CD4+ counts less than 200/mm^3**.
- Differentials for progressive focal brain deficits in HIV include **primary CNS lymphoma** and **PML**. Other focal brain lesions that could occur include **cerebral abscess, subdural empyema, cranial epidural abscess, embolism from infective endocarditis, rupture of mycotic aneurysm, metastatic brain lesions**, or **tumor-like demyelinating lesions**.
- CNS toxoplasmosis is diagnosed by **CT/MRI brain with** and **without contrast**. *Toxoplasma* IgG may be positive in most cases. **Response to antimicrobial therapy** also confirms diagnosis.

- Treatment includes **pyrimethamine, sulfadiazine,** and **folinic acid** or **trimethoprim-sulfamethoxazole.**
- Initial efficacy requires treatment for at least **10–14 days.**
- Secondary prophylaxis required if **CD4+ count is less than 200/mm³.**
- Corticosteroids should be **avoided** if possible until diagnosis confirmed.
- **HAART drugs** should be initiated in HIV-positive patients if **symptomatic, CD4+ count is less than 200/mm³,** or **viral load is greater than 10⁵ copies/mL.**
- Complications of HIV infection should be **identified** and **aggressively treated,** including adverse effects of medications.
- CNS toxoplasmosis is not life threatening if identified and treated aggressively. Mortality is **approximately 40–50%** if untreated or occurs as a late complication of HIV (with **CD4 count <100/mm³**).
- AIDS has a median survival of **46 months** after diagnosis (**11 months** pre-HAART), with **approximately 20%** mortality at **24 months** and **approximately 33%** mortality at **36 months.**
- HIV-infected patients have an **approximately 9% per year** mortality with shift toward **end-organ failure** as the cause of death.
- Patients should be aware of the importance of **pharmacological compliance** and **close follow-up.** Regular testing for **drug resistance, prophylactic therapy** against opportunistic infections, and **counseling** are integral aspects of patient care.

18

Neoplastic Disease

CASE 1

A 57-year-old man with lung cancer for 12 months developed a nonspecific holocranial headache about 3 weeks ago. Over the past 5 days, he complained of double vision, as well as difficulty chewing and swallowing. He had also noticed pain radiating down his left leg to his foot and weakness on that side while walking. Neurological examination revealed an MMSE of 23/30 with deficits in attention/orientation, calculation and multi-stage commands. There was also evidence of bilateral eye abduction paresis, facial diplegia, and tongue weakness. Motor examination revealed weakness in left foot intrinsics, ankle dorsi- and plantarflexion, as well as hip abduction. Sensory examination was significant for reduced pinprick on the left lateral leg, dorsum, and plantar surface of the foot. Left ankle reflex examination was diminished.

Localization

A holocranial headache is nonlocalizing, but may imply meningeal irritation. The deficits on MMSE suggest dysfunction to the frontal and temporal lobes bilaterally. Bilateral eye abduction paresis with diplopia suggests bilateral CN VI nerve dysfunction. These may localize to the pons or their intracranial courses (pontomedullary junction, cavernous sinus, superior orbital fissure) to the lateral recti muscles. Facial diplegia is indicative of bilateral CN VII paresis, localizing to the pons or their intracranial courses (pontomedullary junction, internal auditory canal, geniculate ganglion, stylomastoid foramen) to the muscles of facial expression.

Bilateral tongue weakness implies bilateral CN XII paresis, localizing to the medulla or their intracranial course (via hypoglossal foramina) to tongue muscles. Weakness in the left foot intrinsics, ankle dorsiflexion (tibialis anterior), ankle plantarflexion (gastrocnemius), and hip abduction (gluteus medius and tensor fascia lata), coupled with reduced pinprick in the dorsum and plantar surfaces of the foot and diminished ankle jerk, localize to the left L5–S1 nerve roots. In summary,

From: *Neurology Oral Boards Review:*
A Concise and Systematic Approach to Clinical Practice
By: E. E. Ubogu © Humana Press Inc., Totowa, NJ

the underlying process localizes to the bilateral frontal and temporal lobes and its meninges, the lower brainstem (pons and medulla), and the left L5–S1 nerve roots.

Differential Diagnosis

The most likely diagnosis for a diffuse disorder affecting the cerebral cortex, meninges, multiple cranial nerves (CN VI, VII, and XII), and nerve roots (L5–S1) in a patient with a known neoplasm is *leptomeningeal metastases* (LM, or carcinomatous meningitis). This condition may occur in approximately 5% of cancer patients; seen in about 8% with solid tumors, up to 30% with NHL and up to 70% with leukemia. LM usually occurs in the setting of tumor relapse. Most common causes include breast cancer, lung cancer, melanoma, and GI adenocarcinomas. Primary CNS tumors such as high-grade gliomas and medulloblastoma may also cause LM.

Other etiologies for a meningoradiculitis or meningomyelitis include other *neoplastic conditions* (parenchymal/epidural metastases, paraneoplastic encephalomyelitis), *infections* (*viral*: CMV, VZV, HSV, HIV, Hepatitis B, arborviruses; *spirochete*: Lyme disease, neurosyphilis; *bacteria*: TB; *fungal*: *Cryptococcus*; *parasitic*: cysticercosis, for example), *connective tissue diseases* (SLE, Sjögrens syndrome: causes encephalopathy and dorsal root ganglionopathy; WG, RhA, sarcoidosis, idiopathic vasculitis), *demyelinating diseases* (e.g., MS), and *mitochondrial disorders* (e.g., Leigh disease).

Investigation

CSF analysis is the most important test for LM. Finding malignant cells on cytology establishes the diagnosis. Cytology is positive in approximately 50–60% after initial LP and approximately 90% after third LP. In about 8–10% of patients with LM, cytology is persistently negative. Nonspecific findings on LP include elevated opening pressure, increased CSF protein, and reduced CSF glucose. CSF tumor markers or PCR gene amplification in lymphocytes may be used as adjuncts to establish diagnosis. Neuroimaging (especially MRI brain and/or spinal cord with and without gadolinium: meningeal enhancement in >50%) is useful in supporting or excluding diagnosis and evaluating for hydrocephalus. In atypical cases, further tests may include Lyme titers, HIV titers, RPR/FTA-ABS, CSF viral PCR, CSF cultures, AFB stain, serum ACE levels, ANA titers. EMG/NCS may be useful to document more widespread polyradiculopathies. Meningeal biopsy would be warranted in equivocal cases with normal laboratory results.

Management

The aim of therapy is to improve or stabilize neurologically and prolong survival. The entire neuraxis must be treated. Specific therapy depends on the tumor type, tumor site, and the patient's clinical state. Treatment modalities can be divided into radiation therapy, intrathecal chemotherapy, systemic chemotherapy, and treatment of the underlying tumor.

Radiation therapy is limited to symptomatic areas, sites of bulky disease or CSF blocks (determined by [111]Indium-DTPA CSF flow studies), especially if intrathecal (i.t.) penetration is limited. A dose of about 2000–3000 cGy is administered over 2 weeks in 10–15 fractions. *Intrathecal chemotherapy* includes *methotrexate* (with *leucovorin* to reduce systemic adverse effects, ADRs: aseptic meningitis, leukoencephalopathy, myelosuppression, opportunistic infections), *cytarabine* (with oral dexamethasone to reduce arachnoiditis, ADRs: transverse myelopathy, aseptic meningitis, encephalopathy, headache, seizures with minimal systemic toxicity), and *thiotepa* (ADRs: myelosuppression, carcinogenic potential).

These agents are usually administered twice a week. Slow-release cytarabine is also available for twice a week dosing. Intrathecal drugs are usually administered into the CSF via an intraventricular catheter with a subcutaneous reservoir under the scalp. High dose i.v. therapy (methotrexate or cytarabine) may be used as an alternative to i.t. therapy. Based on the underlying tumor, *concurrent systemic chemotherapy* and any specific measures should be instituted for tumor recurrence. *Symptomatic care* (e.g., nutritional/fluid support, infectious precautions, DVT/GI prophylaxis, adequate analgesia, bladder/bowel hygiene, prevention of decubiti) should be provided.

Prognosis

In untreated patients with LM, median survival is approximately 1–2 months, whereas in treated patients, median survival is approximately 3–6 months; with breast cancer and NHL showing improved survival over other cancers. One-year mortality in breast cancer with LM is approximately 90%, whereas NHL is approximately 75–90%. In LM, death usually occurs secondary to progressive neurological dysfunction (e.g., hydrocephalus, coma) or in treatment responders, secondary to the underlying malignancy. Approximately 50–60% of patients with carcinomas and more than 80% with NHL respond to therapy. Predictors of good treatment response include minimal neurological deficit, good functional status, slowly progressive systemic malignancy with little or no metastases, and a diagnosis of either breast cancer or NHL. In general, fixed neurological deficits on presentation do not improve with therapy, whereas dramatic improvements may be seen with encephalopathy.

Counseling

Patients and their families should be aware of the dismal prognosis. Aggressive therapies with supportive care should be offered to improve survival. Patients should also know the consequences of nonaggressive therapy and should be allowed to make an informed choice. Referral to a neuro-oncologist or general oncologist with special interest in neurological malignancies should be sought early in the disease course. Palliative care should be provided and the necessary referrals should be made to ensure a decent pre-terminal quality of life despite neurological deficits. Adverse drug effects should be managed comprehensively without causing further patient discomfort.

SUMMARY

- **Leptomeningeal meningitis** is a **diffuse disorder** affecting the **meninges** of the **CNS** and **PNS**.
- LM occurs in **about 5%** of cancer patients and is usually associated with **tumor recurrence**.
- Most common causes include **breast cancer, lung cancer, melanoma,** and **GI adenocarcinomas**. Primary CNS tumors such as **high-grade gliomas** and **medulloblastoma** may also cause LM.
- Differentials include other **neoplastic conditions, infections, connective tissue disorders, demyelinating diseases,** and **mitochondrial disorders**.
- **CSF cytology** is the most useful diagnostic test, being positive in **approximately 50–60%** after first LP and **approximately 90%** after third LP. **MRI** is a useful adjunct.
- Treatment modalities include **radiation therapy, i.t. chemotherapy, systemic chemotherapy,** and **treatment of the underlying tumor**. **Supportive care** is also necessary.
- Median survival in untreated patient is **1–2 months,** with that of treated patients **approximately 3–6 months**. Cause of death is **progressive neurological deficit** or **underlying malignancy**.
- Predictors of treatment response include **minimal neurological deficit, good functional status, slowly progressive systemic malignancy,** with little or no metastases, and a diagnosis of either **breast cancer** or **NHL**.
- Referral to **neuro-oncology** may be necessary early in the disease course. **Palliative care** support should be provided.

CASE 2

A 52-year-old right-handed woman presented to the office with a 3- to 4-month history of speaking difficulties. Her husband said that she did not seem to understand him and used words that made no sense. He also believed that her right side was weaker than the left. On examination, there was receptive aphasia with paraphrasic errors and neologisms and mild dysarthria. Visual examination revealed a right superior quadrantanopsia. Right spastic hemiparesis with hyperreflexia and a normal sensory examination were also noted.

Localization

Receptive aphasia with paraphrasic errors and neologisms indicates dysfunction to the dominant (left) temporal lobe. The right superior quadrantanopsia further localizes to the left temporal lobe. Right-sided UMN hemiparesis with dysarthria suggests dysfunction affecting the left frontal lobes, subcortical white matter, cerebral peduncles, or pons above the facial nucleus. However, an expansive lesion in the left temporal lobe is most likely to compress the left cerebral peduncle. In summary, the most likely localization is the left temporal lobe with compression of the left cerebral peduncle.

Differential Diagnosis

The most likely diagnosis for chronic progressive unilateral temporal lobe dysfunction in a middle-aged woman is a *primary brain tumor*. Primary brain tumors that have a predilection for the temporal lobes include *astrocytoma* (e.g., anaplastic astrocytoma, GBM: approximately 20% of all intracranial tumors and approximately 50% of cerebral gliomas; pleomorphic xanthoastrocytoma, pilocytic astrocytoma: both more common in adolescence), *oligodendroglioma* (>50% are calcified; about 5% of cerebral gliomas), and *ganglioglioma* (more common in young adults, consists of neuronal and astrocytic neoplasia). Extradural tumors, such as *meningioma*, or *solitary parenchymal metastasis* are further diagnostic considerations. Other differentials for primary brain tumor include *brain abscess* (*see* pp. 201–204), *subdural empyema, cranial epidural abscess, chronic subdural hematoma*, or *tumor-like demyelinating lesions* (e.g., MS).

Investigations

Investigations include MRI brain with and without gadolinium as the initial diagnostic test with pathological identification after brain biopsy or surgical debulking being confirmatory. CT brain with and without contrast may be utilized when MRI is not relatively available or contraindicated. LP is contraindicated if a mass lesion is suspected. CBC, basic metabolic profile, PT/PTT/INR, and blood type and screen may be required prior to surgery.

Management

Treatment should be tailored toward the underlying cause. If there is any evidence of raised ICP or cerebral herniation, appropriate measures (see pp. 53–54) should be instituted. For GBM, treatment involves surgical debulking, radiation therapy, and chemotherapy. Surgical debulking provides tissue for diagnosis, relieves mass effect, and reduces tumor load. Gross total resection (aiming for >98% of tumor mass removal) could be performed with approximately 3% perioperative mortality and <10% severe neurological morbidity rate.

Radiation therapy should be employed utilizing a limited-field treatment (rather than whole-brain irradiation: increased risk of cognitive decline) to the enhancing tumor with approximately 3.0 cm wide margins with subsequent conedown irradiation to the tumor bed for 5 days a week for 10–12 weeks. Hyperfractionation schemes, stereotactic radiosurgery, radioactive cerebral implants, and radiation with sensitizers have not proven more efficacious than standard therapy.

Chemotherapy may involve the systemic administration of nitrosoureas (e.g., BCNU, CCNU: ADRs include reversible bone marrow suppression and irreversible hepatic and pulmonary toxicity) 3 days a week every 6–8 weeks for a total of 48 weeks, or temozolomide (ADRs: headache, fatigue, nausea, myelosuppression; is relatively well tolerated in comparison to other agents) given orally for 5 days every 28 days for a maximum of 12 cycles. Surgery, radiation therapy, and chemotherapy may result in increased patient survival.

Prognosis

The mean survival of treated patients with GBM is about 1 year, with a mean survival of less than 6 months in untreated patients, from the development of symptoms. These figures have not significantly changed over the last 30 years. The 1-year mortality rate from GBM varies between 55 and 65%, with 2-year mortality rate of approximately 80–90% and 5-year mortality rate of approximately 97%. Factors predictive of poor outcomes include age older than 60 years, poor functional status, lack of surgical debulking, high histological grade (with necrosis), and possibly a noncystic tumor. Death is usually associated with progressive neurological dysfunction with cerebral herniation secondary to raised ICP or tumor bulk.

Counseling

Patients and their families should be aware of the dismal prognosis and the risks and benefits of treatment, including perioperative complications and adverse drug effects. Encouraging informed choice is advisable. Specialist referrals and counseling should be provided as outlined on pp. 215–216. Nursing and emotional support are necessary adjuncts in the care of the primary brain tumor patient.

SUMMARY

- **Primary brain tumors** are a common cause for chronic progressive focal neurological deficit, especially in **middle-aged persons**.
- Neoplastic lesions with a **temporal lobe predilection** include **astrocytoma, oligodendroglioma**, and **ganglioglioma**.
- GBM is the **most common** primary intracranial tumor.
- Differentials include **extradural tumors, solitary parenchymal metastasis, brain abscess, subdural empyema, cranial epidural abscess, chronic subdural hematoma, or tumor-like demyelinating lesions**.

- Diagnosis is made by **MRI brain** and **histopathology**.
- Treatment involves **surgical debulking, radiation therapy**, and **chemotherapy**.
- Mean survival is **approximately 6 months** if untreated or **approximately 12 months** if treated.
- One-year mortality from GBM is **approximately 55–65%**, 2-year mortality is **approximately 80–90%**, and 5-year mortality is **approximately 97%**.
- Poor outcomes are associated with **age older than 60, poor functional status, lack of surgical debulking, high histological grade** (with necrosis), and possibly a **noncystic tumor**.

CASE 3

A 44-year-old man complained of progressive hearing loss in his right ear and difficulty chewing for several months. His co-workers had also noticed asymmetry and reduced facial movements on his right side. On examination, there was a right complete facial paresis with mild buccal dysarthria. Rinne's test was normal with Weber's test localizing to the left ear when performed with a 256 Hz tuning fork.

Localization

Unilateral right facial paresis and buccal dysarthria imply an ipsilateral CN VII lesion, either at the level of the nucleus in the right pons or along its intracranial course (pontomedullary junction [PMJ], IAC, geniculate ganglion, stylomastoid foramen) to the muscles of facial expression. Right-sided sensorineural hearing loss implies dysfunction of the right CN VIII either at the level of the cochlear nucleus at the PMJ or cochlear nerve that travels from the IAC to the brainstem. Both CN VII and VIII transverse at the level of the cerebellopontine angle (CPA) and travel within the IAC. In summary, the underlying process localizes to the right CN VII and VIII, either at the level of the CPA/PMJ or the IAC.

Differential Diagnosis

The most likely diagnosis for a slowly progressive lesion compromising both the right CN VII and VIII is *vestibular schwannoma (acoustic neuroma)*. This is a primary nerve sheath tumor (consists of pure Schwann cell proliferation) of the vestibular portion of the CN VIII that erodes the IAC, occupying the CPA and causes compression of the cochlear portion of CN VIII, as well as CN VII. When present bilaterally, this tumor is virtually diagnostic of *neurofibromatosis type 2* (NF II). Less than 1% of tumors undergo malignant transformation.

Other differentials include *neurofibroma* (proliferation of multiple nerve elements including Schwann cells, fibroblasts, mast cells and perineurial-like cells), *epidermoid cyst* (may be congenital or acquired; more common in young adults and rupture causes granulomatous chemical meningitis), and *meningioma*.

Investigation

MRI brain with and without contrast is the initial diagnostic investigation. Vestibular schwannomas are extradural, extramedullary tumors that enhance with occasional cystic/calcified components. MRI is superior to CT scanning as it provides better resolution and less posterior fossa "beam-hardening" artifact. Histopathological examination following surgical resection is the definitive diagnostic modality.

Management

Small, stable, and symptomatic lesions are followed by serial MRI scans every year. Symptomatic lesions require *microsurgical resection* or *stereotactic radiosurgery* (mortality rate of ~1%, complication rate ~2–3%; risks are related to tumor size and include ipsilateral trigeminal, abducens, or facial nerve injury, deafness, postoperative CSF leak, intracranial hematoma [subdural], CPA, and brainstem or cerebellar edema). Treatment failure rates are approximately 5–8%, with stereotactic radiosurgery being less efficacious for tumors larger than 3.5 cm diameter.

Proton radiosurgery or fractionated stereotactic radiotherapy may control tumor growth without disappearance in approximately 90% of patients (~20% risk of significant hearing loss). With malignant transformation, wide surgical excision with radiotherapy (external beam with or without implants) for residual tumor with or without adjuvant chemotherapy should be considered. Adequate postoperative care (including wound care, speech and language therapy, and facial rehabilitation) should be provided to facilitate recovery.

Prognosis

There is slow progression in tumor size in untreated cases (mean ~1.2 mm per year), with growth more significant for CPA over IAC located tumors. About 65% continue to grow after mean follow-up of 2 years and 80% after mean follow-up of 4 years. Significant growth (>1 mm per year) may occur in approximately 30–40% with little or no growth occurring in approximately 50% over 3 years. About 20% of conservatively managed patients may require surgical intervention within 3 years for worsening symptoms/signs or continuous/rapid tumor growth. There is progressive auditory dysfunction with time irrespective of change in tumor size.

Untreated cases may remain asymptomatic, cause minimal deficit, or progressively cause brainstem compression with consequential morbidity and mortality. About 95% of surgically treated patients are discharged home, with short-term rehabilitation required in about 4% and long-term care in about 1%. Despite adequate surgical treatment, tumor recurrence may occur in 2–5% of patients. Median survival is about 2–5 years after malignant transformation, with tumor recurrence occurring in approximately 50% of these patients within 3 years of treatment. Good prognostic indicators include younger age at diagnosis, small tumor size, and limited extent of required surgical resection.

Counseling

Patients should be aware of the prognostic data as well as the potential risks and benefits of conservative vs surgical treatments based on clinical features, tumor size/growth, and location. Patients should be aware of the potential for irreversible loss of facial sensation, facial paresis, or hearing loss with treated or untreated vestibular schwannomas. In patients with bilateral lesions, genetic assessment and counseling for NF II is necessary.

SUMMARY

- **Vestibular schwannoma** is a **nerve sheath tumor** that commonly occurs in the **IAC or CPA** and causes **CN VII and VIII** compression.
- Differentials include **neurofibroma, epidermoid cyst,** and **meningioma**.
- Diagnosis is made by **MRI brain** with and without contrast and **histopathology**.
- Treatment involves **conservative** and **surgical** (microsurgical resection or stereotactic radiosurgery) modalities. **Malignant transformation** (<1%) may require **wide excision, radiotherapy** with or without **chemotherapy**.
- Perioperative surgical mortality **approximately 1%**, with morbidity of **approximately 2–3%** and **approximately 95%** treatment success. Recurrence rate is **approximately 2–5%**.
- **Progressive auditory dysfunction** occurs irrespective of tumor growth.
- About **30–40%** of tumors significantly grow over **3 years** with **approximately 20%** of conservatively managed patients requiring surgical treatment.
- Median survival of **2–5 years** occurs following malignant transformation with tumor recurrence in **approximately 50%** within **3 years** of initial treatment.

19

Vestibular Disorders

CASE 1

A 63-year-old man complained of attacks of "dizziness" over the past 3 months. He experienced fullness in his right ear, with loss of hearing and a ringing sensation. This was followed by a severe sensation of the room spinning that worsened for about 5 minutes and slowly subsided over about 45–60 minutes. These episodes were usually associated with severe nausea and vomiting, occurring about two to three times a week. Neurological examination showed a normal Rinne's test with localization of sound to the left ear with Weber's test performed with a 256 Hz tuning fork.

Localization

The unilateral hearing loss, tinnitus, and fullness in the ear suggest peripheral dysfunction of the auditory apparatus on the right. The localization of sound to the left ear on Weber's test suggests that there is right-sided sensorineural hearing loss, rather than conductive loss. Sudden vertigo, associated with nausea and vomiting may localize to dysfunction in the vestibular end organs (semicircular canals, utricle, and saccule), vestibular component of CN VIII or vestibular nuclei at the PMJ of the brainstem. The absence of further brainstem signs makes a central cause less likely. In summary, the most likely localization is the right vestibular end organs with associated CN VIII (cochlear component) involvement or isolated CN VIII dysfunction involving both the vestibular and cochlear components.

Differential Diagnosis

The most likely diagnosis for recurrent paroxysmal attacks of hearing loss, tinnitus, and vertigo, associated with ear fullness and spontaneous recovery over hours to days is *Ménière's disease*. This is an idiopathic peripheral vestibular disorder associated with overproduction of endolymph within the semicircular canals (endolymphatic hydrops).

Other differentials include *peripheral vestibulopathy* (labyrinthitis, vestibular neuronitis: presumed viral etiology with isolated involvement of vestibular end

From: *Neurology Oral Boards Review:*
A Concise and Systematic Approach to Clinical Practice
By: E. E. Ubogu © Humana Press Inc., Totowa, NJ

organs or part of a systemic illness, e.g., upper respiratory tract infection, measles, mumps, infectious mononucleosis), *benign paroxysmal positional vertigo* (BPPV; usually induced by a change in head position or movement, with hearing loss, fullness, and tinnitus uncommon), *drug-induced* (e.g., aminoglycoside antibiotics: usually causes progressive imbalance, AEDs, sedative-hypnotics, alcohol, antihypertensives, etc.), and *posttraumatic vertigo* (occurs immediately after head trauma and may be associated with temporal bone fractures with vestibular end-organ damage or cupulolithiasis with BPPV).

Further considerations include *infection* (e.g., bacterial-otitis media, viralherpes zoster: Ramsay-Hunt syndrome, or syphilis), *neoplasm* (e.g., tumor of CN VIII), *degeneration of vestibular end organs* (hereditary or acquired), *ischemia* (from vertebrobasilar disease: rare and usually occurs in association with brainstem ischemia), and *toxic-metabolic* causes (e.g., anemia, polycythemia, DM, hypothyroidism).

Investigations

CBC with differentials, basic metabolic panel, TFT, fasting glucose, and ESR/CRP may be performed in equivocal cases. If syncope were present based on history, further evaluation (*see* p. 177) would be required. Audiological (e.g., audiometry, acoustic reflex, evoked potentials) and vestibular tests (e.g., electronystagmography with bithermal caloric testing, rotational tests, and posturography) should be considered when available to further support a diagnosis of peripheral or central vestibular disorder. The clinical history is paramount in establishing the diagnosis.

Management

The management of Ménière's disease involves treatment of acute attacks and suppressive therapy. Acute attacks may be treated with *antihistamines* (e.g., meclizine, cyclizine) or *benzodiazepines* (e.g., diazepam) with or without an *antiemetic* (e.g., prochlorperazine, promethazine). Suppressive therapy may be divided into lifestyle modifications, medical, and surgical therapies. Lifestyle modifications include low-salt diet (1–2 g per day restriction), avoidance of alcohol, caffeine, nicotine, stress, or any known exacerbating factors. Medical therapy includes diuretics such as *acetazolamide, triamterene-hydrochlorothiazide*, and *furosemide*. Prednisone/methotrexate may be used if an autoimmune etiology is suspected, especially with bilateral disease.

Surgical therapy is usually reserved for medically refractory cases and includes *intratympanic gentamicin injection* (~70–90% with complete or substantial improvement in vertigo, reduction in tinnitus in ~60% with ~30% hearing loss at 2 year follow-up), *endolymphatic sac decompression or shunt surgery*, *vestibular nerve section*, or *surgical labyrinthectomy* (~80–90% improvement in vertigo).

Microvascular decompression of CN VIII may be performed if vascular compression is noted (e.g., vertebrobasilar dolichoectasia [VBD]). The above therapies are empirical and not based on prospective randomized controlled trials, and whether these modalities truly alter the natural history of Ménière's disease is undetermined.

Prognosis

Ménière's disease is incurable but not life-threatening. It can cause progressive disability owing to persistent vertigo and deafness. In general, the disease may be nonprogressive or progressive with bilateral involvement after unilateral onset in about 20% of patients. Spontaneous remissions may occur in a small number of patients, with recurrence after months to years. Substantial reduction or resolution in vertigo may occur in 30–55% of untreated patients after 2 years, with about 70–80% improvement over 6–8 years with greater than 50% complete or near complete hearing loss. Treated patients have substantially higher resolution rates (70–80% at 2 years) with similar long-term rates of vertigo resolution and hearing loss. Untreated patients, however, have higher rates of emotional disability and anxiety in comparison to treated patients with this disease.

Counseling

Patients should be aware of prognostic data and the risks/benefits/complications of medical and surgical therapy. The implications of not treating the disease should also be emphasized. Patients should be advised to actively participate in their care by keeping a diary to help elucidate potential exacerbating factors. Emotional support and reassurance are required as an integral part of patient care. Evaluating for and excluding other potential causes of vertigo or dizziness, including syncope and systemic diseases may be necessary, with early specialist referral suggested, if indicated. Information on patient support groups should be provided as a source of social/emotional support.

SUMMARY

- **Ménière's disease** is a chronic, **idiopathic** peripheral vestibular disorder associated with **endolymphatic hydrops**.
- Differentials include **peripheral vestibulopathy, BPPV, drug-induced, posttraumatic vertigo, infection, neoplasm, ischemia**, and **toxic-metabolic**.
- **Clinical history** is important for the diagnosis. **Audiological** and **vestibular tests** further support a peripheral vestibular disorder.
- Treatment can be divided into **acute attack** and **chronic suppressive therapy**. Suppressive therapy can be divided into **lifestyle modifications, medical**, and **surgical modalities**.

- Acute attacks are treated with **antihistamines** or **benzodiazepines** with or without **antiemetics**.
- The mainstay of suppressive therapy are **lifestyle modifications** and **diuretics**. Surgery is reserved for **medically refractory** cases.
- **Two-year** complete resolution or significant improvement in vertigo occurs in **approximately 70–80%** with treatment and **approximately 30–55%** without treatment.
- Long-term vertigo resolution and deafness rates are **similar** between treated and untreated patients.
- **Emotional support** is a necessary adjunct in treating this disease.

CASE 2

A 59-year-old woman came to the clinic with a complaint of "dizziness" with head movement for 5–6 months. Turning her head down to the left in bed resulted in severe vertigo and nausea. These episodes were worse early in the day. On examination, Dix-Hallpike maneuver showed horizontal-rotatory nystagmus with the fast phase toward the ground with her left ear down, and subjective vertigo. This occurred after about 15 seconds and lasted about 45 seconds with improvement with repeated testing. Neurological examination was otherwise normal.

Localization

Vertigo (an illusion of movement) implies dysfunction in the vestibular apparatus, involving the end organs (semicircular canals, cupula, macula), vestibular portion of CN VIII, or vestibular nuclei at the PMJ of the brainstem. Nystagmus with delayed onset of short duration implies a peripheral etiology (i.e., vestibular end organs or CN VIII). Horizontal-rotatory nystagmus with the fast phase toward the left may imply hyperexcitability of the left vestibular apparatus or reduced function in the right vestibular apparatus. However, reduction in signs and symptoms with repeated testing (i.e., habituation) implies reduction in hyperexcitability in the left vestibular apparatus. In summary, the underlying process most likely involves the left vestibular end organs or the vestibular portion of CN VIII.

Differential Diagnosis

The most likely diagnosis for sudden episodes of vertigo associated with nystagmus and nausea induced by positional change is *benign paroxysmal positional vertigo* (BPPV). This is a chronic peripheral vestibular disorder associated with canalolithiasis or cupulolithiasis, in which otoconia are displaced and free to migrate to the posterior semicircular canals with certain head positions. Patients may have had a preceding history of head trauma or viral labyrinthitis, causing otoconia displacement.

Differentials include *posttraumatic vertigo* (trauma may precipitate BPPV), *peripheral vestibulopathy* (acute phase), *Ménière's disease* (hearing loss, tinnitus more common with reproducible vertigo less common), *infection* (e.g., otitis media), and *neoplasm* (affecting the vestibular apparatus).

Investigations

The clinical history and physical examination (Dix-Hallpike or Epley maneuvers) establish the diagnosis of BPPV. Formal audiological or vestibular studies are not necessary, but could be performed if there are any additional concerns clinically. Evaluation for systemic illness (*see* p. 224) may be considered in equivocal cases when clinically indicated.

Management

The mainstay of therapy for BPPV is canalith repositioning exercise therapy with or without mastoid vibration, such as the Brandt-Daroff, modified Epley or Semont exercises. These procedures involve the rapid movement of individuals from sitting to recumbent positions for a definite amount of time, then to the opposite position and back (one cycle) for 20 cycles twice a day. These procedures can be performed in the office or at home but are relatively contraindicated in patients with cervical or thoracic spine disease. Significant symptomatic relief may occur within 1–2 weeks of treatment, although complete cure may not occur for about 3 months. In rare patients with severely disabling disease refractory to exercise therapy, vestibular nerve section from the posterior semicircular canal could be attempted.

Prognosis

As the name implies, BPPV is not a life-threatening disease and has excellent medical response rates to exercise therapy. There is an 80–95% initial symptom resolution rate within 1–2 weeks of therapy initiation (after an average of 1.1–1.2 maneuvers), with approximately 20% recurrence after 15 months follow-up (mean onset of recurrence is about 4 months) and approximately 35–50% recurrence after 3–5 years follow-up. However, greater than 90% of these patients respond to further canalith repositioning exercise therapy. Prior trauma, viral labyrinthitis, and idiopathic etiologies may predict lower rates of recurrence, whereas associated endolymphatic hydrops or CNS etiology for dizziness may predict higher recurrence rates.

Counseling

Patients should be aware of the excellent prognosis of this disease, and the time delay to achieve complete cure with exercise therapy. Patients should be reassured and encouraged to persist with exercises despite symptom persistence or recurrence. "Vestibular suppressants" (e.g., antihistamines, benzodiazepines) should be avoided, as these agents may reduce the efficacy of canalith repositioning exercise therapy and could prolong the duration of illness.

SUMMARY

- **BPPV** is a benign, chronic peripheral vestibular disorder that is associated with **canalolithiasis** or **cupulolithiasis** in the **posterior semicircular canal**.
- Differentials include **posttraumatic vertigo, peripheral vestibulopathy** (acute phase), **Ménière's disease, infection,** or **neoplasm**.
- Diagnosis is based on **clinical history** and **physical examination** (Dix-Hallpike or Epley maneuver).
- Treatment consists of **canalith repositioning exercise therapy** with or without mastoid vibration. Surgery should be reserved for rare, **severely disabled medically refractory** cases.
- **Approximately 80–95%** initial symptom resolution rate occurs within **1–2 weeks** of therapy initiation.
- Recurrence rates are **approximately 20%** after **15 months** (mean **~4 months**) and **approximately 35–50%** after **3–5 years** of follow-up.
- **Prior trauma, viral labyrinthitis,** and **idiopathic** etiologies may predict **lower** rates of recurrence, whereas associated **endolymphatic hydrops** or **CNS** etiologies may predict **higher** recurrence rates.
- **"Vestibular suppressants"** should be avoided.

20

Pediatric Neurology

CASE 1

A 9-year-old boy was noted by his mother to have become clumsy and unsteady for about a week. This seemed to have occurred suddenly about 5–7 days after an upper respiratory tract infection (URI). On examination, there was mild bilateral end-gaze horizontal nystagmus, truncal ataxia, and bilateral appendicular ataxia with dysmetria. Motor, sensory, and reflex examinations were otherwise normal.

Localization

Bilateral end-gaze nystagmus with truncal ataxia suggests localization to the midline cerebellum (vestibulo cerebellum) or its central connections via the inferior cerebellar peduncles, median longitudinal fasciculus (MLF; for ocular movements) or vestibulospinal tracts (to postural muscles). Bilateral appendicular ataxia with dysmetria may localize to the lateral cerebellar hemispheres (cerebrocerebellum) or their central connections via the superior cerebellar peduncles, red nucleus (and rubrospinal tract), thalamus (ventral anterior nuclei) to the motor cortex (predominantly frontal lobes). In summary, the underlying process most likely localizes diffusely to the cerebellum bilaterally.

Differential Diagnosis

The most likely diagnosis for a diffuse cerebellar disorder in a 9-year-old following an URI is *acute postinfectious cerebellitis*. This is a presumed dysimmune disorder common between ages 2 and 7 years, in which a preceding viral infection may be documented in approximately 50% of cases. Inciting organisms include VZV, EBV, rubeola, coxsackievirus, *Coxiella burneti,* and *Clostridium diphtheria*. However, this is a *diagnosis of exclusion* and other potential causes of acute–subacute cerebellar dysfunction should be evaluated for.

Other differentials include other *postinfectious/autoimmune disorders* such as *Miller-Fisher syndrome* (MFS: GBS variant that is characterized by ataxia, ophthalmoparesis and areflexia with CSF showing albuminocytologic dissociation.

From: *Neurology Oral Boards Review:*
A Concise and Systematic Approach to Clinical Practice
By: E. E. Ubogu © Humana Press Inc., Totowa, NJ

Initial recovery tends to occur within 2–4 weeks after maximal symptoms. Complete recovery is expected within 6 months), *MS* (uncommon in children with variable clinical presentation: truncal/limb ataxia, encephalopathy, hemiparesis, internuclear ophthalmoplegia that may persist for weeks to months), *drug ingestion* (more common in ages <4 years: common agents include alcohol, AEDs, antihistamines, and psychoactive drugs), and *migraine* (*basilar migraine:* recurrent attacks of brainstem/cerebellar dysfunction that peaks in adolescence; *benign paroxysmal vertigo:* positive family history of migraine in 40%, more common in <5 years, with ~20% developing headaches).

Further diagnostic considerations include *neoplasm* (e.g., acute hemorrhage into cerebellar tumors: astrocytoma, medulloblastoma, hemangioblastoma, etc.; paraneoplastic myoclonic encephalopathy: opsoclonus, myoclonus, ataxia, and encephalopathy associated with neuroblastoma, mean onset 18 months with 1–2 week clinical evolution), *infection* (e.g., brainstem encephalitis: commonly secondary to viral infection such as coxsackievirus, adenovirus, echovirus; self-limiting disease associated with multiple cranial nerve dysfunction and leukocytic [monocytic] pleocytosis in CSF), *infarction* (e.g., cerebellar hemorrhage from AVM, angiomas, vertebrobasilar occlusion [procoagulant state or traumatic]: more likely to expect acute, unilateral symptoms at onset, or *vasculitis:* e.g., CTD, Kawasaki disease: fever, conjunctival injection, lymphadenopathy, limb edema, oro-pharyngeal erythema, polymorphic exanthema, treated with aspirin and IVIg).

Based on the clinical history, other differentials may include *trauma* (can cause cerebellar ICH or postconcussion syndrome), *inherited ataxia* (e.g., episodic ataxia (EA) type 1: associated with myokymia and continuous motor unit activity on EMG—K^+ channelopathy; EA type 2: associated with hemiplegic migraines—Ca^{2+} channelopathy; both are inherited in an AD pattern and treated with acetazolamide) or *psychogenic* (conversion reaction, more common in early to mid-adolescence and associated with more immediate life stressors).

Chronic progressive ataxia in a child may imply a *congenital malformation* affecting the cerebellum (e.g., Dandy-Walker malformation, cerebellar/vermal aplasia, Arnold-Chiari malformations: usually present at younger ages and associated with cognitive dysfunction or headaches), *neoplasm* (as above, including supratentorial tumors with cerebellar compression), or *inherited ataxias* such as *Friedreich's ataxia* (AR: most common inherited ataxia caused by trinucleotide repeat in frataxin gene on chromosome 9— onset common between 2 and 15 with diffuse cerebellar dysfunction, peripheral neuropathy, pes cavus, hammertoes, kyphoscoliosis, cardiomyopathy in 50% and DM in 10%), and *ataxia-telangiectasia* (AR: defect in DNA repair gene on chromosome 11—onset after age 2 with cerebellar dysfunction, choreoathetosis, ocular motor dysfunction, polyneuropathy, subpapillary venous plexus telangiectasia with immunodeficiency resulting in sinopulmonary infections and neoplasms-glioma, leukemia, and lymphoma that cause death by age 20).

Additional causes for chronic progressive ataxia include *abetalipoproteinemia* or *Bassen-Kornzweig syndrome* (AR: defect in microsomal triglyceride transfer protein on chromosome 4: present from birth with fat malabsorption and vitamins A,D, E, and K deficiencies, psychomotor retardation, cerebellar dysfunction, peripheral neuropathy, pigmentary retinopathy, acanthocytosis by age 10: treated with dietary fat restriction and vitamin E replacement), *juvenile GM$_2$ gangliosidosis* (hexosaminidase deficiency: age of onset usually before 15 with progressive cerebellar syndrome), *autosomally dominant ataxias* (spinocerebellar ataxia syndromes: more commonly present in early adulthood, e.g., SCA1-3, DRPLA) or *x-linked ataxias* (e.g., *Leber's hereditary optic neuropathy:* mitochondrial multisystemic disorder affecting several respiratory chain enzymes that is more common in males, and *adrenoleukodystrophy*—defect in perioxisomal acylcoenzyme A synthetase: *see* pp. 242–246).

Investigations

Investigations should be tailored toward potential etiologies. For acute or chronic ataxias, CT/MRI brain with and without contrast should be performed to exclude cerebellar mass or structural lesions, including congenital malformations. Noncontrasted T$_2$-weighted MRI brain may show hyperintense cerebellar gray matter signal changes in acute postinfectious cerebellitis. LP for CSF analysis can be helpful in diagnosing MS, MFS, or brainstem encephalitis.

Serum/urine toxicology may be useful in cases of suspected drug ingestion. Serum Ig (ataxia-telangiectasia), vitamins A, D, E, K, lipid panel, CBC, and blood smear (abetalipoproteinemia), lactate/pyruvate (mitochondrial disorders), very long-chain fatty acids (adrenoleukodystrophy), enzyme levels (in blood or fibroblasts), genetic tests ("ataxia panel") for inherited ataxias, or urine organic acids can be performed based on clinical suspicion. EMG/NCS may help in characterizing an associated peripheral neuropathy, but is nondiagnostic (e.g., in inherited ataxias).

Management

The treatment for acute or chronic progressive ataxias should be tailored toward potential etiologies. For acute postinfectious cerebellitis, there is no particular treatment apart from supportive care. This also holds true for brainstem encephalitis and most inherited ataxias. Complications of chronic progressive inherited ataxias (e.g., DM, cardiomyopathy in Friedreich's ataxia, sinopulmonary infections in ataxia-telangiectasia) should be identified and managed aggressively.

MFS may be treated with IVIg (also Kawasaki's disease) or PE. MS exacerbation and myoclonic encephalopathy-neuroblastoma can be treated with corticosteroids. Cerebellar hemorrhage is a neurological emergency, and warrants prompt treatment (*see* p. 23).

If a neoplasm is identified, appropriate confirmatory diagnosis and therapy (surgical debulking, radiotherapy, chemotherapy should be undertaken). Antiplatelet therapy may be useful in Kawasaki's disease and other rare procoagulant causes for posterior circulation infarction. If a migraine-variant is identified, then appropriate prophylactic therapy should be initiated. Cessation of drug ingestion and spontaneous elimination would be the mode of treatment for drug-induced ataxias unless severe cardiorespiratory compromise warrants dialysis with ICU support.

Prognosis

The prognosis of an acute or chronic ataxic disorder of childhood depends on its etiology. The prognosis for acute postinfectious cerebellitis and brainstem encephalitis is excellent, as these are self-limiting diseases with no residual sequelae. Rarely, death or residual sequelae may occur secondary to hydrocephalus or edema-induced cerebellar herniation. MFS usually resolves completely within 6 months. MS could be relapsing-remitting or chronic progressive (*see* pp. 181–184).

In general, structural etiologies (especially acute hemorrhage) are potentially life-threatening and residual symptoms may persist despite treatment. Neoplasms may confer a reduced or normal 5-year survival rate based on the type of neoplasm and response to therapy. Prevention of neurological sequelae or cessation of progression may occur with early treatment of abetalipoproteinemia (vitamin E replacement).

Death by age 20 occurs in patients with ataxia-telangiectasia, whereas survival into the fourth and fifth decades may occur with Friedreich's ataxia. Autosomally dominant inherited ataxias are slowly progressive with death in the fifth to seventh decades. Cerebellar infarctions usually result in near complete or complete recovery over several months. Ataxia associated with postconcussive syndrome usually resolves within 1 month. Mental retardation is a common sequelae of congenital malformations and early-onset metabolic ataxias.

Counseling

Families and patients should be made aware of the prognostic information, dependent on the underlying etiology. Emotional support and reassurance are important in assisting patients and their parents cope with the self-limiting acquired ataxias. For inherited ataxias, more extensive family history should be ascertained and genetic counseling should be provided based on the mode of inheritance, disease penetrance, potential sequelae, and availability of prenatal testing. Psychological support is necessary for patients with psychogenic ataxia. Safety advice should be provided in cases of accidental drug ingestion, including the use of childproof bottles and cabinets for medications.

SUMMARY

- **Childhood ataxias** can be divided into **acute** and **chronic progressive** ataxias.
- Etiologies for acute ataxias include **postinfectious/autoimmune, drug ingestion, migraine, hemorrhage into neoplasm, paraneoplastic, infection, infarction, trauma, inherited,** or **psychogenic.**
- Etiologies for chronic ataxias include **congenital malformations, neoplasms,** and **inherited** (AR, AD, or x-linked).
- Investigations should be tailored toward clinical suspicion. **CT/MRI brain, CSF analysis, serum toxicology, vitamin, enzyme,** and **Ig levels, lipid profile, CBC, genetic tests,** and **urine organic acids** may be useful in establishing a diagnosis.
- Treat the underlying cause. No treatment is required in **acute postinfectious cerebellitis, brainstem encephalitis, postconcussive ataxia,** and **mild cases of MFS.**
- **Prompt treatment** should be instituted for potentially treatable or reversible disorders.
- Prognosis is **excellent** for self-limiting acquired childhood ataxias where no treatment is indicated. **Neoplasms, cerebellar ICH, severe drug ingestion,** and **ataxia-telangiectasia** confer a worse prognosis.
- **Mental retardation** is a common sequelae of **congenital malformations** and **early-onset metabolic ataxias.**

CASE 2

A 21-month-old girl was brought to the ER by her mother, who stated that she had been behaving strangely for several hours. She was less cooperative, irritable, and did not respond to her name or simple commands. Her mother was concerned that she may have ingested some of her sleeping pills. On examination, vitals signs were normal. Neurological examination showed an irritable, agitated child who did not respond to her mother's comfort or questioning. No deficits on cranial nerve (limited ocular examination), motor, or sensory examinations were elicited.

Localization

An acute confusional state is nonlocalizing, with irritability, agitation, and inability to respond to name or simple commands being indicative of bilateral cerebral hemispheric dysfunction. Normal cranial nerve, motor and sensory examinations further support the lack of localizing features.

Differential Diagnosis

The differential diagnoses for an acute encephalopathy in a 21-month-old child are numerous. Based on the concern of ingestion, a highly likely differential is *drug/toxin exposure. Accidental drug/toxin exposure* is a relatively common cause for childhood encephalopathy. Drugs commonly implicated include AEDs, antidepressants, sedative-hypnotics, antipsychotics, and analgesics. Common household products such as cleaning solvents, insecticides, or alcohol may also cause an encephalopathy associated with initial emesis. Substances of abuse (e.g., opiates, hallucinogens, cocaine, or amphetamines) could also be implicated through accidental or forced exposure.

Other differentials include *metabolic encephalopathy* (e.g., hypo-/hyperglycemia, hypo-/hypernatremia, hypo-/hypercalcemia, uremia, hepatic failure), *endocrine disorders* (e.g., hypo-/hyperthyroidism, hypo-/hypercortisolemia, hypoparathyroidism), and *infections* (e.g., *bacterial* such as *cat scratch disease*: rare encephalopathy, seizures, or combative behavior with lymphadenopathy proximal to scratch caused by *Bartonella henselae*; septicemia, Gram-positive/Gram-negative meningitis like *S. pneumoniae*; *viral* such as HSE, measles, aseptic meningitis, arboviral encephalitis; *spirochetes* such as Lyme disease: early erythema chronicum migrans and later mild aseptic meningitis/encephalitis associated with cranial nerve palsy or chronic encephalopathy caused by *B. burgdoferi* and most common in northeastern United States).

Further diagnostic considerations includs *postinfectious* (e.g., post-viral demyelinating encephalomyelitis, *Reye's syndrome*: systemic mitochondrial disorder associated with viral illness, precipitated by salicylates intake, causing hepatocellular dysfunction), *seizures* (e.g., absence SE or complex partial seizures), *inherited metabolic defects* (e.g., heterozygotes for *urea cycle defects, mitochondrial disorders* such as *Leigh's disease, Menkes syndrome*: cherubic facies with kinky hair and myoclonic seizures; *primary carnitine deficiency*; e.g., medium-chain acyl-CoA dehydrogenase deficiency with attacks of encephalopathy and emesis induced by fasting or systemic illness), and *vascular disease* (e.g., posttraumatic SAH, SLE, vasculitis).

Investigations

Investigations should be tailored toward potential etiologies, so a thorough history is important to direct evaluation. Child abuse should be suspected with multiple injuries. When history is nonrevealing, a broad screen is necessary. Laboratory tests may include CBC with differential, comprehensive metabolic panel (includes LFTs), serum ammonia, lactate/pyruvate, TFT, ESR/CRP, blood cultures, serum/urine toxicology.

CT of the brain should be performed to exclude SAH and LP would be necessary if infection is suspected or the cause of encephalopathy is unclear. CSF cultures, viral PCR, and Lyme titers may be required based on history. If seizures are suspected, EEG would be diagnostically useful. EEG may also show nonspecific slowing in encephalopathy. If Reye's syndrome is suspected, liver biopsy is diagnostic. Specific enzyme analyses can be performed for inherited metabolic deficits.

Management

Treatment for drug/toxin exposure depends on the agent ingested and severity of poisoning suspected based on the amount and time from ingestion to presentation. Caution is required, as children may rapidly progress from a confusional state to a potentially life-threatening coma requiring emergency intubation. Admission for close cardio-respiratory monitoring should be considered, and i.v. access obtained. Telemetry should be considered for continuous EKG.

Gastric lavage may be considered for noncorrosive substances, activated charcoal may reduce absorption, and forced diuresis or hemodialysis may facilitate drug clearance. The specific antidote should be administered early if available; e.g., pralidoxime for organophosphates, *N*-acetylcysteine for acetaminophen, naloxone for opiates, and flumazenil for benzodiazepines. Metabolic derangements should be corrected and supportive nursing care provided.

Prognosis

In general, there is a less than 1% mortality rate in children with accidental drug/toxin exposure, however, the risk is dependent on the ingested agent. Early recognition is necessary in order to provide pharmacological reversal or supportive care. Rare fatalities are most likely caused by cardiac arrhythmias. Patients are usually left without any appreciable sequelae if treated early.

Counseling

Parents should be advised on ensuring that drugs and toxins are always out of reach for children, and safe cabinets and child-proof bottles should be used for prescription medications. Children less than 4 years of age are at the highest risk for accidental drug exposure, so good parental supervision is paramount. In adolescence, suicidal intent is an important cause for toxic drug ingestion, and this should be thoroughly evaluated for, including co-morbid psychiatric illness and social stressors. Child protection services should be consulted if child abuse (traumatic or forced drug ingestion) is suspected.

SUMMARY

- **Accidental drug/toxin exposure** is a **relatively common** cause of acute childhood encephalopathy.
- Potential agents include **AEDs, antidepressants, sedative-hypnotics, antipsychotics, analgesics, common household products**, and **substances of abuse**.

- Differentials for acute childhood encephalopathy include **metabolic, endocrine, infectious, postinfectious, seizure, inherited metabolic deficit**, and **vascular** disorders.
- Investigations should be tailored toward potential etiologies. A general screen should include **CBC, comprehensive metabolic panel, serum/urine toxicology, ammonia, TFTs, ESR/CRP, blood cultures,** and **neuroimaging.**
- Treatment for drug/toxin exposure depends on the **agent ingested** and **severity of poisoning. Reduction in systemic absorption, enhancement of clearance, specific antidote** (if available), and **supportive care,** including cardio-respiratory monitoring should be provided.
- Mortality is **less than 1%** in children with accidental drug exposure. Cause of death is usually **cardiac arrhythmias.**
- Risk of ingestion is highest in children **less than 4 years** of age.
- **Prevention of drug/toxin exposure** (safe cabinets and childproof bottles) and **good parental supervision** are paramount in preventing recurrences.

CASE 3

A 13-year-old girl complained of blurred vision for more than 2 weeks. This developed suddenly without any clear precipitating events and progressed rapidly over 3–5 days. Her left eye was initially affected with subsequent involvement of her right eye 2–3 days later. On examination, visual acuity was 20/100 on the right and 20/200 in the left, with bilateral relative afferent pupillary deficits. Bilateral large central scotomata were present on confrontation visual field assessment. Fundoscopy revealed bilateral disk swelling with mild hemorrhages. The remainder of the neurological examination was normal.

Localization

Bilateral loss in visual acuity implies bilateral retinal or optic nerve dysfunction. A relative afferent pupillary deficit implies dysfunction to the anterior pathways of the pupillary reflex (retina, optic nerve, optic chiasm, optic tracts prior to synapse in the midbrain). However, papillitis on fundoscopic examination bilaterally makes lesion most likely to involve the optic nerves. In summary, the underlying process most likely localizes to the bilateral optic nerves.

Differential Diagnosis

The most likely cause for acute bilateral monocular visual loss in a child is *demyelinating optic neuropathy* (*optic neuritis*). This could be an idiopathic disorder, or part of the spectrum of *multiple sclerosis* (*see* pp. 181–184 and 230) or *Devic's disease* (neuromyelitis optica: bilateral painful optic neuritis with transverse myelitis).

Other differentials include *toxic optic neuropathy* (e.g., secondary to drugs such as ergotamine, streptomycin, sulfonamides, isoniazid, barbiturates, digoxin), *nutritional deficiencies* (e.g., vitamins B_1, B_2, B_6, B_{12} and folic acid), *ischemia* (anterior ischemic optic neuropathy secondary to hypotension or vascular disease: relatively rare in children, but more common in older adults, e.g., associated with DM or temporal arteritis), *trauma* (history of preceding head injury is usually present and visual loss may be immediate or delayed), and *neoplasm* (if there is acute hemorrhage, e.g., optic glioma commonly associated with neurofibromatosis; retinoblastoma in infants; pituitary adenoma and craniopharyngioma with optic chiasmal compression and secondary optic atrophy).

Hereditary causes include *Leber's hereditary optic neuropathy*: usually progressive, but symptoms of painless unilateral blurred central vision may be perceived subacutely and progress rapidly to permanent binocular blindness. This is a mitochondrial disorder with defects in respiratory chain complexes, more common in young males and inherited maternally; and *Wolfram's syndrome* (DIDMOAD: **d**iabetes **i**nsipidus, **d**iabetes **m**ellitus with **o**ptic atrophy and bilateral sensorineural **d**eafness: mutation on chromosome 4 with rapid incomplete visual loss in adolescence).

Investigations

Formal perimetry and indirect ophthalmoscopy may be performed as extensions of the physical examination. Visual evoked potentials may be useful in confirming demyelinating optic neuropathies. MRI of the orbits is useful to demonstrate showing optic nerve swelling and demyelination, as well as exclude neoplasms. MRI of the brain and spinal cord with or without contrast should be considered if more diffuse demyelination is clinically suspected. If multiple lesions are identified on MRI, LP should be considered to establish a diagnosis (*see* pp. 182 and 231). A careful drug history and serum/urine drug screens may be useful, in addition to serum B vitamins and RBC folate levels. Genetic testing would be warranted if there is a suggestive family history.

Management

The mainstay of treatment for demyelinating optic neuropathy (optic neuritis) is corticosteroids. Intravenous methylprednisolone 250 mg every 6 hours for 72 hours followed by oral prednisone 1 mg/kg per day for 10–14 days with steroid taper is a standard approach. Supportive care (e.g., personal hygiene, nutritional, and emotional support) is a necessary adjunct during the acute phases of the disease. For patients subsequently diagnosed with MS or Devic's disease, the efficacy of prophylactic immunomodulating agents in children is unknown.

Prognosis

In general, the prognosis of demyelinating optic neuropathy is very good, with complete recovery expected in approximately 70% at 2–3 year follow-up and approximately 75–90% of individuals over a mean follow-up of 9 years. Visual evoked potentials normalize in about 60% of patients. There is about a 10% risk of recurrence of optic neuritis in children. Lifelong risk of subsequently developing MS is 0–15% with isolated optic neuritis, and approximately 100% if diffuse CNS involvement is initially present or recurrence occurs within 1 year of initial attack. Monocular optic neuritis confers a higher (approximately twofold) risk of MS than bilateral disease. Neuromyelitis optica could be potentially life-threatening and may result in residual sequelae such as visual loss, urinary incontinence, or paraplegia. Corticosteroids increase the rate of recovery from demyelinating optic neuropathy.

Counseling

Patients and their families should be aware of the prognostic data, especially the recovery rates and the future risk for developing MS. Reassurance is necessary to alleviate fears of permanent residual blindness, although this may occur in about 10% of patients or individuals with Devic's disease. The risks and benefits of short-term high-dose corticosteroids in optic neuritis should be discussed at length.

SUMMARY

- **Demyelinating optic neuropathy (optic neuritis)** could be **idiopathic** or secondary to **MS** or **Devic's disease**.
- Other differentials for an acute bilateral monocular visual loss in a child include **toxins, nutritional deficiency, ischemia, trauma, neoplasm**, and **hereditary** etiologies.
- **Visual evoked potentials** and **MRI of the orbits** are useful in documenting demyelination. Further tests should be tailored toward clinical suspicion.
- Treatment involves the administration of **high-dose corticosteroids**.
- Corticosteroids **increase** the rate of recovery from demyelinating optic neuropathy. Role of immunomodulating drugs is **unknown**.
- Complete recovery is expected in **approximately 70%** at **2–3 year** follow-up and **approximately 75–90%** of individuals over a mean follow-up of **9 years**.
- **Approximately 10%** have permanent residual visual loss.
- **Approximately 10%** recurrence occurs in children with optic neuritis.
- Neurological residual **more common** with **Devic's disease**.
- Lifelong risk of MS **approximately 0–15 %** with isolated disease and **approximately 100%** with diffuse CNS disease on presentation or recurrence **within 1 year**. **Monocular optic neuritis** confers higher risk than bilateral disease.

CASE 4

A 5-month-old boy was noted by his parents to have frequent "muscle spasms." These are described as rapid flexion of the neck, trunk, and arms with contractions that sometimes last about 10 seconds. These were most noticeable on awakening. His parents were also concerned that he does not seem to laugh or babble like his older sister did. Cutaneous examination showed multiple hypomelanotic macules with a raised skin plaque over the buttocks. No distinct neurological deficits were elicited on examination.

Localization

Infantile spasms (myoclonic seizures) are highly suggestive of diffuse cerebral (gray matter) dysfunction. The perceived delay in language development may also suggest dysfunction in the dominant frontotemporal lobe or associated subcortical white matter, but could also imply bilateral hearing loss. Hypomelanotic macules and skin plaques over the buttocks suggest an associated cutaneous disorder. In summary, the underlying disorder diffusely affects the cerebral hemispheres with associated cutaneous involvement.

Differential Diagnosis

In cases of infantile encephalopathy (i.e., <2 years of age), it is important to ascertain if the child was normal at birth (with normal milestones: *progressive encephalopathy*) or not (with delayed milestones: *static encephalopathy*). Static encephalopathies may seem progressive if the child develops seizures, hydrocephalus or a movement disorder.

A neurocutaneous (NC) disorder characterized by myoclonic seizures, early mild developmental delay, hypomelanotic (ashleaf spots) and raised buttock skin plaques (Shagreen patch) in a 5-month-old boy is most consistent with *tuberous sclerosis (TSC)*. This is an AD-inherited disorder with variable phenotypic expression associated with mutations in the *TSC 1* (chromosome 9) or *TSC 2* (chromosome 16) genes. About 40–50% of cases are spontaneous mutations without any family history. Patients may develop retinal hamartomas, cortical tubers (dysplasia), subependymal nodules, or subependymal giant cell astrocytomas.

Other NC disorders to consider include *NF 1* (AD-inherited [chromosome 17] with café-au-lait spots [more than six of >5 mm diameter], subcutaneous neurofibromas [more than two] and axillary/inguinal freckles), *Chediak-Higashi syndrome* (defective pigmentation in skin and hair associated with MR, seizures, peripheral neuropathy (including dysautonomias) and recurrent infections secondary to neutrophil dysfunction), and *incontinentia pigmenti* (x-linked dominant disorder that is usually lethal in males: neonatal seizures associated with erythematous skin bullae that evolve into pigmentary whorls, and residual MR).

Other differentials to consider for progressive infantile encephalopathy with early seizures (suggestive of gray matter disease) include *poliodystrophies* (e.g., *early infantile neuronal ceroid lipofuscinosis* (NCL) or *Santavori-Haltia disease*: more common in Finland and presents with visual loss, myoclonus, psychomotor regression, and ataxia secondary to mutation in PPT enzyme on chromosome 1; *Rett's syndrome*: x-linked dominant mutation in *MCBP-2* gene that occurs in females characterized by developmental arrest and regression starting between 6 and 18 months, seizures: tonic-clonic or myoclonic, loss of purposeful hand movements, and disorganized breathing), *mitochondrial disorders* (e.g., *Menkes disease*: x-linked recessive disorder in intestinal Cu^{2+} absorption with secondary deficiency in Cu^{2+}-dependent mitochondrial enzymes: developmental arrest after 3 months, myoclonic seizures, cherubic facies, sparse, poorly pigmented kinky hair, and low plasma Cu^{2+} and ceruloplasmin levels; *Leigh disease* or *subacute necrotizing encephalomyelopathy*: deficiency in multiple mitochondrial enzymes including cytochrome *c* oxidase, patients are usually normal for first 6–12 months, then developmental delay, failure to thrive, paralysis of deglutition, hypotonia, seizures with subsequent movement disorder, ocular dysmotility, and respiratory pattern abnormalities develop), and *infections* (e.g., *AIDS*: secondary to transplacental or perinatal transmission of HIV: progressive loss of milestones, microcephaly, dementia, spasticity, ataxia, seizures, and opportunistic infections in ~10%, death occurs within a few months).

Further diagnostic considerations include *metabolic* (e.g., *phenylketonuria*: AR deficiency in phenylalanine hydroxylase on chromosome 12 [most common]: musty skin odor, developmental delay/regression after 3 months, behavioral disturbance, eczema, and seizures in ~30%; *Lesch-Nyhan disease*: x-linked deficiency in HGPRT enzyme with delayed motor development within first 3 months, compulsive self-mutilation with aggression, spasticity, and choreoathetosis), *lysosomal storage disorders* (e.g., *Tay-Sach's disease* or *infantile GM_2 gangliosidosis*: AR deficiency in hexosaminidase A on chromosome 15, more common in Ashkenazi Jews, abnormal startle at age 3–6 months, macula cherry-red spot, motor delay/regression, progressive macrocephaly, seizures and death by age 5; *mucopolysaccharidosis type 1* (MPS 1) or *Hurler disease*: AR deficiency in α-L-iduronidase on chromosome 4: developmental arrest with slow regression after 12 months, corneal clouding, coarse facies, hepatosplenomegaly, bony deformities with dwarfism, and death by age 10), and *endocrine disorders* (e.g., *congenital hypothyroidism*: defects in multiple genes encoding the synthesis of thyroxine, causing large babies at birth, macroglossia, generalized edema, widened fontanelles, constipation, and early MR within weeks of birth. Incidence is very low in the United States secondary to neonatal testing and early treatment).

Investigations

In suspected NC syndromes, MRI of the brain should be performed as a diagnostic aid (e.g., cortical tubers, subependymal nodules in TSC; optic gliomas in NF 1;

vestibular schwannoma ,or meningiomas in NF 2). Hydrocephalus can also be seen with MRI. The diagnosis of TSC is clinically based with the combination of two major features or one major and two minor features being definitive diagnostic. Genetic testing for TSC 1 or 2 could be performed as well. In patients with infantile spasms, EEG may show hypsarrythmia. Screening CT/MRI of the lungs or kidneys (for cysts or tumors) or echocardiography for cardiac rhabdomyomas may also be performed on initial evaluation. In atypical cases, diagnostic evaluation should be tailored toward clinical presentation. For example, enzyme analysis in serum, fibroblasts, or WBCs, genetic tests, lactate/ pyruvate, Cu^{2+} and ceruloplasmin levels, HIV titers (including PCR), TFT, and tissue biopsy (e.g., skin biopsy for fingerprint/curvilinear bodies in NCL, muscle biopsy for mitochondrial disorders) may be required.

Management

Developmental arrest/regression is progressive and usually not amendable to therapy. Seizure frequency in TSC may be reduced (but not completely eliminated) by pharmacotherapy such as *adrenocorticotrophic hormone* (ACTH; first choice for infantile spasms), *prednisone, AEDs* such as *clonazepam, vigabatrin* (ADR: retinal toxicity), *VPA* (risk of fatal hepatotoxicity in children <2 years), *levetiracetam,* or *surgical resection of epileptogenic foci* (tumor or focal cortical dysplasia) if functional neuroimaging suggests such localization. Pooled data only confirms the efficacy of ACTH and possibly vigabatrin in the short-term treatment of infantile spasms. Supportive care, including symptomatic treatment for renal failure, cardiac dysfunction, orthopedic complications, and neuropsychiatric disturbances should be provided.

Prognosis

Life expectancy is reduced in TSC. About 10% of individuals affected die from the disease by age 40. Causes of death include progressive renal failure (most common), cardiac failure, SE and bronchopneumonia with severe MR, and brain tumors causing hydrocephalus. MR occurs in about 50–60% of patients; intractable seizures before age 1 and CNS lesions being predictive factors. Learning difficulties may occur in more than 90% of children with TSC, including those with normal intelligence.

Autism or pervasive developmental delay may occur in 20–70% of cases by age 5, with features of hyperactivity or attention deficit disorder being present in as many as 60–90% of patients. Aggressive behavior may be present in approximately 15 % of patients. Infantile spasms may progress to Lennox-Gastaut syndrome (MR, multiple seizure types and 1.5–2 Hz spike and wave discharge on EEG). There is insufficient evidence to support the, hypothesis that treatment of infantile spasms improves long-term outcomes in TSC.

Counseling

Parents should be informed about the severity of their child's disease: irreversible neurological and mental impairments, with poor prognosis. Provision should be made for parents doubting the diagnosis and its associated implications. The systemic nature of TSC should also be emphasized. Genetic counseling is paramount, as there is a 50% risk of having another child with TSC if a parent is affected. Referral to developmental specialists and special educational facilities is appropriate. Support groups and provision of additional resources to assist the family in coping with the child's disease (e.g., handicap benefits for infants, home nursing care) should be offered. Routine screening CT/MRI of the brain and viscera should be performed every 1–3 years to identify asymptomatic tumors that could benefit from early treatment.

SUMMARY

- **TSC** is a **systemic neurocutaneous disorder** characterized by **MR, seizures** (infantile spasms) and several cutaneous lesions such as **ashleaf spots, Shagreen patches, angiokeratomas**, and **subungual fibromas**.
- TSC is AD-inherited with a **40–50%** spontaneous mutation rate.
- Other causes of progressive infantile encephalopathy with early seizures include other **neurocutaneous syndromes, poliodystrophies, mitochondrial disorders, infections, metabolic, lysosomal storage**, and **endocrine disorders**.
- Diagnosis of TSC is based on **clinical** and **radiological** features. Screening CT/MRI of the brain, lungs and kidneys may show asymptomatic lesions.
- Treatment of infantile spasms includes **ACTH**, prednisone, AEDs (clonazepam, **vigabatrin**, VPA, levetiracetam) or **surgical resection**.
- **Approximately 10%** of TSC patients die by age **40**. **Renal failure** is the most common cause of death.
- Sequelae include **MR** (50–60%), **learning difficulties** (>90%), **autistic spectrum** (20–70%), **hyperactivity-attention deficit** (60–90%), **aggression** (~15%), and **Lennox-Gastaut syndrome**.
- **Intractable seizures** and multiple **CNS lesions** predict MR in TSC.
- Parents should receive **emotional support and adequate resources** and should undergo **genetic counseling**.

CASE 5

A 7-year-old boy had been socially withdrawn for several months for no apparent reason. His academic performances had been declining as well. About 1 month ago, his parents noticed a lack of coordination in his arms and legs with difficulty walking. He had recently complained of difficulty with his vision. MMSE revealed deficits in attention, orientation, calculation, short-term memory, and multi-stage commands with relative preservation of naming and praxis. Visual examination revealed 20/200 acuity on the right and 20/100 on the left, with pale discs on fundoscopy. There was truncal and appendicular ataxia in all limbs with generalized hyperreflexia. Increased skin pigmentation, especially in skin creases, was noted.

Localization

Social withdrawal and poor academic performance are nonlocalizing, but may imply diffuse cerebral dysfunction. Relative sparing of language and praxis on MMSE may indicate a subcortical dementia. Bilateral truncal and appendicular ataxia imply dysfunction in the midline and lateral cerebellar hemispheres (vestibulo- and cerebrocerebellum). Reduced visual acuity implies disease of the anterior visual pathways (lens, retina, optic nerve) bilaterally. Pale discs on fundoscopy make optic nerve disease most likely.

Hyper reflexia suggests UMN dysfunction (brain or spinal cord). Increased skin pigmentation indicates increased melanocyte production that could be secondary to activation of the pro-opiomelanocortin gene in the anterior pituitary. This could be indicative of a primary adrenal insufficiency. In summary, the underlying process diffusely affects the bilateral cerebral (possibly subcortical) and cerebellar hemispheres and optic nerves with activation of the anterior pituitary gland secondary to possible adrenal disease.

Differential Diagnosis

A progressive childhood encephalopathy characterized by early cerebellar ataxia and visual loss without seizures is most consistent with a *leukodystrophy* (LD). Possible primary adrenal insufficiency in a 7-year-old boy with LD is most suggestive of *adrenoleukodystrophy* (ALD). This is an x-linked inherited disorder secondary to a deficiency in perioxisomal acyl coenzyme A synthetase, causing an accumulation of very long-chain fatty acids (VLCFA) in tissues and plasma. Approximately 60% of affected patients have the cerebral form, approximately 25% have adrenomyeloneuropathy (central and peripheral form; more common in adults), and approximately 15% have Addison's disease (primary adrenal insufficiency) only or are asymptomatic.

Further considerations (without skin changes) include other *juvenile LD* such as *metachromatic LD* (AR deficiency in arylsulfatase A on chromosome 22: mild mental regression with slowly progressive dementia, prominent appendicular ataxia and speech disturbances with death in second decade), *globoid-cell LD* (AR deficiency in galactosyl-ceramide β-galactosidase on chromosome 14: mental regression, cortical blindness, and spasticity without peripheral neuropathy), and, *infections*, for example, *AIDS* (*see* pp. 207–211); and *SSPE* (chronic measles encephalitis with patients usually exposed to virus by age 2, presents with personality changes [social withdrawal and reduced academic performance], pigmentary retinopathy, myoclonic seizures [with EEG showing periodic sharp wave complexes]; movement disorders and dementia).

Firther diagnostic considerations include *lysosomal storage disorders,* for example, *Niemann-Pick disease type C* (AR deficiency in sphingomyelinase on chromosome 18: normal early milestones, then cerebellar ataxia, dystonia, apraxia of vertical gaze, dementia, spasticity and seizures); and *Gaucher's disease type III* (AR deficiency in glucocerebrosidase on chromosome 1: hepatosplenomegaly, mental regression, myoclonic seizures, ataxia, CN dysfunction, spasticity and positive Gaucher's cells on bone marrow biopsy); and *mitochondrial disorders*, for example, *MERRF* (maternally inherited defect in mt-DNA-Leu affecting cytochrome *c* oxidase/complex IV: cognitive decline, cerebellar ataxia/action myoclonus, seizures, myopathy, and hearing loss).

In certain cases polyodystrophies may resemble LD clinically. *Polyodystrophies* to consider include *NCL-late juvenile form* or *Spielmeyer-Vogt disease*: AR inheritance on chromosome 16; visual loss, dementia, psychosis, parkinsonism, mild seizures/ myoclonus; and *Huntington's disease* (AD trinucleotide repeat disorder on chromosome 4, usually paternally inherited in childhood cases with >50 repeats; 5% of affected children with onset before 14; cerebellar dysfunction in ~25%, seizures in ~50% and death within an average of 8 years from onset. *See* pp. 154–158).

Investigations

Basic metabolic panel may reveal low Na^+ and high K^+; serum cortisol may be reduced with inadequate response to ACTH stimulation test (indicative of primary adrenal insufficiency). Serum VLCFA is usually elevated. Enzyme levels and genetic tests may be assessed. MRI brain shows high intensity T_2-weighted signal changes in the periventricular and subcortical white matter that usually starts posteriorly (parieto-occipital) that spares subcortical U-fibers. In equivocal cases, further tests may be performed as directed by the clinical history, for example, enzyme analyses in WBC/fibroblasts, viral antibody titers, gene analyses, and tissue biopsies (e.g., muscle for ragged red fibers in mitochondrial disorders, bone marrow for Gaucher's cells in Niemann-Pick disease, skin for fingerprint or curvilinear bodies in NCL) may be required.

Management

The mainstay for treatment in ALD is corticosteroid replacement. This caters to the endocrine and metabolic consequences of ALD. However, the nervous system complications progress unrelentlessly. AEDs are administered to treat seizures. Baclofen or muscle relaxants could be used symptomatically for spasticity. Bone marrow-derived allogenic hematopoietic stem cell transplantation (HSCT) should be administered to males with early clinical involvement and MRI evidence of CNS demyelination as this improves outcomes (~85% engraftment rate at median follow-up of 11 months, with ~12% graft-vs-host-disease [GVHD]) in comparison to untreated patients. Lorenzo's oil should be administered to neurologically asymptomatic males less than 6 years of age, as this may reduce the probability of developing CNS disease in later life.

Prognosis

Mortality occurs in ALD usually between 2 and 5 years (mean 3 years) after symptom onset. The 5-year survival rate is less than 40% with 15-year survival of 0%. With HSCT, estimated 5- to 8-year survival is approximately 55%. The survival rate is approximately 90% in individuals with minimal neurological deficit and mild MRI changes prior to treatment. Prognostic indicators include age at onset (older having a better prognosis), baseline neurological or neuropsychiatric function, degree of disability (mild impairment indicative of better prognosis), and neuroradiological status (early cerebellar or corticospinal tract demyelination confers better prognosis than early parieto-occipital or frontal demyelination—more common in childhood ALD). In ALD, death is caused by disease progression, with evolution to a vegetative state prior to demise.

Counseling

Parents should be aware of prognostic data and genetic counseling should be offered to families. Sisters of affected individuals have a 50% chance of carrier status and transmitting ALD to their male offspring if heterozygous. VLCFA may be abnormal in more than 80% of female carriers and this could serve as an initial screening test. Supportive care should be provided (including information on family support groups) and adequate resources (e.g., financial, nursing, rehabilitative) should be made available to assist parents in coping with the physical and mental impairment of their child. Specialist referral to a hematologist with expertise in childhood HSCT should be considered, particularly for individuals with early, mild disease.

SUMMARY

- **Adrenoleukodystrophy** is an **x-linked** juvenile LD secondary to deficiency in **perioxisomal acyl coenzyme A synthetase**, causing accumulation of **VLCFA** in tissues and plasma.
- Differentials include other **leukodystrophies** (e.g., metachromatic and globoid-cell LD), **infections** (e.g., AIDS, SSPE), **lysosomal storage disorders** (e.g., Niemann-Pick disease type C, Gaucher's disease type

III), **mitochondrial disorders** (e.g., MERRF), and **poliodystrophies** (e.g., NCL, Huntington's disease).

- **MRI brain** usually shows **posterior-dominant demyelination** of **periventricular** and **subcortical white matter**. Serum tests for **VLCFA**, **basic metabolic panel**, and **ACTH-stimulation test** are useful.
- The mainstay of treatment is **corticosteroid** replacement therapy. In neurologically asymptomatic patients, **Lorenzo's oil** may be useful and **HSCT** should be considered in **early disease**.
- HSCT has **approximately 85%** engraftment rate at **11 months** with about **12% GVHD**.
- Mortality usually occurs within **2–5 years** (mean **3 years**) from onset. Five-year survival is **less than 40%** with 15-year survival **0%**.
- With **HSCT**, an estimated 5- to 8-year survival rate is **approximately 55%**, with **92%** survival rate in patients with minimal neurological deficits and mild MRI findings.
- Prognostic indicators include **age, baseline neurological/neuropsychiatric function, degree of disability**, and **neuroradiological status**.

CASE 6

A 9-year-old girl has had difficulty hearing for several months. Her parents think that her hearing had been reduced since she recovered from acute meningitis a year ago. Her school performance had started to decline in the recent months. On examination, there was reduced bone conduction in comparison to air conduction on performing Rinne's test and failure to perceive vibration with Weber's test performed with a 256 Hz tuning fork bilaterally. Otoscopic examination revealed no distinct abnormalities.

Localization

Loss of hearing or hearing impairment may indicate dysfunction in the external or middle ear (ossicles) for conductive loss or the inner ear, auditory nerve, cochlear nucleus (pontomedullary junction), superior olive (pons), lateral lemniscus, inferior colliculus (midbrain), medial geniculate body (thalamus), or auditory cortex (temporal lobe) for sensorineural hearing loss. The findings on Rinne's test could be normal or indicate sensorineural hearing loss bilaterally. The abnormal Weber's test confirms bilateral sensorineural hearing loss. Central causes for bilateral hearing loss would require bilateral cerebral cortex, diencephalic or brainstem dysfunction, with associated signs and symptoms. The absence of these additional features on examination suggests that the inner ear or auditory nerve is the most likely localization bilaterally.

Differential Diagnosis

The most likely diagnosis for bilateral sensorineural hearing loss following acute meningitis is *postmeningitis deafness*. Initial hearing loss may occur during the acute bacterial infection (e.g., *Streptococcus pneumoniae, Neisseria meningitides, Haemophilus influenzae,* and *M. tuberculosis*), with organisms entering the inner ear or affecting the auditory nerve via the subarachnoid space. This is the most common cause for acquired hearing loss in children. Other infectious causes include *otitis media* (causes transient conductive hearing loss and could lead to meningitis), *viral encephalitis,* and *viral exanthemas* (such as VZV, measles, or mumps).

Other differentials to consider include *drug-induced ototoxicity* (e.g., aminoglycoside antibiotics, vancomycin, furosemide, NSAIDs), *tumor* (e.g., *bilateral vestibular schwannomas; see* pp. 219–221; virtually diagnostic of NF 2: AD inheritance on chromosome 22, associated with meningiomas and paucity of peripheral neurofibromas) *cholesteatoma*: erosive keratinous lesion secondary to chronic middle ear infections, causing inner and middle ear fistula formation with subsequent hearing loss and vertigo with raised external canal pressure or Valsalva maneuver; should be visualized on otoscopic evaluation and is usually unilateral), *trauma* (e.g., fracture to petrous portion of temporal bone; vestibular function more affected), and *mitochondrial disorders* (e.g., MELAS, MERRF, Leigh's disease).

Herditary disorders to consider include *Refsum's disease* (AR inheritance on chromosome 10–phytanoyl-CoA hydroxylase deficiency: presents with pigmentary retinopathy, polyneuropathy, cerebellar ataxia, and hearing loss, ichthyosis; treated with phytanic acid and plasmapheresis), *xeroderma pigmentosa* (AR inheritance on chromosome 9: a neurocutaneous disorder of photosensitive dermatitis, psychomotor retardation, microcephaly, sensorineural hearing loss, and spinocerebellar ataxia), or *Wolfram's disease* (DIDMOAD; *see* p. 237).

In children born with failure to develop adequate hearing, *developmental deficits, congenital chromosomal deficits, genetic disorders* (including osteogenic disorders), *intrauterine (TORCH) infection* and *maternal substance abuse* should be considered. Dysmorphic features would be clinically expected in most of these disorders.

Investigations

Audiological tests should be performed to better characterize the nature and extent of the hearing deficits. Such tests include pure-tone audiometry, speech discrimination test, speech reception threshold, and brainstem auditory-evoked potentials. MRI of the brain would be useful to exclude cerebellopontine angle tumors. LP would be diagnostically useful in the acute phase of meningitis or encephalitis. If fracture is suspected, plain radiographs of the skull should be performed. In equivocal cases or if the clinical presentation is nonsuggestive, further tests (e.g., lactate/pyruvate levels, genetic tests, muscle biopsy) should be considered in order to elucidate the etiology for hearing loss.

Management

Postmeningitis hearing loss is an irreversible sequelae of acute bacterial meningitis. The mainstay of treatment include speech and language therapy (including sign language), use of communicative devices, hearing aids, and for more severe cases, cochlear implantation (~2.5% major surgical complication rate, ~15% minor complication rate with mean follow-up of 4 years. Minor complications include eardrum perforation, hematoma, flap swelling, wound infection, and temporary facial weakness. Major complications include severe flap infection requiring explantation, cholesteatoma, and persistent eardrum perforation). In experienced centers, 0% major perioperative or early postoperative complications (i.e., within 1 week of surgery) have been reported.

Prognosis

Postmeningitis hearing loss may account for approximately 50% of acquired hearing loss in children. Irreversible hearing loss may occur as long-term sequelae of acute bacterial meningitis unilaterally or bilaterally in 10% of patients. Early use of corticosteroids in the management of childhood meningitis reduces the risk of deafness (*see* pp. 58–59).

In general, language development and recovery of hearing are less likely with prelingual hearing loss in comparison to perilingual forms. Early identification with formal detection of postmeningitis hearing loss within 6 weeks from discharge from hospital following acute bacterial meningitis and early institution of therapy results in better long-term outcomes. In patients undergoing cochlear implants, subjective assessment of hearing and language performance suggests improvement with maximum benefit observed within the first 12 months.

Counseling

Patients and their families should be provided with emotional support for coping with the bad news of irreversible hearing loss. Early intervention is clinically recommended, but it should only be initiated when the affected patient and family members are fully knowledgeable and emotionally ready. Different communicative options should be provided through the aid of pediatric speech and language therapists. Encouragement should be provided throughout the treatment course. It is essential for family members to be actively involved and to learn novel means of communication with the patient. For severe cases that may require cochlear implants, the risks and benefits of surgery should be discussed in depth, facilitating informed decision making. Formal audiological tests should be considered as part of the routine predischarge evaluation of children with acute bacterial meningitis.

SUMMARY

- **Post meningitis hearing loss** is the **most common** cause of acquired childhood deafness, complicating **10%** of acute bacterial meningitis.
- Direct infection of the **inner ear** or **auditory nerve** by spread of organism through the **subarachnoid space** is the most likely cause.
- Differentials for progressive childhood hearing loss include other **infectious** etiologies, **drug-induced ototoxicity, tumors, trauma, mitochondrial disorders**, and **inherited** causes.
- Evaluation primarily consists of **formal audiological tests**.
- The mainstay of treatment includes **speech and language therapy, use of communicative devices, hearing aids**, and **cochlear implantation**.
- **Approximately 2.5%** major complication and **approximately 15%** minor complication risk occurs with cochlear implants with mean **4** years follow-up.
- Early **corticosteroid** administration during the treatment of acute childhood bacterial meningitis **reduces** risk of postmeningitis deafness.
- **Early identification** via formal detection of postmeningitis hearing loss **within 6 weeks** from discharge from hospital following acute bacterial meningitis and **early institution of therapy** result in better long-term outcomes.
- **Emotional support, involved family participation, patient and family encouragement**, and **informed choice** are important in the care and long-term prognosis of childhood hearing loss.
- Formal **audiological tests** should be considered as part of the routine **predischarge evaluation** of children with acute bacterial meningitis.

CASE 7

A 6-year-old boy developed right-sided jerky upper extremity movements about 3 weeks ago. This had progressed to affecting all the extremities as well as his face over the last week. His school performance had been declining for several months and his teachers were concerned about his poor "language." On examination, there were migratory jerky and writhing movements affecting the upper greater than lower extremities; right worse than left, with abnormal oro-facial jerky movements that the patient tried to incorporate into normal movements. Cranial nerve examination revealed mild dysarthria that affected the buccal, palatal, and lingual components.

Localization

Choreoathetosis (in contrast to myoclonus that is not incorporated into normal movements) implies basal ganglia dysfunction (caudate-putamen). The initial right-sided symptoms imply dysfunction in the left caudate-putamen, with subsequent bilateral generalization. Mild dysarthria affecting all bulbar components could imply UMN dysfunction (perisylvian area of frontal cortex, descending corticobulbar tracts at the level of the internal capsule, cerebral peduncles, or pons), LMN dysfunction (CN VII, X, XII or their nuclei in the pons or medulla, respectively) or loss of extrapyramidal modulation of corticobulbar output from the basal ganglia or cerebellum.

Reduction in school performance could be secondary to the intrusive effects of the choreoathetosis or be a nonspecific symptom of diffuse CNS dysfunction. In summary, the underlying process most likely involves the bilateral basal ganglia (caudate-putamen), their central projections, or both, with initial involvement on the left.

Differential Diagnosis

The most likely diagnosis for a progressive choreoathetoid movement disorder in a 6-year-old boy is *rheumatic (Sydenham) chorea* (RhC). This is part of the spectrum of **p**ediatric **a**utoimmune **n**europsychiatric **d**isorder **a**ssociated with **s**treptococcus infection (PANDAS). It is most likely secondary to crossreactive antibodies to the basal ganglia produced after exposure to group A β-hemolytic streptococcal infection (commonly pharyngitis) in genetically susceptible children. This usually occurs about 3–4 months after initially untreated infection.

Other diagnostic considerations include *connective tissue disorders* (e.g., SLE: clinically indistinguishable from RhC, may occur 7 years before to 3 years after systemic symptoms and lasts about 12 weeks with ~25% recurrence rate), *endocrine* (e.g., hyperthyroidism: rare manifestation that could affect face, trunk, and limbs with resolution after adequate treatment), *drug-induced* (e.g., AEDs, antidopaminergic agents such as neuroleptics, antiemetics, oral contraceptives, stimulants, theophylline), and *metabolic disorders* (e.g., high Na^+, low Ca^{2+}, low PTH, vitamin B_{12} deficiency).

Further diagnostic considerations include *pregnancy* (chorea gravidarium: occurs between the second and fifth months of gestation, but could occur postpartum; most likely secondary to aPL antibodies: need to consider in postpubertal teenage girls; spontaneous recovery occurs within weeks to months), *vascular* (usually unilateral; e.g., infarction to the basal ganglia secondary to stroke: arterial, venous, or vascular malformations), *neoplasm* (e.g., astrocytomas affecting the basal ganglia), *cardiopulmonary bypass surgery* (~1–10% of children with congenital heart disease undergoing surgery; mechanism unknown), and *infections* (e.g., bacterial meningoencephalitis, viral encephalitis: cognitive changes predominate movement disorders).

Hereditary causes of choreoatherosis in this age group may include *abetalipoproteinemia* (*see* p. 231), *ataxia-telangiectasia* (*see* pp. 230–231), *Wilson's disease* (AR inheritance on chromosome 13 affecting hepatic Cu^{2+} transporter, with liver failure [common in age <10] with or without neurological signs. Neurological signs include dysarthria, cerebellar dysfunction [including wing-beating tremor], bulbar dystonia, chorea, psychiatric disturbances and Kayser-Fleischner rings in cornea; *see* pp. 163–166), *Huntington's disease* (*see* pp. 154–158 and 244), *familial paroxysmal choreoathetosis* (also known as *paroxysmal nonkinesiogenic dyskinesia*: sporadic inheritance, episodic attacks of dystonia, choreoathetosis or dystonia with intact consciousness that last several hours or days precipitated by alcohol or caffeine. Treated at the onset of attack with clonazepam or gabapentin), and *Hallervorden-Spatz disease* (progressive rigidity, choreoathetosis, dysarthria-clenched teeth expression, pigmentary retinopathy, seizures in ~25% and death within 5–10 years. This is due to AR defect in pantothenate kinase 2 gene with iron deposition in the basal ganglia, mainly globus pallidus).

Investigations

RhC is diagnosed clinically as ASO titers are usually normal or only slightly elevated at the disease onset. Other causes of childhood chorea (particularly SLE and drug-induced) should be excluded. Laboratory tests should be tailored toward clinical suspicion. Such tests may include ESR/CRP, ANA profile, anti-ds-DNA, TFT, aPL antibodies, serum/urine toxicology, urine β-hCG (in females of childbearing age), basic metabolic profile, CBC with differential, RBC smear for acanthocytes, Cu^{2+}/ceruloplasmin, vitamin B_{12}, and E levels, lipid profile, genetic tests or enzyme assays, LP (if meningitis or encephalitis suspected), or MRI brain (to exclude stroke or neoplasms with unilateral signs: increased T_2 signal in putamen may occur in RhC during illness). Blood cultures and echocardiography should be considered to evaluate for rheumatic valvular heart disease.

Management

In children with significant choreoathetosis, pimozide (first choice for its non-sedating effects), benzodiazepines, or neuroleptics (including haloperidol) should be administered for symptomatic relief. There is no benefit of corticosteroids in RhC, but IVIg/TPE may be useful in medically severe cases refractory to symptomatic therapy. High-dose penicillin should be given for 10 days with prophylactic oral therapy until the age of 21. In penicillin-allergic patients, erythromycin or cephalosporin (use with caution, as there is 10–20% cross-reactivity with penicillin) should be given.

Prognosis

Most patients with RhC recover completely without residual sequelae. Gradual improvement occurs over several months. In untreated patients, about

33% develop rheumatic heart disease (85% involve mitral valve with risk of cardiac failure or arrhythmias, 45% involve aortic valve and can be asymptomatic; both can cause stroke via septic thrombophlebitis). Recurrences may occur in approximately 25–40% of patients 3 months to 10 years after initial episode and depend on compliance with prophylactic antibiotics. Supportive care (e.g., for feeding, toileting, and ambulation) may be required in the early stages of this disorder, to facilitate resumption of school activities and ADLs.

Counseling

Patients and their families should understand that RhC is one of the major diagnostic features of rheumatic fever (and include carditis, polyarthritis, erythema marginatum, and subcutaneous nodules) and requires acute and chronic antibiotic therapy to prevent recurrence and valvular heart disease. Prognostic information for recovery should be highlighted and used as a tool for encouragement and compliance with chronic antibiotic therapy. Parental and patient reassurance are important facets in the provision of care of a patient with this disorder.

SUMMARY

- RhC is a **post-streptococcal autoimmune disorder** of the CNS that is part of the spectrum of **PANDAS**.
- Other causes of childhood choreoathetosis include **connective tissue disorders, endocrine, drug-induced, metabolic, pregnancy, vascular, neoplasm, cardiopulmonary bypass surgery, infections,** and **inherited disorders**.
- Diagnosis is established **clinically**. Other potential diagnoses (**SLE** and **drug-induced**) should be excluded with laboratory investigations.
- Treatment includes **symptomatic** (e.g., pimozide, benzodiazepines, neuroleptics), **therapeutic** (IVIg/TPE and/or high-dose **penicillin**), and **prophylactic** (penicillin until age **21**).
- Recovery is gradual over **several months** and occurs in **most** patients.
- **Approximately 33%** of patients develop rheumatic heart disease if untreated.
- **Approximately 25–40%** of patients relapse **3 months to 10 years** after initial episode. **Non-compliance** with prophylaxis increases the risk of relapse.
- **Reassurance** and **emotional support** are important facets in the care of patients with RhC.

CASE 8

A 6-month-old male infant was brought to the clinic by his parents. They were concerned that he felt "floppy" and did not seem to move around like his older brother did at that age. On examination, he was interactive with the examiner and responded appropriately to social cues with symmetrical facial expressions. His coughing and sucking abilities were normal. Further examination revealed generalized hypotonia. He was unable to hold his head up or sit independently. There were reduced active movements predominantly affecting the proximal limb muscles. Facial grimacing was symmetrical to noxious stimuli and reflexes were absent.

Localization

Generalized hypotonia with weakness and areflexia imply a disorder affecting the LMN (AHC, nerve roots, plexi, peripheral nerve, NMJ, or muscle) in the cervical and lumbosacral myotomes. Normal cough (CN IX, X) and suck (CN VII, X, XII) exclude significant craniobulbar dysfunction. Normal sensory responses to noxious stimuli makes cervical and lumbosacral nerve roots, brachial or lumbosacral plexi or peripheral neuropathy less likely.

Preferential generalized proximal muscle weakness is usually indicative of a myopathy or NMJ disorder, although AHC disease may present similarly. The reduced ability to hold the head up or to sit independently suggests a gross motor developmental delay secondary to cerebral dysfunction or could indicate proximal muscle disease involving axial muscles. Normal alertness and interaction observed during the examination makes the former less likely. In summary, the underlying process is a diffuse disorder affecting the AHC, NMJ, or muscles of the cervical and lumbosacral myotomes with associated axial muscle involvement.

Differential Diagnosis

The most likely diagnosis for a progressive, diffuse disorder of the motor unit in a 6-month-old child with relatively spared cerebral and craniobulbar function is *spinal muscular atrophy* (SMA). This is an AR-inherited AHC disorder involving the SMN gene on chromosome 5. Three types of childhood SMA have been described based on age of onset. SMA I (Werdnig-Hoffman disease) is a more fulminant form with onset from birth to age 6 months, SMA II has an onset from 3 to 12 months, with a less fulminant course, whereas SMA III (Kugelberg-Welander disease) develops after 18 months.

Other differential diagnoses include *NMJ transmission disorders* such as *familial infantile MG* (predominantly AR inheritance, with slow channel disease being AD) in which defects in presynaptic ACh synthesis, packaging or release or postsynaptic deficiency in AChR, defects in kinetics of AChR or endplate AChE deficiency, with negative antibodies to AChR: may present with respiratory insufficiency, ptosis, generalized weakness with relatively spared extraocular movements; and *infantile botulism* (*see* pp. 43–45).

Muscular dystrophies (MD) should be considered in this age group. These usually involve defects in the structural framework of myofibers, such as *congenital dystrophinopathies* (x-linked inheritance), *merosin-deficient MD, Bethlem myopathy* (a slowly progressive limb girdle MD associated with collagen type VI gene on chromosome 21). Other myopathic conditions in this age group include *congenital myopathies* (developmental skeletal muscle disorders) such as *nemaline-rod myopathy* (AD inheritance of tropomyosin-3 gene on chromosome 1 or nebulin gene on chromosome 2: presents with severe neonatal respiratory insufficiency and death or mild hypotonia, motor developmental delay with facial muscle weakness), and *central core disease* (AD inheritance on chromosome 19, allelic for malignant hyperthermia with increased risk for rhabdomyolysis with inhalational anesthetics).

Further considerations include *metabolic myopathies* such as *acid-maltase deficiency* (*Pompe's disease*; AR inheritance on chromosome 17, with more fulminant disease occurring at younger ages), *myophosphorylase deficiency* (*McArdle's disease*: AR inheritance on chromosome 11, may present with slowly progressive myopathy in childhood or rarely as a neonate), *mitochondrial myopathies* (enzyme defects in respiratory chain, such as cytochrome *c* oxidase deficiency, Leigh's disease, and MERRF.) and *congenital polyneuropathies* such as *congenital hypomyelinating neuropathy* (usually sporadic with diffuse weakness, distal atrophy and areflexia with relatively spared sensation), *HMSN types I to III* (especially type III: *Dejerine-Sottas syndrome*), or *leukodystrophies* (e.g., *Krabbe's disease*: look for combined CNS and PNS involvement).

In children with hypotonia from birth with global developmental delay, *cerebral causes* such as static encephalopathies secondary to *congenital malformations, in utero disease,* and *perinatal injury,* or progressive disorders such as *cerebrohepatorenal (Zellweger's) syndrome, oculocerebrorenal (Lowe) syndrome,* and *infantile GM_2 gangliosidosis,* should be considered. In older children with progressive proximal muscle weakness, *inflammatory myopathies* such as *dermatomyositis* or *polymyositis,* or *endocrine myopathies* (thyroid, adrenal, PTH disease) should be included as potential etiologies.

Investigations

If myopathy is suspected, serum CK should be checked. CK levels can be markedly elevated in inflammatory myopathies and MD, moderately elevated in congenital myopathies and mildly elevated (two- to fourfold above the upper limit of normal) in SMA. Edrophonium (Tensilon®) test should be administered if MG is suspected. In older children, serum electrolytes, TFTs, Ca^{2+}, PO_4^{3-}, cortisol levels, may be used in evaluating for endocrine myopathies. EMG/NCS would be useful in ascertaining if the underlying etiology is neuropathic (as in SMA) or myopathic.

A muscle biopsy would be useful in establishing the diagnosis for congenital myopathies, MD, metabolic and mitochondrial myopathies. A nerve biopsy would be useful if congenital hypomyelinating neuropathy or HMSN is suspected. For SMA, the diagnosis can be readily confirmed via commercially available genetic tests, obviating the need for muscle biopsy. In equivocal cases, enzyme levels in WBC, fibroblasts, or muscle can be performed as part of the diagnostic evaluation.

Management

The mainstay of therapy for SMA is supportive. Physical and occupational therapy should be encouraged as these could improve functional capabilities, aid in milestone development early in the disease and reduce muscle contractures, disuse atrophy and increase time to non-ambulation (wheel-chair bound). Dietary counseling may be required in older children to prevent obesity. Orthotic devices, such as splints, may be required to maintain the joints in neutral or functional positions, as well as prevent contractures. Respiratory (invasive or noninvasive) and nutritional support would be required for patients that develop progressive bulbar dysfunction or restrictive lung disease.

Prognosis

The prognosis of SMA is dependent on the age of onset. The most common cause of death is respiratory failure secondary to aspiration pneumonia, with restrictive respiratory failure being less common. In infants with SMA I, death usually occurs between ages 6 and 12 months. Survival beyond 2 years is rare in patients with onset before 2 months of age or without respiratory support. Early tracheostomy may increase mean survival to 72 months, whereas noninvasive ventilatory support and cough-assist devices may increase mean survival to about 40 months.

SMA II patients usually develop ability to sit independently, but fail to walk. Death may occur in childhood, although survival into adulthood commonly occurs. Five-year survival in SMA II is about 98.5%, with 25-year survival of 62.5%. SMA III patients have different prognoses depending on the age of onset. In patients with onset before age 3, 70% are ambulatory 10 years after onset, whereas only 20% are ambulatory 40 years after onset. In patients with onset after age 3, 97% are ambulatory 10 years after onset with 60% remaining so 40 years after onset. A normal life expectancy is expected in SMA III.

Counseling

Prognostic data should be provided to families. There is clinical heterogeneity in SMA, so prognostic data should be used as a guide and not as an absolute predictive tool. Affected children should be offered rehabilitation and respiratory support if needed as these modalities reduce morbidity and improve survival. Parents should be given the necessary support and appropriate referrals to medical and non-medical specialists, including support groups. Genetic counseling should be provided to all affected families. Because of the common AR pattern of inheritance, parents should be aware of the 25% risk of having another child with SMA. Chorionic villous sampling can be performed for intrauterine diagnosis, if required, with associated risks.

SUMMARY

- **SMA** is an AR-inherited disorder affecting AHC associated with defects in the **SMN gene** on **chromosome 5**.
- Three childhood forms are described based on age of onset: **SMA I, SMA II**, and **SMA III**.
- Differentials include **NMJ transmission disorders, muscular dystrophies, congenital myopathies, metabolic myopathies, mitochondrial myopathies**, and **congenital polyneuropathies**.
- **Cerebral** disease should be considered with **neonatal** presentation.
- **Inflammatory/endocrine myopathies** are possible in older children
- Diagnosis of SMA can be confirmed with **genetic testing**. CK may be normal or mildly elevated (two- to fourfold) and EMG/NCS shows a **neuropathic** pattern.
- Management is **supportive. Rehabilitation** is useful early to improve functional capabilities, aid in motor milestone development and prevent contractures. **Respiratory and nutritional support** would be required in more severely affected patients.
- Prognosis depends on **age of onset** of disease.
- In **SMA I**, death usually occurs between **6 and 12 months** with survival longer more than 2 years unlikely with onset **less than 2 months** of age and **no respiratory support**.
- Mean survival is **approximately 72 months** with invasive and **approximately 40 months** with noninvasive respiratory support in SMA I.
- In SMA II, **98.5%** are alive at **5 years**, with **62.5%** alive at **25 years**.
- In SMA III, life expectancy is **normal**. With onset **before 3 years, 70%** are ambulatory at **10 years** and **approximately 20%** at **40 years** from onset. With onset **after 3 years, 97%** are ambulatory at **10 years** and **60%** at **40 years**.
- **Genetic counseling** should be provided to all affected families.

CASE 9

A pediatrician saw an 18-month-old infant girl for the first time for routine evaluation and immunizations. Her head circumference was greater than the

98th percentile for her age and sex. Her weight was on the 75th percentile and her height, the 50th percentile. A neurological opinion was sought. Her parents stated that she had achieved normal developmental milestones and seemed healthy. Physical examination did not reveal any significant findings apart from the enlarged head circumference.

Localization

An enlarged head circumference (macrocephaly) implies one of the following: enlargement of the cerebral hemispheres (megalencephaly), excessive CSF in the ventricles (hydrocephalus) or increased skull thickening. The normal physical examination reduces the likelihood for cerebral or ventricular disease, but these are by no means excluded. Disorders of increased skull thickness usually result in craniofacial dysmorphisms (abnormal facies). The assumed absence of dysmorphisms on examination makes such a disorder unlikely in this child. In summary, the underlying process most likely affects the cerebral hemispheres or ventricles diffusely.

Differential Diagnosis

The lack of significant physical findings on examination, coupled with a normal weight and height for age and sex make a diagnosis of *benign familial megalencephaly* (BFM) very likely. This is a probably a multi-genetically inherited condition in which the head circumference is 2–4 cm greater than 2 standard deviations (s.d.) above normal for age and sex. This is associated with normal mental and neurological functioning and lack of dysmorphic features. Macrocephaly in either one or both parents further supports the diagnosis. However, this is a diagnosis of exclusion, so other potential differentials need to be considered. These can be divided into causes of megalencephaly and hydrocephalus.

Megalencephaly can be divided into *anatomical* or *metabolic* etiologies. Anatomical etiologies include *Soto's syndrome* (AR/AD inherited megalencephaly with gigantism: infants exhibit excessive growth in head circumference, height and weight until age 3, associated with mild craniofacial dysmorphisms), *neurocutaneous syndromes* (e.g., tuberous sclerosis, neurofibromatosis, incontinentia pigmenti; *see* pp. 239–242), and *achondroplasia* (AD inherited on chromosome 4, associated with high rate of spontaneous mutations and most common cause of short-limbed dwarfism).

Metabolic etiologies include *leukodystrophies* (e.g., *Alexander's disease*: AR chromosome 11 deficiency in nicotinamide adenine dinucleotide-ubiquinone oxidoreductase flavoprotein-1; *Canavan's disease*: AR chromosome 13 deficiency in aspartoacyclase; *metachromatic LD*: AR chromosome 22 deficiency in arylsulfatase A), *lysosomal storage disorders* (e.g., gangliosidoses, MPS) and *aminoacidopathies* (e.g., *glutaric academia type I*: AR deficiency in glutaryl-coenzyme

A dehydrogenase: megalencephaly, acute encephalopathy, seizures and progressive dystonia and choreoathetosis; *maple syrup urine disease* [MSUD]: AR chromosome 19 deficiency in branched chain ketoacid dehydrogenase: protein ingestion-induced encephalopathy, fluctuating ophthalmoplegia, seizures, cerebral edema, and neonatal death if untreated. Leucine, isoleucine and valine are elevated in serum with positive 2,4-dinitrophenylhydrazine urine test).

Hydrocephalus can be divided into *communicating (nonobstructive)* or *noncommunicating (obstructive)* forms. Communicating hydrocephalus can be secondary increased CSF production or reduced absorption. Causes include *meningitis, meningeal carcinomatosis, choroid plexus papilloma, post-SAH,* and *benign enlargement of the subarachnoid space* (BESAS: more common in male infants and most likely paternally inherited with normal physical examination and enlarged subarachnoid space on CT scan).

Noncommunicating hydrocephalus is secondary to obstruction to the ventricular flow of CSF. For example, *aqueductal stenosis* (acquired secondary to infections, tumor, hematoma, etc. or inherited as an x-linked trait), *Arnold-Chiari malformation* (type II or III: causes hydrocephalus via aqueductal stenosis or fourth ventricular obstruction secondary to cerebellar herniation), *Dandy-Walker malformation* (embryonic failure of formation of Foramen of Magendie with associated agenesis of the cerebellar tonsils, cystic dilatation of posterior fossa in communication with the fourth ventricle and hydrocephalus), or *mass lesions* (e.g., neoplasms, hematoma: SDH, epidural hematoma [EDH], intraparenchymal; cerebral abscess, vascular malformations: vein of Galen malformation, a midline AVM that rarely ruptures but causes high-output cardiac failure in infants).

Investigations

Review of previous growth charts would be important (if available), as sudden changes in growth percentiles are more concerning for pathology. Head circumference measurement should be repeated to ensure accuracy. CT scan of the head would be important to exclude ICH and mass lesions, as well as to demonstrate increased skull thickness or increased ventricular size. CT scan is normal in BFM. MRI better delineates intraparenchymal lesions, cerebral malformations, posterior fossa anomalies, and leukodystrophies. Guided by clinical suspicion, genetic/chromosomal analysis, enzyme assays in WBC/fibroblasts/urine, serum and urine organic acids and LP (in communicating hydrocephalus), may be performed to establish the diagnosis.

Management

Treatment is not required for BFM or BESAS, as these are considered normal anatomic variants. Anatomic megalencephalies are not usually amenable to direct therapy, however, symptomatic therapy may be required, for example,

AEDs for seizures, and hormonal treatment for Soto's syndrome. Certain metabolic megalencephalies may benefit from dietary restriction (e.g., MSUD) or hemodialysis, with symptomatic treatment provided for seizures or movement disorders.

Noncommunicating hydrocephalus can be treated with ventricular shunting and removal of the obstructive mass lesion if possible. Cerebral herniation is a neurological emergency, requiring aggressive treatment (*see* pp. 50 and 53). Communicating hydrocephalus would be less amenable to ventricular shunting, so the underlying cause should be identified and treated appropriately.

Prognosis

BFM and BESAS have normal prognoses. In general, the prognosis of macrocephaly would depend on the underlying disorder, with noncommunicating hydrocephalus and metabolic megalencephaly having poorer prognoses if untreated. Communicating hydrocephalus may also have a poor prognosis dependent on the underlying cause (e.g., malignancy or infection) or raised ICP.

Counseling

Parents should be reassured that their child is normal if BFM or BESAS is diagnosed. These are diagnoses of exclusion, so adequate evaluation (including neuroimaging) should be performed, especially if there are parental concerns with the mental, developmental, or neurological status of the child. For other causes of macrocephaly, counseling would be tailored toward underlying diagnosis.

Genetic counseling should be offered if an inherited disorder is identified. For patients with noncommunicating hydrocephalus, the risks, benefits, and complications of ventricular shunting should be discussed in depth and neurosurgical consultation sought. For pathological causes of macrocephaly, parental support and participation in specialized support groups (e.g., for neurocutaneous disorders) should be offered and encouraged.

SUMMARY

- **Macrocephaly** could be secondary to **megalencephaly** (increased brain size), **hydrocephalus** (increased ventricular CSF), or **thickened skull**.
- **Megalencephaly** can be divided into **anatomic** and **metabolic** causes. If there are no associated signs or symptoms, **BFM** should be considered (especially with parental macrocephaly).
- Hydrocephalus can be divided into **communicating** and **noncommunicating** forms. If there are no associated signs or symptoms, **BESAS** should be considered.
- Investigations should include **CT/MRI scan of the brain**. Depending on clinical suspicion, genetic/chromosomal analyses, enzyme assays,

serum/urine organic acids, and LP may be required to establish the diagnosis. **Previous growth charts** and **parental head circumference** should be obtained.

- Management depends on the underlying cause. BFM and BESAS are normal anatomic variants and do not require therapy. **Symptomatic therapy** and **ventricular shunting** may be required for other causes of macrocephaly. Cerebral herniation is a **neurological emergency** that requires prompt treatment.
- Prognosis is dependent on the **underlying cause**. BFM and BESAS have normal prognoses without any mental or neurological sequelae. **Noncommunicating hydrocephalus** and **metabolic megalencephaly** have poorer prognoses in general.
- Counseling should be tailored toward potential diagnoses and their etiologies. **Supportive care** is important for pathological macrocephaly.

CASE 10

A 16-month-old boy has had an URI for 2 days. About 1 hour ago, he developed generalized convulsions affecting his head and limbs, associated with unresponsiveness. This episode lasted about 30–60 seconds and was followed by sleep. On arrival to the ER 30 minutes ago, temperature was 39.4°C, HR 120 per minute, BP 100/55 mmHg, and RR 28 per minute. Neurological examination revealed an alert, interactive infant, who was socially appropriate with his parents, but reluctant to have medical evaluation. Cranial nerve, motor, sensory, and reflex examinations were within normal limits.

Localization

Generalized convulsions imply global hyperexcitability of the cerebral cortex, involving at least, the frontal lobes bilaterally. The normal neurological examination afterwards implies that no residual global or focal neurological deficits persisted. In summary, the underlying process is of transient duration and localizes diffusely to the cerebral hemispheres bilaterally.

Differential Diagnosis

The most likely diagnosis for a generalized convulsive seizure of brief duration in a 16-month-old child associated with a febrile illness is *simple febrile seizure* (FS). FS occur in approximately 5% of all children with incidence highest between 6 months and 5 years of age. Complex FS is defined as prolonged (>5–10 minutes), multiple, or focal seizures associated with a febrile illness. Of patients with FS, 20–45% have a positive family history. FS may be inherited as an AD condition with incomplete penetrance.

Other differentials include *nonfebrile seizures* (may be associated with post-ictal fever of <38°C: associated conditions include congenital malformations, neonatal seizure disorders, in-born errors of metabolism, drug intoxication/withdrawal, poliodystrophies, and positive family history of epilepsy), and *meningitis/encephalitis* (~20–25% of children with bacterial/viral meningitis experience GTC seizure: would expect prolonged post-ictal unresponsiveness, nuchal rigidity, or complex FS pattern).

Further considerations include *syncope* (with reflex anoxic convulsions, e.g., *cyanotic syncope*: cessation of breathing in expiration associated with crying, causing tonic posturing of body and brief limb convulsions with complete resolution; or *pallid syncope*: loss of consciousness following sudden, unexpected noxious stimuli with initial hypotonia, followed by limb hypertonia and clonic movements) and *rigors* (repetitive episodes of generalized stiffness, trembling of the limbs and chattering of teeth associated with high fevers without unresponsiveness).

Investigations

In a child less than 2 years of age (in whom signs of CNS infection may be subtle), LP should be performed to exclude meningoencephalitis (especially HSE). Further indications include complex FS, prolonged post-ictal unresponsiveness or neurological deficit, pretreatment with oral antibiotics or history of irritability, reduced feeding, or lethargy before seizure onset.

CBC with differential, comprehensive metabolic panel, urinalysis, blood/urine cultures, and serum/urine toxicology, may be considered on an individualized basis, guided by the clinical history. EEG should be performed if the child is not neurologically normal after the seizure or there is a positive family history of epilepsy. MRI of the brain (with and without gadolinium) with thin cuts through the temporal lobes should be performed in infants with prolonged focal (complex). This may show mesial temporal sclerosis or hippocampal atrophy.

Management

No treatment is required for simple FS. The underlying cause for the febrile illness should be identified and treated appropriately (e.g., antipyretics, antimicrobials, fluid, and nutritional support). For prolonged or multiple (complex) FS, rectal diazepam can be administered to induce seizure termination. Seizures refractory to diazepam should be treated as febrile SE (*see* pp. 34–35 for treatment of SE).

Prophylactic AED therapy is not indicated in simple or complex FS, as there is no objective evidence that these measures significantly reduce the risk for recurrent FS or development of epilepsy. However, children with a history of FS can be given rectal diazepam as soon as, or before a seizure occurs if there is a low threshold for FS following a febrile illness.

Prognosis

FS does not confer an increased risk of mortality (including febrile SE: occurs in ~25% of FS cases) or morbidity. FS has no association with sudden infant death syndrome. There is no concrete evidence supporting the later development of neurological deficits, cognitive decline or memory impairment in FS patients. The risk of recurrent FS is approximately 33%, with 50% occurring within the first year and 90% within 2 years after initial FS. Risk factors for recurrence include age less than 18 months at first FS, positive family history of FS in first-degree relative, initial FS at temperature less than 40°C and multiple FS with single initial febrile illness.

The risk of developing epilepsy (nonfebrile seizures) is increased fourfold in FS patients compared with the general population, however, only about 2–4% of FS patients develop nonfebrile seizures by age 7. Risk factors for developing epilepsy in FS patients include positive family history of epilepsy, complex FS, and early onset of neurodevelopmental abnormalities.

Counseling

Parents should be aware of the prognostic data and reassured that the risk of brain damage and epilepsy are very low with FS. Parents should be taught how to administer rectal diazepam and advised to call emergency services for febrile SE. Because the incidence of meningitis is about 2–5% in children with FS, parents should have a low threshold to seek emergent neurological evaluation if their child has a prolonged post-ictal phase following an FS.

SUMMARY

- **Simple FS** are **GTC seizures** of **brief** duration associated with febrile illness. **Complex FS** could be **prolonged, multiple,** or **focal.**
- Incidence is highest between **6 months** and **5 years** of age and affects **approximately 5%** of all children.
- Differential diagnoses include **nonfebrile seizures, meningitis/ encephalitis, syncope,** and **rigors.**
- **LP** should be considered in FS if **age is less than 2 years, complex FS, prolonged post-ictal unresponsiveness** or **neurological deficit, pretreatment with oral antibiotics** or history of **irritability, poor feeding,** or **lethargy.**
- **EEG** should be considered in patients with **residual neurological deficits** after seizure or **positive family history of epilepsy.**
- Treatment is **not required** for FS. Underlying febrile illness should be treated.

- **Rectal diazepam** can be given for prolonged FS. Seizures refractory to diazepam should be treated as **febrile SE**.
- Prophylactic AED therapy is **not indicated** in simple or complex FS.
- Risk of mortality or morbidity is **not increased** with FS.
- The risk of recurrent FS is **about 33%**, with **50%** occurring within the **first year** and **90%** within **2 years** after initial FS.
- Risk factors for recurrent FS: **age less than 18 months at first FS**, **positive family history of FS in first-degree relative**, initial FS at temperature **less than 40°C**, and **multiple FS** with single initial febrile illness.
- Only **about 2–4%** of FS patients develop nonfebrile seizures by **age 7**.
- Risk factors for developing epilepsy following FS: **positive family history of epilepsy, complex FS**, and **early onset of neurodevelopmental abnormalities**.
- Parents should be reassured that risk for developing **brain damage** or **epilepsy** is **very low** with FS. Education on the administration of rectal diazepam is required for all parents.

CASE 11

A 7-year-old girl was brought to the clinic by her parents. They were concerned that she was not paying attention in school or at home. They described 10- to 15-second periods of staring during activities with return to that activity as if nothing had happened. These seemed to occur at least 20 times a day. Neurological examination was normal. Hyperventilation induced in the office resulted in a 10-second period of a vacant stare with bilateral rhythmic eyelid flickering without confusion afterward.

Localization

Poor attention, staring, and loss of awareness of the surroundings may imply dysfunction in the frontotemporal and parietal lobes bilaterally. This global cerebral dysfunction could be the result of reduced input from the reticular-activating system in the brainstem or thalamus. Bilateral rhythmic eyelid flickering could imply hyper-excitability of the frontal cortex providing input to the levator palpebrae superioris muscles (CN III nuclei in midbrain). In summary, the underlying process localizes diffusely to the cerebral cortex bilaterally with possible frontal hyper-excitability.

Differential Diagnosis

The most likely diagnosis for a 7-year-old child with paroxysmal staring spells induced by hyperventilation is *childhood absence seizures*. This is a generalized epilepsy syndrome that is transmitted as an AD trait with onset between 6 and 8 years of age. *Juvenile absence seizures* have an onset between ages 10 and 16. Alterations in thalamic T-type Ca^{2+} channels are thought to contribute to the pathogenesis of absence seizures. Other epilepsy syndromes in which absence seizures occur include *juvenile myoclonic epilepsy* (JME) and *epilepsy with grand mal on awakening*.

Other differentials include *complex partial seizures* (usually last >1 minute, may have an aura, automatisms and followed by post-ictal confusion, aphasia, or lethargy), *pseudoseizures* (associated with significant neuropsychological disturbances, but rare in pre-adolescent children), and *daydreaming* (transient phase of slow-wave sleep. A form of escapism that may be difficult to break and associated with unresponsiveness to verbal but usually not tactile stimuli).

Investigations

EEG is pathognomonic for the diagnosis of absence seizures. Inter-ictal EEG is normal with ictal EEG showing 3 Hz spike and wave discharges, activated by hyperventilation (in ~90%) with maximal amplitude in the frontocentral regions. EEG can be used to differentiate absence seizures from complex partial seizures, pseudo-seizures and daydreaming. No further diagnostic work-up is required if absence seizure is diagnosed. If the inter-ictal EEG is abnormal (diffuse slowing, focal or multifocal spike discharges), cerebral dysfunction should be suspected and evaluated for (e.g., developmental, metabolic, infectious, degenerative disease).

Management

There are insufficient clinical studies guiding initial choice of AED for absence seizures. Initial choice is based on perception of tolerability, potential cognitive side effects, potential systemic toxicity, and need for rapid control. The most common AED of choice for treating childhood absence seizures is *ethosuximide* (ADRs: nausea, gastric irritation, abdominal pain) owing to lower incidence of side effects. Other options include *VPA* (ADRs: nausea, hyperammonemia, hepatoxicity, thrombocytopenia, pancreatitis) and *lamotrigine* (ADRs: rash, ataxia, dizziness, headache: requires slow titration to therapeutic doses).

Each of these agents is equally effective as monotherapy, with complete seizure relief in about 70–80% of children. These drugs can be used in combination for patients refractory to monotherapy. *Clonazepam* can also be used for refractory absence seizures. Carbamazepine should be avoided as it can worsen seizures and precipitate absence SE. A clinical approach is to use ethosuximide for absence seizures and substitute with VPA if tonic-clonic seizures recur after initial AED treatment. EEG can be used to document treatment success and seizure-free state.

Prognosis

Patients with childhood absence seizures are neurologically normal, without long-term neurological sequelae or increased risk of mortality. Patients with absence seizures may have poorer psychosocial outcomes compared to age-matched children. About 60% become seizure-free (>2 years) without need for prophylactic AED therapy lifelong. About 50% of children with absence seizures have at least one GTC seizure. This does not change the prognosis in untreated patients, however, in treated patients, this (as well as myoclonic seizures) predicts lack of remission and progression to JME, requiring lifelong AED therapy.

Counseling

Patients and their parents should be aware of the prognostic data and relatively benign nature of this disorder. School performance can be improved by the use of AEDs, as seizure frequency reduction or cessation can be achieved. The risks and benefits of different AEDs should be discussed. Withdrawal of AEDs should be considered if the patient is seizure-free for 2–3 years without other seizure types being present.

SUMMARY

- **Childhood absence seizures** are a **generalized epilepsy syndrome** with onset between **ages 6 and 8**, inherited as an **AD trait**.
- Absence seizures may also occur in other epilepsy syndromes: **juvenile absence seizures, juvenile myoclonic seizures,** and **epilepsy with grand mal on awakening**.
- Differentials include **complex partial seizures, pseudoseizures,** and **daydreaming**.
- **EEG** is pathognomonic for absence seizures: **ictal 3 Hz spike and wave discharges** with **normal inter-ictal EEG**.
- Treatment includes **ethosuximide, VPA,** or **lamotrigine**. These AEDs have about a **70–80%** success rate as **monotherapy**. In refractory cases, **combination therapy** or **clonazepam** can be used.
- **Ethosuximide** is a common drug of choice for initial therapy owing to **low incidence** of major side effects.
- **Carbamazepine** should be **avoided** in absence seizures.
- EEG is used to document **treatment success** and **seizure-free state**.
- **Approximately 60%** of patients become seizure-free lifelong, without need for AEDs.
- **GTC seizures** occur in **about 50%** of patients with absence. If present during treatment, this predicts **lack of remission** and **development of JME**.

• Parents should be aware of the **benign** nature of childhood absence seizures and its response to AED therapy. Potential **psychosocial complications** may occur in their children.

CASE 12

A 13-year-old boy was brought to the urgent care clinic by his parents several hours after having a witnessed GTC seizure. He stated that he has had uncontrollable short-duration, repetitive flexion jerks in his upper extremities in the mornings that last for 2–3 minutes while brushing his teeth. These have been ongoing for several months. The GTC seizure had occurred on awakening from the previous night's sleep. Neurological examination was normal.

Localization

A GTC seizure implies diffuse hyper-excitability of the cerebral cortex bilaterally. The repetitive upper extremity myoclonic jerks may localize to the bilateral frontal (motor) cortices without generalized spread (as consciousness is retained). In summary, the underlying process diffusely involves the cerebral cortex bilaterally with possible independent bifrontal involvement.

Differential Diagnosis

The most likely diagnosis for myoclonic epilepsy associated with GTC seizures on awakening in a 13-year-old boy with a normal neurological examination is *juvenile myoclonic epilepsy* (JME). This is an AD-inherited epilepsy syndrome, localized on chromosome 6. Males and females are equally affected with onset of myoclonic seizures between 12 and 18 years. Most patients develop GTC seizures, with approximately 33% also experiencing absence seizures.

Other differentials include causes for progressive myoclonic epilepsy: *neurodegenerative, mitochondrial*, or *lysosomal storage disorders*. Neurodegenerative causes include *juvenile NCL* (*Spielmeyer-Vogt disease*: AR chromosome 16: visual failure, ataxia, dementia and seizures; most common childhood neurodegenerative disorder, *see* pp. 239–240,244), *Unverricht-Lundborg disease* (Baltic myoclonus: AR chromosome 21: myoclonic seizures, ataxia, dementia; common in Finland), *Lafora's disease* (AR chromosome 6: dementia, ataxia, myoclonic seizures, death by age 20; common in southern Europe with characteristic intracytoplasmic basophilic bodies in brain or eccrine sweat glands), *juvenile neuroaxonal atrophy* (AR trait: myoclonus or choreoathetosis, dementia, ataxia and neuropathy) and *DRPLA* (rare trinucleotide repeat disorder on chromosome 12: chorea, ataxia, dementia, myoclonus; most common in Japan).

Mitochondrial causes include *MERRF* (maternal inheritance of mutation to t-RNA-lysine: myoclonus/myoclonic epilepsy, myopathy with ragged red fibers, neuropathy, deafness, optic atrophy, ataxia) and MELAS (*see* p. 269).

Lysosomal storage disorders include *sialidosis* (*type I*: AR chromosome 20 deficiency in neuraminidase: severe myoclonus, visual failure, ataxia without dementia, or *type II*: AR chromosome 10 deficiency in neuraminidase and β-galactosidase: type I features, corneal clouding and coarse facies), *Gaucher's disease type III* (AR chromosome 1 deficiency in glucocerebrosidase β-glucosidase: myoclonus, supranuclear gaze palsy, pancytopenia, splenomegaly without dementia) and *juvenile GM$_2$ gangliosidoses* (AR chromosome 15 deficiency in hexosaminidase: myoclonus, dementia without cherry-red macula spot).

Investigations

Interictal EEG shows 3.5–6 Hz bilateral symmetrical spike and polyspike and wave discharges, maximal in the frontocentral regions. A normal neurological examination does not warrant further evaluation. However, neurological deficits on examination or background slowing on EEG require evaluation for causes of progressive myoclonic epilepsy. This should be tailored towards the clinical suspicion, for example, enzyme assays in WBCs or fibroblasts for lysosomal storage disorders, genetic tests for inherited disorders, EMG/NCS for juvenile neuroaxonal atrophy and MERRF, skin biopsy for curvilinear/fingerprint bodies in NCL, eccrine sweat gland biopsy for Lafora's disease, muscle biopsy for MERRF, nerve biopsy for juvenile neuroaxonal atrophy (axonal spheroids at nerve endings), or bone marrow biopsy for Gaucher's disease.

Management

VPA is the drug of choice for treating JME, with complete seizure relief in about 75% of patients. Other options include lamotrigine monotherapy (*see* pp. 168–169 for ADRs of both AEDs). In females, there is a putative concern for polycystic ovarian syndrome (PCOS: infertility, weight gain, hirsutism, oligomenorrhea, or amenorrhea) associated with chronic VPA therapy. Topiramate (ADRs: fatigue, altered cognitive state, renal stones) can be used as adjunctive therapy in refractory cases. Other potential adjunctive agents include levetiracetam (no appreciable hepatic metabolism, ADRs: somnolence, fatigue, dizziness), and zonisamide (ADRs: drowsiness, anorexia, altered cognition, hypohidrosis). Treatment is required lifelong despite seizure-free status.

Prognosis

If treated, JME does not carry an increased risk of mortality or neurological morbidity. With adequate AED therapy, about 40% of patients are seizure-free within 1 year, with approximately 80% without GTC seizures over the same time period. Less than 10% of patients without AED therapy become seizure-free within 1 year. The rate of seizure relapse is associated with AED withdrawal. Seizures are often precipitated by sleep deprivation, alcohol ingestion, and awakening from nocturnal or daytime sleep. The natural history of JME involves recurrent seizures of one type or another that could occur several years after being "seizure-free," so lifelong AED therapy is warranted.

Counseling

Patients and their parents should be aware of the prognostic data and need for lifelong AED therapy. The risks and benefits of AED therapy should be discussed at length and encouragement offered, especially to adolescent patients. The importance of medication compliance should be stressed to patients. Sleep deprivation and alcohol ingestion should be avoided. The issues surrounding PCOS and chronic VPA use should be discussed in depth with pubertal and postpubertal females and referral to a reproductive endocrinologist may be warranted.

SUMMARY

- **JME** is an **AD-inherited generalized epilepsy syndrome** with an onset between **12 and 18 years** of age.
- Most patients have **GTC seizures on awakening** and **about 33%** have **absence seizures**.
- An abnormal neurological examination suggests a **progressive myoclonic epilepsy** disorder.
- Progressive myoclonic epilepsy can be divided into **neurodegenerative, mitochondrial** and **lysosomal storage disorders**.
- EEG shows interictal **3.5–6 Hz** bilateral, symmetrical, **spike, and polyspike and wave discharges**, maximal in **frontocentral** regions in JME.
- **VPA** is the drug of choice for treating JME. Other options include **lamotrigine** and **topiramate** (as adjunctive therapy only).
- Initial treatment response is **approximately 75%** with VPA.
- Treatment is required **lifelong**.
- **Approximately 40%** of patients are seizure-free and **about 80%** are GTC seizure-free within **1 year**, compared **less than 10%** without treatment.
- Patients should be counseled on the importance of **medication compliance** and should **avoid potential precipitants** such as **sleep deprivation** and **alcohol ingestion**.

CASE 13

A 9-year-old right-handed boy suddenly developed right-sided weakness while playing soccer at school this morning. His teammates also noticed that his speech was "slurred." He was brought to the ER several hours later. On examination, he was alert with expressive aphasia. Further examination revealed mild right hemiparesis affecting the face (forehead sparing) and upper extremities (MRC 3/5) worse than the lower extremity (MRC 4/5). There was also right hemisensory deficit to pinprick and light touch with diminished right-sided reflexes and an extensor plantar response of the right hallux.

Localization

Expressive aphasia, right hemiparesis (face and arm > leg) and multimodal right hemisensory loss imply involvement of the left frontoparietal cortex. Expressive aphasia would not be expected with subcortical etiologies, although transcortical and conductive aphasias could be secondary to subcortical white matter lesions. Diminished reflexes could occur early with UMN lesions or with LMN lesions. The positive Babinski sign verifies an UMN cause for the patient's weakness. In summary, the lesion most likely localizes to the left frontoparietal cortex supplied by the left MCA.

Differential Diagnosis

The most likely diagnosis for the sudden development of a left frontoparietal lesion in an otherwise healthy 9-year-old boy is *acute cerebral infarction or stroke*. This could be due to cerebral ischemia secondary to thrombo-occlusive or embolic disease of the left MCA or ICH. In this age group, in the absence of trauma, this scenario most likely implies *acute cerebral ischemia secondary* to a *hypercoagulable disorder* (accounts for about 30% of all childhood strokes; e.g., congenital coagulation defects, sickle-cell disease/anemia, aPL syndrome, lupus anticoagulant, drug-induced thrombosis, malignancy, and thrombocytopenic purpura). If trauma has been suggested, epidural, subdural, or subarachnoid hemorrhages would be potential diagnoses, although it may be expected that the child would be less alert secondary to raised ICP. Trauma could also result in carotid or vertebral arterial dissection with subsequent cerebral ischemia.

Other potential etiologies for childhood stroke include *cardiac disease* (accounts for about 40% of all childhood strokes; e.g., rheumatic heart disease, bacterial endocarditis, cardiomyopathies, cyanotic heart disease, cardiac arrhythmias), *vasculitis* (e.g., associated with sympathomimetic drug abuse, PACNS, CTDs e.g., SLE, Kawasaki disease; *see* p. 230), and *infection* (e.g., bacterial meningitis, viral encephalitis, VZV: subcortical small vessel infarcts, carotid infection).

Further considerations include *vasculopathies,* such as *MELAS*: maternal inheritance of mutation to mitochondrial tRNA-leu: recurrent migraine-like headaches, seizures (myoclonic, GTCs), stroke (initially occipital lobes) and encephalopathy; *Fabry's disease*: x-linked recessive deficiency in α-galactosidase

A: lancinating limb pains, skin angiokeratoma of buttocks or groin, stroke, and renal failure; *homocystinuria*: AR chromosome 21 deficiency on cystathionine β-synthase: Marfinoid habitus, downward lens dislocation (ectopia lentis), optic atrophy, mental retardation, seizures, and stroke with increased methionine and homocysteine in serum; *Moyamoya disease*: chronic progressive idiopathic noninflammatory vasculopathy with recurrent headaches, stroke (hemiparesis, hemianesthesia, aphasia, etc.) or TIAs, and *vascular malformations* such as AVM, fibromuscular dysplasia: rare idiopathic segmental nonatheromatous disorder of ICA; *Osler-Weber-Rendu syndrome* or *hereditary hemorrhagic telangiectasia*: AD trait with angiomas of skin, CNS, GI tract, GU tract and mucous membranes with cerebral hemorrhage secondary to increased blood vessel wall mechanical fragility.

Other differentials for sudden unilateral neurological deficit include *hemorrhage into a brain tumor, migraine* (complicated or familial hemiplegic migraine: usually associated with a preceding aura and concurrent frontotemporal throbbing headache), or *seizure* (ictal event as in focal inhibitory or hemiparetic seizure or post-ictal Todd's paralysis: usually evolves over minutes with spontaneous resolution over hours).

Investigations

Noncontrasted CT head should be performed to exclude ICH. MRI head (with and without DWI), MRA (intra- and extracranial)/MRV should also be performed for anatomical localization and etiology determination. Fat-suppression images should be included with the MRA if dissection is suspected. "Thrombophilia screen" should be performed: CBC with differential, ESR, protein C, protein S, factor V Leiden, activated protein C resistance, plasminogen, fibrinogen, aPL antibodies and lupus anticoagulant.

Other tests to consider include Hb electrophoresis (especially in African Americans), lipid profile, serum homocysteine, blood cultures, lactate/pyruvate levels and serum/urine toxicology. EKG and echocardiography should be performed to exclude cardiac etiologies and four-vessel cerebral angiography may be required for equivocal cases or where the pathology is below the resolution of MRA (e.g., vasculitis) or prior to surgery (e.g., AVM).

Management

The patient should be admitted to the general pediatric or neurology floor for continued care. The initial management of an acute ischemic stroke is outlined on pp. 100–101 and is based on adult studies/experience and small pediatric case studies. Depending on the etiology, additional treatment may be required, for example, aggressive hydration, oxygen administration, and RBC transfusion to keep HbS level less than 30% in sickle cell vaso-occlusive crises, corticosteroids for vasculitis, antibiotics for rheumatic heart disease, bacterial endocarditis and meningitis, dietary restriction of methionine, with vitamin B_6, vitamin B_{12} and cysteine supplementation in homocystinuria, aspirin for Kawasaki disease, and surgery (stereotactic radiosurgery or microsurgery) for AVMs.

Patients with identifiable hypercoagulable disorders would require treatment of the underlying disease (for secondary causes such as malignancy) and often require lifelong anticoagulation. Rehabilitation (speech and language, physical and occupational) should be initiated early, once the patient is clinically stable, and continued on discharge to improve functional capabilities and facilitate recovery.

Prognosis

Prognosis is dependent on the underlying cause. No underlying cause is identified in 20–35%. In general, for childhood stroke, about 5–15% of patients die either during the acute phase or during follow-up related to the initial stroke and only 10–30% completely return back to normal. About 60% have residual neurological deficits including hemiparesis, hemisensory, hemivisual deficit or residual aphasia. About 10–20% are severely handicapped as a consequence of the stroke. About 30% develop epilepsy secondary to the initial stroke.

Approximately 50–65% develop neuropsychological deficits, with behavioral problems occurring in as many as 30–40%. Poorer prognosis is predicted by infarct volume greater than 10% of intracranial volume or seizures on presentation. There is a 20–40% risk of recurrence, with recurrences more common with Moyamoya disease, vasculitis, homocystinuria, aPL antibody syndrome, and lymphopenia.

Counseling

Patients and their families should be aware of the prognostic data. Chronic anticoagulation for cardiac sources of embolic should be suggested based on adult data. Role for chronic antiplatelet or anticoagulation therapy for noncardiac acquired or inherited coagulopathies has not been fully elucidated, but should be advised in order to reduce risk of stroke recurrence. Parents should be aware of the neuropsychological sequelae of stroke. Support should be provided, especially for educational and social purposes.

SUMMARY

- **Childhood stroke** could be secondary to **cerebral ischemia** or **hemorrhage**.
- Differentials include **hemorrhage into a tumor, migraine**, or **seizure**.
- Etiologies for childhood stroke include **hypercoagulable disorders, trauma, cardiac disease, vasculitis, infection, vasculopathies,** and **vascular malformations**.

- Diagnosis requires **noncontrasted CT head** to exclude ICH, **MRI, MRA, MRV, "thrombophilia screen," EKG, echocardiography,** possible **cerebral angiography,** and other laboratory tests tailored to clinical presentation.
- Initial management is directed based on **adult** stroke experience. Specific measures may be required for certain disorders.
- In general, mortality is **5–15%, approximately 60%** have residual neurological deficits, **approximately 10–20%** are severely handicapped, **approximately 50–65%** develop neuropsychological deficits, and only **10–30%** completely return to normal.
- **Aproximately 30%** develop epilepsy secondary to initial stroke.
- Poor prognosis is predicted by infarct volume **greater than 10%** of the intracranial volume or **seizure** on presentation.
- There is an **approximately 20–40%** risk of recurrence. Recurrence is more common with **Moyamoya disease, vasculitis, homocystinuria, aPL antibody syndrome,** and **lymphopenia.**
- There are **no established studies** guiding the use of chronic antiplatelet or anticoagulation in childhood stroke, but use is advised in order to **reduce recurrent rates** based on adult studies.

CASE 14

A 13-year-old girl was brought to the clinic by her mother for "fainting" spells. These episodes had been going on for about 3 months and were precipitated by severe anxiety. She felt lightheaded, dyspneic, and nauseous for about 1 minute before losing awareness of her surroundings. Her mother had noticed that she falls to the ground, looks pale, and feels cold, but recovers in less than 1 minute. Her mother was concerned that she had convulsions associated with these spells recently. General physical and neurological examinations were normal.

Localization

Symptoms of lightheadedness, dyspnea, and nausea are nonspecific but could imply diffuse brain dysfunction, involving the cerebral cortex or brainstem (medulla) bilaterally. Loss of consciousness implies diffuse cerebral dysfunction or dysfunction of the brainstem reticular-activating system (pons and medulla). Loss of muscle tone could imply bilateral UMN (motor cortex, subcortical white matter, posterior limb of internal capsule, cerebral peduncles, basis pontis, pyramids, or spinal cord) or LMN (AHC, nerve roots, lumbosacral plexi, multiple peripheral nerves, NMJ, or multiple muscles) dysfunction. The rapid onset and recovery in tone makes UMN dysfunction more likely.

Convulsions may indicate global cerebral cortical hyper-excitability or occur as brainstem-release phenomena associated with lack of cortical inhibition. In summary, the underlying process most likely localizes diffusely to the cerebral cortex and brainstem (particularly medulla) bilaterally.

Differential Diagnosis

The clinical description is most consistent with a diagnosis of *syncope with associated anoxic convulsions*. Other differentials include *seizures* (pale, cold, and clammy skin not expected), *cataplexy*, or *cerebrovascular drop attacks* (*see* p. 177). The most likely diagnosis for syncopal episodes in an otherwise healthy 13-year-old girl provoked by severe anxiety is *vasovagal syncope*. This is a reflex neurocardiogenic syncope, whereby transient disturbances in the autonomic control of BP (vasodepressor type), HR (cardioinhibitory type), or both (mixed type) occur with emotional stress, anemia, crowded/poorly ventilated environments dehydration, hunger, physical exhaustion, or recent illness, in an upright position. This is the most common type of childhood syncope, with peak ages between 12 to 24 months and 9 to 14 years of age.

Other causes for neurocardiogenic or neurally mediated syncope include *postural orthostatic tachycardia syndrome* (POTS: type of orthostatic intolerance characterized by excessive tachycardia and decreased cerebral blood flow in the upright position), *pure autonomic failure* (inherited or acquired), and *MSA* (more common in elderly individuals).

Cardiac causes of syncope include *arrhythmias* (e.g., long Q-T syndrome, ventricular/supraventricular tachycardias), *vascular* (e.g., valvular aortic stenosis, hypertrophic obstructive cardiomyopathy), and *myocardial disease* (e.g., dilated cardiomyopathy, *muscular dystrophies*, myocarditis, ischemia, Kawasaki disease). Non-cardiac causes include *migraine* (especially basilar migraine), *drug/toxin exposure, metabolic derangement* (e.g., hypoglycemia, hyperammonemia), *hyperventilation, psychogenic* (clinical evaluation during witnessed event does not reveal any autonomic or cardiovascular compromise and episode may be prolonged despite being in a recumbent position), *situational* (e.g., cough, micturition, defecation, swallow, stretch; i.e., neck hyperextension, and hair grooming), *carotid sinus hypersensitivity*, and *idiopathic*.

Investigations

The clinical history and physical examination are extremely important for the diagnosis of recurrent syncope and direct investigative choice. Initial evaluation should include CBC, serum electrolytes, and EKG. If drug ingestion is suspected, serum/urine toxicology should be performed. If the history is suggestive of a noncardiac cause or vasovagal syncope and the initial evaluation is normal, further syncope evaluation is usually not necessary. If the history is suggestive of arrhythmia and the EKG is normal, holter or cardiac event monitors can be used for short- and longer-term evaluation. If the history is suggestive of myocardial disease (e.g., chest pain, exercise-induced, nonvasodepressor, or abnormal cardiac examination), echocardiography with or without exercise-stress testing should be performed.

Evaluation for neurally mediated syncope may involve tilt-table testing (period of supine rest, followed by tilt to 60–80° for at least 40 minutes: sensitivity ~50%, specificity 80–100%) if the diagnosis is not obvious in children older than age 6 or cardiac event monitoring in younger children. EEG (continuous monitoring is more sensitive) and neuroimaging should be reserved for atypical cases that are highly suggestive of seizures or cerebrovascular compromise.

Management

This is usually reserved for recurrent or severe cases of syncope. Treatment should be directed toward the underlying etiology. For neurocardiogenic syncope, known precipitants or triggers of the syncopal attack should be avoided. When presyncopal symptoms are experienced, maneuvers such as crossing the legs and folding the arms, reverting to a supine position or placing head below the level of the heart in a stooped forward posture may reduce the severity, or completely prevent the syncopal attack. Patients should also be advised to keep well hydrated and increase dietary salt intake.

Refractory patients may require pharmacotherapy with agents such as fludrocortisone (a mineralocorticoid: ADRs: fluid retention, weight gain), β-blockers (first-line drugs), SSRIs, midodrine, or atropine (use limited by anticholinergic side effects). Biofeedback techniques, such as tilt training or active tension, can be used as adjuncts or alternatives to drug therapy. Cardiac syncope could be treated with anti-arrhythmics, β-blockers, Ca^{2+} channel antagonists, permanent cardiac pacemakers, or surgery, depending on the etiology.

Prognosis

About one in five children will experience syncope before age 15. Most cases are isolated and benign. In fact, childhood syncope does not confer a higher risk of mortality (including sudden death) or morbidity in comparison to the normal population. However, the rare cardiac causes of syncope may cause sudden death in as many as 5–15% of affected patients, warranting careful, thorough evaluation, and early institution of therapy, including permanent pacemakers.

Counseling

Reassurance of the patient and family is important. This plays an important therapeutic role in vasovagal syncope. The benign and common nature of most childhood syncope should be emphasized. The importance of precipitant or trigger avoidance, and preventative and therapeutic maneuvers should be stressed. If a rare cardiac cause for syncope is suspected, referral to a pediatric cardiologist should be offered as soon as possible due to its potential risks for sudden death.

SUMMARY

- **Childhood syncope** can be divided into **neurocardiogenic, cardiac**, and **non-cardiac** etiologies.
- Differentials include **seizures, drop attacks**, and **cataplexy**.
- The most common etiology is **vasovagal syncope**, a reflex neurocardiogenic syncope commonly associated with **emotional stress**.
- The **clinical history and examination** are paramount for the diagnosis and direct investigation.
- **CBC, electrolytes**, and **EKG** should be performed initially.
- **Holter** or **cardiac event monitoring, echocardiography**, and **tilt-table testing** should be reserved for certain clinical situations.
- Management of neurally mediated syncope includes **conservative measures, avoidance of triggers, preventative maneuvers**, or **pharmacotherapy** with or without **biofeedback** for refractory patients.

Index